Bedside Critical Care Manual

Second Edition

EDWARD D. CHAN, MD
Assistant Professor of Medicine, National Jewish Medical and Research Center, Division of Pulmonary Sciences and Critical Care Medicine, University of Colorado School of Medicine, Denver, Colorado

LANCE S. TERADA, MD
Associate Professor of Medicine, Division of Pulmonary and Critical Care Medicine, University of Texas Southwestern and Dallas VAMC, Dallas, Texas

JOHN KORTBEEK, MD
Clinical Associate Professor, Department of Surgery, Director, Calgary Regional Trauma Services, Foothills Medical Centre, Calgary, Alberta, Canada

BRENT W. WINSTON, MD
Assistant Professor, Faculty of Medicine, University of Calgary, Departments of Medicine and Biochemistry and Molecular Biology, Division of Critical Care Medicine and the Immunology Research Group, Calgary, Alberta, Canada

HANLEY & BELFUS, INC. / Philadelphia

Publisher: HANLEY & BELFUS, INC.
Medical Publishers
210 South 13th Street
Philadelphia, PA 19107
(215) 546-7293; 800-962-1892
FAX (215) 790-9330
Web site: http://www.hanleyandbelfus.com

Note to the reader: Although the information in this book has been carefully reviewed for correctness of dosage and indications, neither the authors nor the editors nor the publisher can accept any legal responsibility for any errors or omissions that may be made. Neither the publisher nor the editors make any warranty, espressed or implied, with respect to the material contained herein. Before prescribing any drug, the reader must review the manufacturer's current product information (package inserts) for accepted indications, absolute dosage recommendations, and other information pertinent to the safe and effective use of the product described.

Library of Congress Cataloging-in-Publication Data

Bedside critical care manual / edited by Edward D. Chan . . . [et al.].—2nd ed.
p. ; cm.
Includes bibliographical references and index.
ISBN 1-56053-431-1 (alk. paper)
1. Critical care medicine—Handbooks, manuals, etc. I. Chan, Edward D., 1959–
[DNLM: 1. Critical Care—methods—Handbooks. 2. Critical Illness—therapy—Handbooks. WX 39 B413 2001]
RC86.8 .B43 2001
616'.028—dc21

2001039369

BEDSIDE CRITICAL CARE MANUAL, 2nd ED ISBN 1-56053-431-1

Last digit is the print number: 9 8 7 6 5 4 3 2 1

Contents

Foreword

The management of critically ill patients has become increasingly important in the modern medical system. At the same time that the number of intensive care beds in hospitals has grown, the complexity of the medical problems and the severity of illness in critically ill patients has also increased. Multiple organ system dysfunction is the common denominator in the critically ill population now occupying intensive care units and demands appropriate diagnosis as well as management of the pathophysiologic processes involving multiple organ systems. A key issue concerning diagnostic procedures and therapies aimed at a single organ system is their effects on other organs. For example, antibiotics directed toward pneumonia may well have renal or hepatic toxicities. The management of a critically ill patient therefore represents a continual balancing act in which the risks and benefits of diagnostic procedures and interventions must be carefully weighed.

The *Bedside Critical Care Manual* represents a comprehensive approach to the multiplicity of clinical issues involved in the management of critically ill patients. Both underlying pathophysiologic issues and practical diagnostic and therapeutic approaches are covered. It represents a valuable addition to the literature on the critically ill in that it provides an important bridge between comprehensive textbooks and relatively short, therapeutic monographs. This manual provides information of fundamental importance in an accessible manner and should be of great utility to all those responsible for the care of critically ill patients.

Edward Abraham, MD
Professor of Medicine
Head of Critical Care
University of Colorado
School of Medicine
Denver, Colorado

Contributors

Marcie M. Chase, RD
Clinical Nutritionist, Denver Veterans Administration Medical Center, Denver, Colorado

Kim Milevic, RRT
Respiratory Therapist, Foothills Medical Centre, Calgary, Alberta, Canada

Preface to the First Edition

Our principal aim in writing this book is to provide a usable manual for the clinician managing critically ill patients. We have attempted to focus on highly practical information and to present it in a succinct fashion. Initially intended for pulmonary and critical care fellows, it may also serve the medical resident as well as more seasoned physicians. We dedicate this manual to the faculty of the Division of Pulmonary Sciences & Critical Care Medicine at the University of Colorado School of Medicine and to Marvin I. Schwarz, M.D., for providing a challenging and academic environment. We especially thank the fellows in the division, from whom we learn. Finally, we are grateful to budding artists Mallory and Michael Chan, who provided the spider figures.

Preface to the Second Edition

It is an old maxim of mine that when you have excluded the impossible, whatever remains, however improbable, must be the truth.

Sherlock Holmes in Arthur Conan Doyle's *The Sign of Four*.

In this second edition of *Bedside Critical Care Manual*, we have attempted to update the topics based on current state-of-the-art medicine. To this end, we are indebted to the following talented physicians for their time and input: Drs. Mary Bessesen, Sarah Faubel, Ed Gill, Kathy Hassell, Konnen Heard, Stu Linas, David Lynch, Mark Powis, Diana Quan, and Tom Truijillo. The nutrition chapter was completely rewritten by Marcie Chase, RD, and the mechanical ventilation section was substantially revised by Kim Milevic, RRT. We thank Barry Kushner, BSP, for proof-reading. Three new chapters on surgical aspects of critical care were added by coauthor John B. Kortbeek, MD. We again dedicate this manual to the faculty of the Division of Pulmonary Sciences & Critical Care Medicine at the University of Colorado School of Medicine and to Marvin I. Schwarz, M.D., James C. Campbell Professor of Medicine, and Edward Abraham, M.D., Roger S. Mitchell Professor of Medicine, for providing a nurturing environment. We especially thank the fellows in the division, from whom we continue to learn. EDC is also grateful to Gerard M. Turino, M.D., John H. Keating Sr. Professor of Medicine, Columbia University College of Physicians and Surgeons, and Director of the James P. Mara Center for Lung Disease, St. Lukes-Roosevelt Hospital, New York City, for inspiring the former into the field of pulmonary medicine. We also dedicate this edition to the hard working members of the Department of Critical Care Medicine at the University of Calgary: physicians, nurses, respiratory therapists, physical and occupational therapists, and nutritionists. We are very thankful to growing artists Mallory and Michael Chan for providing the improved spider figures, and to William Lamsback, executive editor for Hanley and Belfus, for his continued patience and help. We also thank Dr. Polly E. Parsons, whose insight resulted in the fruition of the original edition.

Edward D. Chan, MD, DWNP
Lance S. Terada, MD
John B. Kortbeek, MD
Brent W. Winston, MD

General Issues in the Intensive Care Unit

1. Daily chest x-rays in any patient with a pulmonary artery (PA) catheter or an endotracheal tube.
2. Obtain x-ray to confirm placement of gastric or feeding tubes if unsure of placement.
3. Check the x-ray **yourself**, and confirm the name of the patient on the x-ray after endotracheal intubation or central line placement.
4. Deep venous thrombosis (DVT) prophylaxis recommended for every patient.
5. Stress ulcer prophylaxis for every patient (especially patients on ventilator for over 24 hrs or with coagulopathy).
6. Use adequate analgesia, especially in intubated patients.
7. There is no difference, either ethically or legally, between withholding and withdrawing support.
8. Sometimes it is more prudent to rely on clinical assessment rather than take an unstable patient to the radiology suite.

Pulmonology

Conventional Mechanical Ventilation (Kim Milevic, RRT)

I. **Definitions**

Tidal volume (V_T): the volume delivered by the ventilator per breath. In measurement of compliance using V_T, it is important to use the exhaled V_T rather than the set V_T.

Peak airway pressure (Ppk): the maximal airway pressure at any time during inspiration. It is a function of the inflation volume, airways resistance, and the compliance of the lungs and chest wall. Increases in Ppk are an indication of decreased lung compliance, increased airways resistance, or both. It is thus important to determine the contribution to the elevated Ppk by measuring the plateau pressure (Pplat).

Static airway pressure or plateau pressure (Pplat): the airway pressure that is measured when the V_T is held in the lungs after end-inspiration, preventing the lungs from deflating. It reflects the elastic recoil pressure of the lungs and thoracic cage. If the Pplat is high, elastic recoil of the lung is great, i.e., low compliance such as seen in acute respiratory distress syndrome or fibrotic lung disease.

Dynamic compliance (Cdyn): compliance is the change in volume associated with a given change in pressure required to overcome the resistance of flow through the airways and the elastance of the lungs and chest wall. The dynamic compliance is the exhaled V_T/Ppk. The product of Cdyn and negative inspiratory pressure (NIP) is an estimate of vital capacity.

Static compliance (Cstat): static compliance reflects the distensibility of the lungs and chest wall. It is defined as the exhaled V_T/Pplat. The normal range is ~ 50–70 ml/cmH_2O in intubated patients without lung disease. In spontaneously breathing subjects, the normal Cstat is > 90 ml/cmH_2O. Compliance measurements are useful when obtained serially to evaluate changes (improvement or deterioration) in lung or chest wall disease in patients on mechanical ventilation.

Positive end-expiratory pressure (PEEP): the maintenance (by the ventilator) of positive pressure throughout exhalation. PEEP is used to help maintain adequate oxygenation at lower FiO_2 to help prevent O_2 toxicity (generally, FiO_2 is believed to have toxic effects when > 0.60%). PEEP increases PaO_2 primarily by augmenting mean airway pressure. Other potential benefits include recruitment of collapsed alveoli, increased functional residual capacity, and improvement in ventilation-perfusion matching.

Mean airway pressure: the average of the airway pressures throughout one respiratory cycle.

Minute ventilation $\dot{V}_E$: the sum volume of air exhaled in 1 minute. Normal values are **4–8 L/min.** $\dot{V}_E$ >> or << normal is not a good sign in a patient on mechanical ventilation and suggests that the patient is not a candidate for weaning.

Maximal inspiratory pressure (PI_{max}) or negative inspiratory pressure (NIP): a measure of the strength of the diaphragm and other respiratory muscles. It is measured by first having the patient exhale fully, followed by maximal inspiration against a closed valve. **Normal PI_{max} cmH_2O:** males: > –70 cmH_2O (i.e., more negative than –70 cmH_2O).

Inspiratory flow rate ($\dot{V}$insp): the flow rate set on the ventilator in L/min. The $\dot{V}$insp may be increased to decrease the time it takes to give the tidal volume and thus is used principally to increase expiratory time. A commonly used initial $\dot{V}$insp is 60 L/min.

II. **Controlled mechanical ventilation (CMV)**
 1. **Description**: A V_T is applied to the lungs with positive pressure. The operator sets respiratory rate, V_T, and a flow rate. It is one of the earlier forms of mechanical ventilation. There are no patient-triggered breaths. Each breath delivered results in delivery of the full set V_T to the patient.
 2. **Initial settings**: V_T, 6–10 cc/kg ideal body weight; respiratory rate (RR), 10–15/min; $\dot{V}_E$, 8–10 L/min; FiO_2, 100%; $\dot{V}$insp, 60 L/min; and PEEP, 0.
 3. The rate and volume are totally controlled. Patient triggering or spontaneous breathing is not possible.
 4. This form of ventilation is used in surgery for paralyzed patients.

III. **Assist-control ventilation (ACV)**
 1. **Description**: A V_T is applied to the lungs with positive pressure. The operator sets respiratory rate, V_T, and a flow rate. It is one of the earlier forms of mechanical ventilation. Any patient-triggered breaths result in delivery of the full set tidal volume to the patient.
 2. **Initial settings**: same as above.
 3. The set rate on the ventilator is the **minimal** number of full V_T breaths delivered by the ventilator (mandatory breath). Each patient-initiated breath is also assisted by the ventilator with a full set V_T. The inspiratory time is set secondarily, based on RR, V_T, and $\dot{V}$insp.
 4. Patient initiates each assisted breath by decreasing the airway pressure (P_{aw}) by 1–2 cmH_2O to open a unidirectional valve.
 5. The diaphragm does not stop contracting after the machine breath is initiated, but, overall, ACV decreases work of breathing for the respiratory muscles.
 6. **Advantages**
  a. Ideal mode for patients who are apneic or who do not have an intact respiratory drive.
  b. ACV delivers consistent V_T and mandatory minimal $\dot{V}_E$.
  c. ACV is used in conjunction with PEEP.
 7. **Disadvantages**
  a. Peak airway pressures vary with changes in pulmonary compliance. As a result, when ventilating patients with poorly compliant lungs, high peak airway pressures are difficult to avoid.
  b. ACV can be uncomfortable for the awake patient, resulting in patient-ventilator asynchrony.
  c. ACV is a poor mode from which to wean a patient from ventilation.
  d. Like virtually all forms of mechanical ventilation, much of the V_T delivered will go to the most compliant area of the lung, leaving the noncompliant areas of the lungs hypoventilated and resulting in V/Q mismatching.

IV. **Intermittent-mandatory ventilation (IMV)**
 1. **Description**: Volume control breaths are applied to the lungs with the set rate on the ventilator, resulting in the maximal number of machine breaths delivered. Patients are, however, able to take their own breaths between the set rate. The V_T of the patient-initiated breaths depends on patient effort.
 2. **Initial settings**: same as above.
 3. **Advantages**
  a. Lower airway pressure can be achieved, with decreased incidence of barotrauma and increased cardiac function.
  b. IMV may be useful in patients with respiratory alkalosis because $\dot{V}_E$ may decrease.
 4. **Disadvantages**
  a. In some patients, IMV may increase the work of breathing, thus contributing to CO_2 production. Therefore, if IMV is used, it is generally recommended

that a pressure support of 5–10 cmH_2O be added to decrease the work of breathing imposed by the endotracheal tube.

b. The ventilator-initiated breaths are not in synchrony with the patient-initiated breaths; hence, the development of SIMV (see below).

V. **Synchronized intermittent-mandatory ventilation (SIMV)**

1. **Description**: Volume control breaths (either ventilator- or patient-initiated) with the opportunity for the patient to breathe spontaneously with pressure support breaths between SIMV breaths. The IMV breaths are initiated by the patient within certain tolerances. Pressure support is an optional adjunct.
2. In addition to the basic IMV mode, the ventilator senses when a voluntary effort is made to initiate a breath (within a certain period) and assists the patient's breath if it is time for a machine-delivered breath.
3. Thus, SIMV is more in synchrony with the patient's own respiratory effort and avoids breath stacking; there is less work of breathing with SIMV than with IMV alone.
4. **Advantages**
   a. SIMV challenges the patient when the operator increases the work of breathing either by decreasing the frequency of the SIMV breaths or by decreasing the magnitude of the pressure support.
   b. Ideal for patients who are making the transition from full ventilation support to breathing spontaneously (e.g., a patient who is coming off sedation).
   c. Increased comfort for the conscious patient compared with assist control.
5. **Disadvantages**
   a. If the operator sets the frequency or the minute ventilation too high, the patient may rely on the set rate and not breathe above that rate (i.e., SIMV becomes like ACV).

VI. **Continuous positive airway pressure (CPAP)**

1. **Description**: CPAP is a baseline pressure that can be provided by the ventilator and is present throughout the respiratory cycle.
2. CPAP is a spontaneous breathing mode in which airway pressure is kept constant throughout the respiratory cycle.
3. The respiratory rate, V_T, and inspiratory time are determined by the patient; CPAP provides PEEP for the spontaneously breathing patient (i.e., PEEP occurs on machine breaths). In the CPAP mode, the ventilator delivers a constant pressure.
4. Most commonly used as a weaning technique but also may be administered with a nasal or face mask in nonintubated patients.

VII. **Pressure support ventilation (PSV)**

1. **Description:** Pressure support is commonly used with CPAP to provide a boost of positive pressure for patient-initiated breaths. The level of pressure support can be varied by the operator to optimal levels for each patient.
2. PSV assists an intubated patient's spontaneous inspiratory efforts with a preselected amount of positive airway pressure. The machine controls only the P_{aw} limit and FiO_2; because the patient controls $\dot{V}insp$, V_T, RR, and inspiratory time, PSV has been called a modified form of spontaneous ventilation. Thus, patients with abnormal respiratory drives (e.g., drug overdose, stroke, head trauma, encephalopathy) should **not** receive PSV as the sole mode of ventilation because there is no back-up rate.
3. Every breath is augmented by a set level of inspiratory pressure; thus, work of breathing is decreased. The machine shuts off pressure (ends inhalation) when (1) inspiratory flow drops below a set minimum (e.g., 5 L/min or 5–25% of peak flow), signaling the onset of expiration; (2) P_{aw} transiently rises above a set maximum, which occurs during a cough (e.g., 1.5 × set pressure or 3 cmH_2O

above set pressure; or (3) inspiration lasts beyond a set maximal time (e.g., 5 sec or > 80% of respiratory cycle time). If inspiratory time is excessively long, it may mean a leak in the circuit, or the set pressure may be too low for patient's lung compliance. PSV is often combined with SIMV to decrease the work of breathing.

4. The amount of pressure to use initially in PSV can be estimated by one of the following three methods although it is usually adjusted based on patient comfort and respiratory rate:
   a. PS to create a desired V_T (e.g., 8–10 cc/kg)—usually 15–25 cm
   b. PS = Ppk – Pplat
   c. PS = Maximal inspiratory pressure/3
5. **Advantages**
   a. Patients controls their own respiratory rate, and their own effort impacts the size of the V_T they receive.
   b. Increased comfort for patients who are awake compared with ACV.
   c. PSV as the primary mode of ventilation has been shown to decrease the level of auto-PEEP in patients with airflow obstruction, primarily by decreasing the RR.
   d. The combination of CPAP and PSV is an excellent transition mode and facilitates weaning to extubation.
6. **Disadvantages**
   a. There is no guarantee of consistent ventilation. For example, hypoventilation may result in patients receiving in-line continuous bronchodilator nebulization because the additional flow through the nebulizer makes it more difficult for the patient to generate the negative pressure required to initiate PS breath.
   b. An intact respiratory drive is required.
   c. Clinicians must be careful with levels of sedation, and paralytics cannot be used in conjunction with this mode. With no fixed $\dot{V}_E$, $\dot{V}_E$ may fall in patients with decreased respiratory drives.
   d. Alveolar recruitment maneuvers may be required to prevent atelectasis for patients who are ventilated on pressure support for prolonged periods.
   e. With no periods of sustained negative intrathoracic pressure, venous return to the right heart may be decreased.

VIII. **Pressure control ventilation (PCV)**

1. **Description**: Pressure-limited, time-cycled ventilation in which the operator sets a respiratory rate, ventilation pressure, inspiratory time, and I/E ratio. V_T is allowed to vary with changes in pulmonary compliance.
2. The following values are set on the ventilator: PEEP, driving pressure (above PEEP), respiratory rate, and inspiratory time.
3. The ventilator delivers an approximately square pressure waveform (not flow), and the magnitude of the pressure wave is determined by the master rate and % inspiratory time (the inspiratory:expiratory [I:E] ratio will vary if the patient breathes above the set rate because the ventilator will assist the inspiration if the patient initiates the breath). The flow profile and therefore the V_T are secondary to the time constant of the lung, which may change over time. (This is opposite to volume control ventilation, in which the flow profile and V_T are set and the inspiratory time and pressures are secondary variables.)
4. **Advantages**
   a. Facilitates increases in mean airway pressure without significant increases in peak airway pressure.
   b. Decreases the risk of barotrauma.
   c. Allows more even distribution of ventilation in patients with variable levels of compliance within the lung due to disease processes.

d. I/E ratios can be readily inversed to increase mean airway pressure.
e. Peak airway pressures are reduced, as well as the pressure gradient, resulting in less leakage in patients with a persistent air leak or bronchopleural fistula.

5. **Disadvantages**
a. Decreased patient comfort, particularly when inverse I/E ratios are used. Sedation and paralytics are required to achieve adequate patient compliance.
b. V_T can be inconsistent. V_T and therefore $\dot{V}_E$ are not set; they may vary with time and depend on the mechanical properties of the lungs and chest wall. It is thus imperative that the V_T and $\dot{V}_E$ be monitored constantly (at least every 1 hr). For example, if the resistance of the lungs and chest wall rises (due to decrease or discontinuation of neuromuscular blockers), V_T and $\dot{V}_E$ may markedly decrease.
c. Mean airway pressure increases as inspiratory time is prolonged and may cause hemodynamic compromise.
d. Increased inspiratory time also may increase auto-PEEP and decrease V_T.
e. PCV is not available on all ventilators.

IX. **Volume support ventilation**

1. **Description**: Similar to pressure support but with a volume guarantee. If the patient's inspiratory effort is insufficient to generate V_T as set by the operator, the ventilator compensates with an increase of pressure to give the desired V_T.
2. **The following are set**: PEEP, master rate, % inspiratory time, V_T, and pressure bracket, as with PRVC (see below). In this case, however, the patient rate is essentially set at zero (the master rate and % inspiratory time determine the absolute inspiratory time). The ventilator now acts like pressure support except that a guaranteed V_T is delivered. Patients set their own rate.
3. **Advantages**
a. The operator knows that the patient will always get the appropriate V_T.
b. Volume support ventilation is a good weaning tool because it acts like pressure support except that the pressure is adjusted to achieve a desired V_T.
4. **Disadvantages**
a. Can be less effective as a weaning tool because the ventilator automatically takes over some of the work of breathing for the patient.
b. Volume support is not available on all ventilators.
c. Patients must have an intact respiratory drive, because they need to initiate the breath.

X. **Pressure-regulated volume control (PRVC) ventilation**

1. **Description**: A control mode of ventilation whereby the ventilator delivers the set V_T but automatically dials down the pressure so that the V_T is delivered with the least amount of pressure necessary. It is similar in effect to the AutoFlow adjunct on the Evita ventilator, whereby the pressure at peak inspiration is slightly reduced.
2. **The following are set**: PEEP, master rate, and % inspiratory time, as with PCV. Instead of setting driving pressure, set V_T and acceptable pressure range. The ventilator senses the return V_T and adjusts its driving pressure up or down for the next breath, until it is delivering the desired V_T. If the pressure required to deliver the set V_T falls above or below the set pressure range, the machine alarms.
3. **Advantages**
a. The beneficial effects of the pressure-flow profile of PCV are achieved, but you have control over the V_T.
b. Lower peak inspiratory pressure decreases the risk of barotrauma.
c. Increased patient comfort.

4. **Disadvantages**
   a. PRVC is not available on all ventilators.
   b. As the lung's time constant changes with the disease, the pressure required to achieve the set V_T will change and the machine will alarm. If the gas exchange is still acceptable, simply adjust the pressure bracket.
   c. Because pressures are moderated, V_T is not as consistent as with traditional volume control ventilation.

XI. **Inverse ratio ventilation (IRV)**
1. IRV is not a specific ventilator mode (e.g., it may be used with ACV or PCV) but rather a strategy in which I:E ratio is prolonged to 1:1 or greater (e.g., 2:1).
2. It is a means to improve oxygenation in adult respiratory distress syndrome but requires heavy sedation (and possibly paralysis) because it is quite uncomfortable.

XII. **Mandatory Minute Ventilation**
1. **Description**: A minimum minute ventilation is set, and the patient breathes on pressure support. If the patient's spontaneous minute ventilation should be less than the level of minute ventilation set, the ventilator delivers the set minute ventilation to the patient with assist control breaths until the patient's own spontaneous minute ventilation exceeds the level set by the operator. If the patient's spontaneous minute ventilation exceeds the set minute ventilation, the patient will continue to breathe spontaneously with pressure-supported breaths.
2. **Advantages**: An excellent transition mode for postoperative patients who will go from control to spontaneous ventilation as the sedation wears off.
3. **Disadvantages**: Not a desirable mode for patients who require the operator to be active or aggressive in increasing the patient's work of breathing.

XIII. **Airway Pressure Release Ventilation (APRV)**
1. **Description**: The ventilator provides the patient with two pressure levels: high and low. Both levels are time-cycled and ventilator-initiated. The patient can breathe spontaneously at any point in the high/low pressure cycle. The high pressure is maintained for the majority of the respiratory cycle. The pressure is allowed to decrease to the low level for a short duration, usually < 1 second, to allow exhalation and gas exchange to take place. APRV is most commonly used in patients with severe lung injury progressing to ARDS.
2. **Advantages**
   a. Alveolar recruitment. APRV increases functional residual capacity in poorly compliant lungs.
   b. Inverse I/E ratios can be achieved without the use of paralytic medication.
   c. The patient can breathe spontaneously throughout the respiratory cycle. (It is hard to say whether this translates to improved patient comfort.)
   d. Decreases the disadvantages created from the extended use of paralytics.
3. **Disadvantages**
   a. The inverse ratios can create air trapping and a hyperinflation picture in patients with airway obstruction.

Nonconventional Mechanical Ventilation

I. **Proportional assist ventilation (PAV)**
1. **Description**: A relatively new mode of ventilation in which the pressure, flow, and volume are proportional to the patient's effort. Spontaneous respiratory effort is required for PAV. The airway pressure produced by the ventilator

depends on: (1) the amount of flow and volume demanded by the patient and (2) the amount of assist set by the operator. The operator dials in the amount of flow assist to overcome resistive load and the amount of volume assist to overcome lung elastance (compliance) load.

2. **Advantages**: ideal for spontaneously breathing patients in whom one desires to base the degree of assistance on the patient's pulmonary characteristics.
3. **Disadvantages**
   a. PAV can be used only as a mode of assisted ventilation (i.e., an intact respiratory drive is mandatory).
   b. In the presence of auto-PEEP it may be more difficult for the patient to trigger the ventilator.
   c. In patients in whom compliance changes rapidly, the ventilator setting must be adjusted accordingly.
   d. PAV does not tolerate leaks in the system very well, including pneumothorax.

II. **High-frequency ventilation (HFV).** Several forms of HFV have been developed over the years in which ventilatory frequencies are substantially greater (60–2000 breaths per minute) and tidal volumes less (1–5 ml/kg) than those of conventional modes of ventilation. Some studies suggest that HFV may be beneficial in patients with bronchopleural fistula, although this condition is relatively rare and is not significantly associated with increased mortality.

1. **High-frequency positive pressure ventilation (HFPPV).** In HFPPV the respiratory frequencies are 60–120 bpm, and the tidal volumes are 3–5 ml/kg, yielding an I:E ratio of < 0.3. HFPPV has been used successfully in upper airway surgery because it allows access to tracheal and laryngeal surgical fields.
2. **High-frequency jet ventilation (HFJV).** In HFJV a small volume of gas (2–5 ml/kg) is delivered into the airway at high pressure (15–50 psi) through a small bore canula (14–18 gauge) at frequencies normally ranging from 100–600 bpm, resulting in an I:E ratio of 1:2–1:8. The variables that alter alveolar ventilation include driving pressure, frequency, and I:E ratio. Increasing driving pressure or frequency tends to increase gas trapping. HFJV has been used successfully for unilateral ventilation during pneumonectomy and resection of abscess and for treatment of patients with bronchopleural fistulas.
3. **High-frequency oscillations (HFO).** In HFO 1–3 ml/kg of gas is delivered at a frequency of 1–60 Hz (60–3600 cycles per minute), and both inspiratory and expiratory phases are active. O_2 supply and CO_2 removal require a bias gas flow. There is no proven clinical advantage to this form of ventilation, which currently is used primarily in neonates. Results of animal and pediatric studies using HFO are encouraging, but further work is necessary to determine the value and optimal use of HFO in adults with acute lung injury and acute respiratory distress syndrome. Few adult ventilators are on the market.

III. **Extracorporeal membrane oxygenator (ECMO)**. ECMO uses an artificial lung to oxygenate blood and remove CO_2 without using the gas exchange surface of the lungs. Large arterial and venous cannulas are required so that enough cardiac output can be directed through the membrane to allow adequate oxygenation and CO_2 removal. Risks of bleeding, clotting, and infection are significant.

IV. **Low-frequency positive-pressure ventilation with extracorporeal CO_2 removal (LFPPV-ECCO$_2$R).** This mode of ventilation allows reduced lung motion (using 100% O_2 into the trachea), and CO_2 is eliminated by the extracorporeal circuit.

Key References: Krishman JA, Brower RG: High-frequency ventilation for acute lung injury and ARDS. Chest 118:795–807, 2000; Pilbeam SP: Mechanical Ventilation: Physiological and clinical applications, 3rd ed. St. Louis, Mosby, 1998; Tobin MJ: Respiratory monitoring during mechanical ventilation. Crit Care Clin 6:679–709, 1990.

Pressure-Time Curves

I. **Pressure-time curves provide information about:**
   1. The type of breath delivered to the patient
   2. Timing and adequacy of expiration and inspiration
   3. Adequacy of flow rate
   4. Results of static mechanics

II. **Ventilator-initiated mandatory breath (VIMB).** The lack of a negative pressure deflection at the onset of inspiration identified the VIMB.

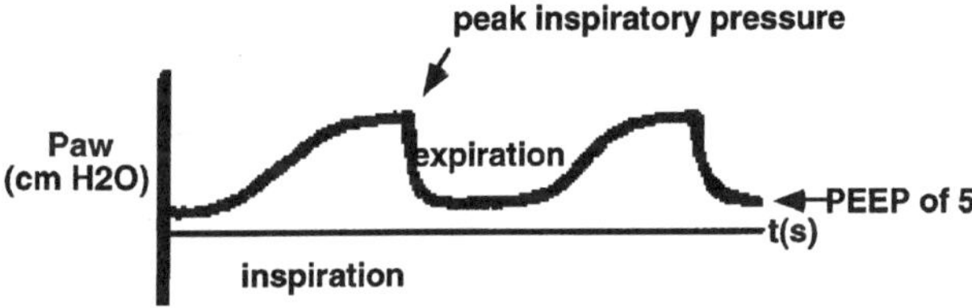

III. **Patient-initiated mandatory breath (PIMB).** In contrast to the VIMB, there is a negative pressure deflection in the PIMB.

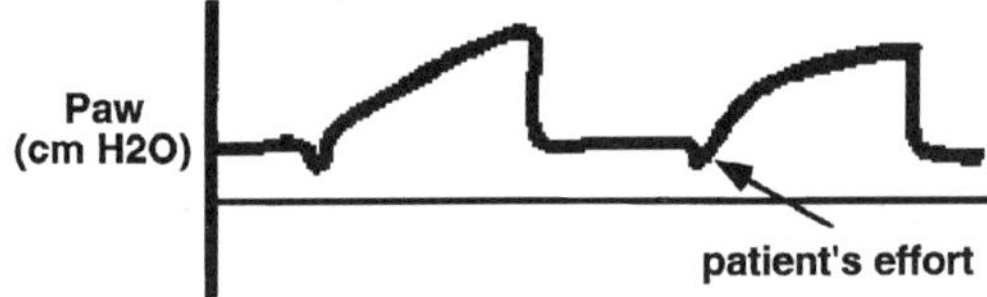

IV. **Spontaneous breath.** Note that with spontaneous ventilation, there is no assistance by the ventilator with each inspiration. The baseline is above the x-axis because PEEP is set on the ventilator. Thus, this is an example of CPAP ventilation.

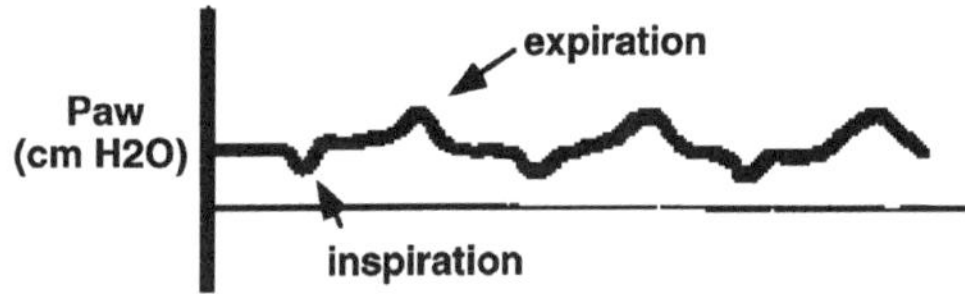

V. **Evaluating respiratory events.** When pressure does not return to the baseline before the next inspiration, expiratory time is inadequate. Measures to increase expiratory time include increased $\dot{V}$insp, decreased RR, and decreased V_T.

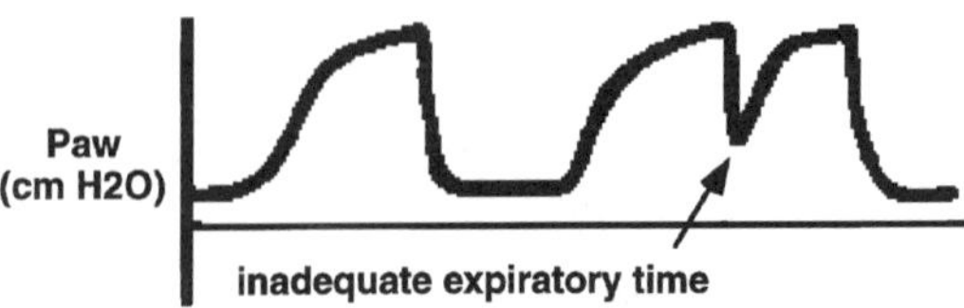

VI. **Adjusting peak flow rate ($\dot{V}$insp).** In volume-assisted ventilation, the rate of rise in pressure (slope) is related to the peak flow setting.

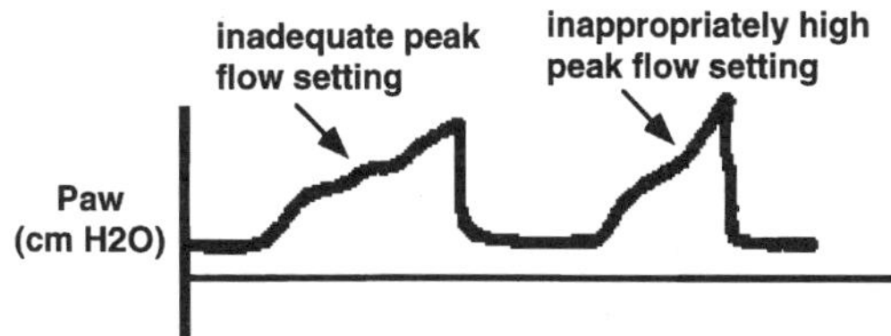

VII. **Measuring static mechanics.** The difference between Ppk and Pplat represents the pressure due to flow resistance in the patient's airway and the endotracheal tube (ETT).

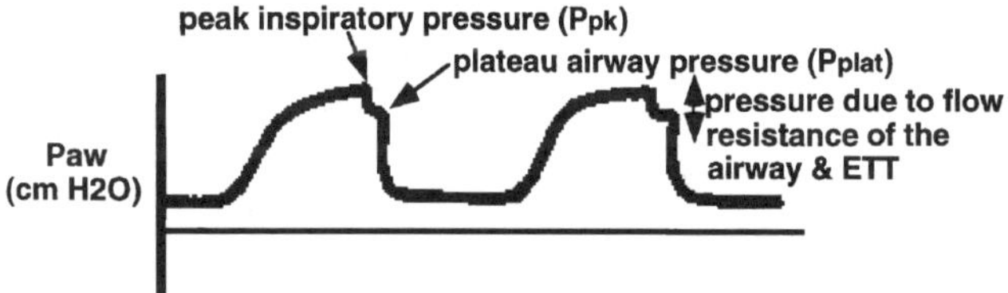

Key Reference: Adapted from Waveforms. Puritan Bennett, 1991, pp 3–9, with reference to MacIntyre NR, Hagus CK: Graphical Analysis of Flow, Pressure, and Volume. Riverside, CA, Bear Medical Systems, 1989.

Flow-Time Curves

I. Flow is defined as the volume of gas displaced in a given time (L/min). Inspiratory flow is arbitrarily set as (+) and expiratory flow is arbitrarily set as (–). Flow-time curves are useful for detecting:
   1. Type of breath delivered to the patient
   2. Presence of auto-PEEP
   3. Patient's response to bronchodilators
   4. Adequacy of ventilatory time in pressure-control ventilation

II. **Detecting type of breathing**

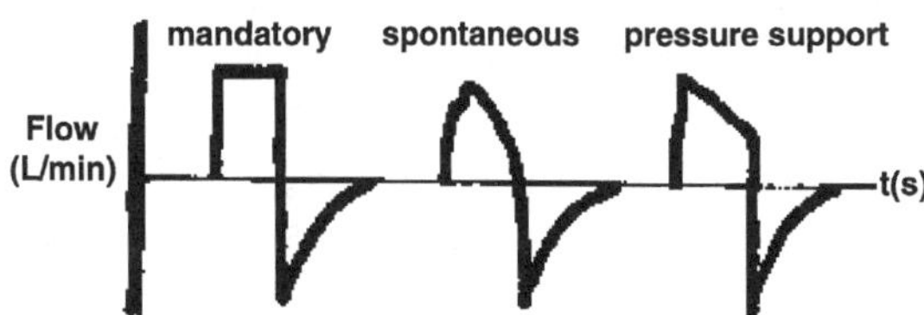

III. **Determining the presence of auto-PEEP.** Surrogate marker is the presence of an expiratory flow that does not return to zero before the next inspiration: the higher the end expiratory flow, the higher the auto-PEEP.

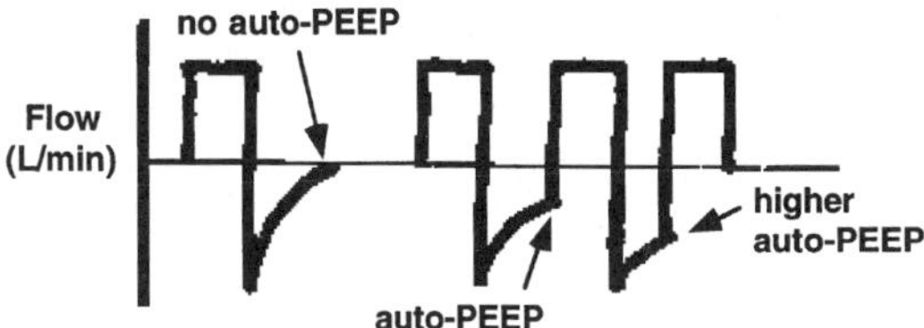

IV. **Evaluating bronchodilator response.** After bronchodilator, peak expiratory flow is greater, and the expiratory time to reach zero flow is less (y < x).

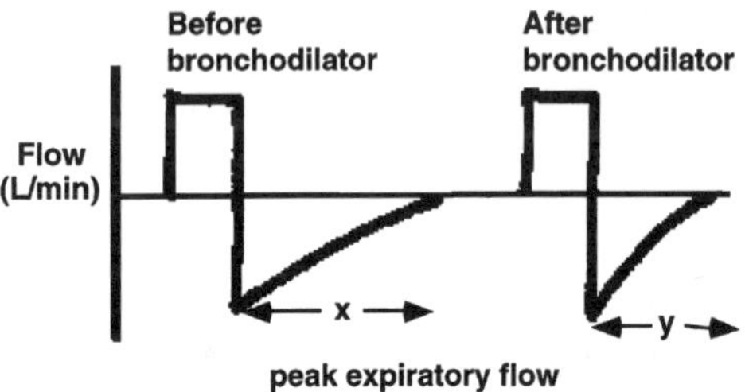

V. **Evaluating inspiratory time in pressure control ventilation.** Inspiratory flow rates that return to zero usually indicate adequate inspiratory (I) time. If inspiratory flow does not return to zero, increasing the I time results in increased tidal volume without increasing the inspiratory pressure.

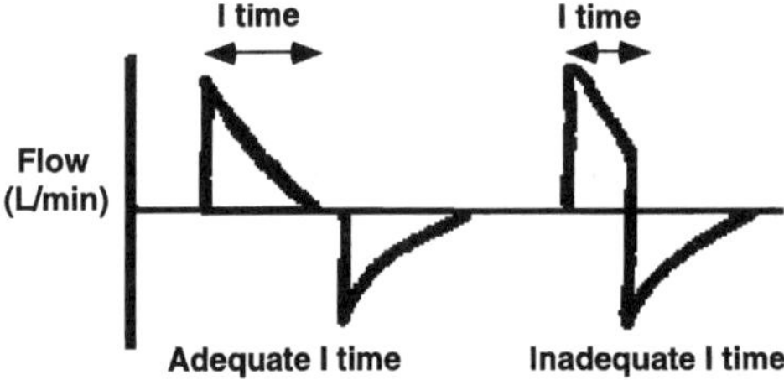

Key Reference: Adapted from Waveforms. Puritan Bennett, 1991, pp 11–16, with reference to MacIntyre NR, Hagus CK: Graphical Analysis of Flow, Pressure, and Volume. Riverside, CA, Bear Medical Systems, 1989.

Weaning

I. The ability to wean depends on the severity of the underlying problems and not necessarily on the method of weaning. When the underlying disease is corrected, which should be the major focus, a patient's chance of successful weaning is increased.

II. In addition to treatment of the underlying disorder, other factors (summarized by the acronym **WEANS NOW**) should be addressed in assessing suitability of extubation:

Weaning parameters (see below)
Endotracheal tube size/**e**lectrolyte (phosphate)
Arterial blood gas (ABG); optimize acid–base status (e.g., avoid overcorrection of $PaCO_2$ in patients with previous chronic stable respiratory acidosis)
Nutrition (either malnutrition and overfeeding may make weaning more difficult)
Secretions
Neuromuscular status (any drugs inhibiting neuromuscular function)
Obstruction of airways
Wakefulness (and adequate sleep).
Other factors: motivation and volume status.

III. **Standard criteria for weaning.** Many weaning parameters (spontaneous ventilatory parameters [SVP]) have been evaluated as objective criteria for weaning.

Patients do not need to satisfy every parameter, but the traditional ones are negative inspiratory force (NIF), minute ventilation ($\dot{V}_E$), and forced vital capacity (FVC) in a patient who is alert and oxygenating with an $FiO_2 < 40–50\%$. More recently, it has been shown that a frequency/V_T ratio < 100 (the lower the better) is predictive of successful extubation.

V_T (spontaneous) > 5 ml/kg*	f/V_T < 100 breaths/min/L
FVC > 10 ml/kg*	CROP index > 13 ml/breath/min†
NIF < –30 cmH_2O	$P_{0.1} < 4$ cmH_2O‡
$\dot{V}_E$ < 10–12 L/min	$V_D/V_T = (PaCO_2 - P_ECO_2)/PaCO_2 < 0.5$
Respiratory rate < 25/min	Shunt ≈ AaO_2 on 100%/20 < 30%
C_{stat} > 30 ml/cmH_2O	$PaO_2/P_AO_2 \geq 0.35$
$FiO_2 \leq 40–50\%$	
No PEEP	
No abdominal paradox or respiratory alternans	

* Applicable to postoperative patients or patients with neuromuscular disease, but not necessarily to patients with severe lung disease.

† CROP is an acronym for compliance, rate, oxygenation, and pressure:
CROP = [dynamic compliance × PImax × (PaO_2/P_AO_2)]/respiratory rate.

‡ $P_{0.1}$ is the airway occlusion pressure. It is an estimate of neuromuscular respiratory drive. It is not widely used as a weaning parameter because of conflicting data about its utility.

IV. **Weaning methods**

1. **T-piece.** This method of weaning is based on a circuit design in which a constant flow of oxygen-rich gas passes by the end of the endotracheal tube (ETT), forming a T-shaped circuit. The patient spontaneously breathes through the ETT without assistance but is able to entrail the oxygen-enriched gas.
   a. Ideal for uncomplicated postoperative patients and patients who have recovered from an uncomplicated drug overdose because it is a simple and fast mode of weaning.
   b. For more complicated patients in the ICU who are candidates for weaning, use a flow-by circuit ± CPAP (5 cmH_2O) mode for ventilator monitoring instead of the T-piece so that V_T, respiratory rate, and $\dot{V}_E$ may be monitored. Flow-by circuit is a sensitivity setting in which a small flow change results in opening of the demand valve, thus lessening the work of breathing.
2. **IMV wean.** A weaning method in which the IMV mode of ventilation is used. The support given by the ventilator is gradually withdrawn from the patient as tolerated.
   a. Major criticism: the work of breathing may increase.
   b. Begin with a high V_T (10–15 ml/kg) and decrease the machine breaths by 2 breaths/min every 2 hr.
   c. If ABG and clinical status are acceptable at IMV 4, extubation is possible.
3. **Pressure support (PS) wean.** A weaning method using the PS mode of ventilation. Because it is a spontaneous mode, it is a good method for patients who are prone to breath-stacking by the ventilator, leading to auto-PEEP, and hyperinflation (e.g., patients with COPD and asthma).
   a. Start with a PS level to give a V_T 8–12 ml/kg (but < 50 cmH_2O), but the patient's comfort should be ensured by adjustments of the pressure support at the bedside. PS is often combined with CPAP to counteract auto-PEEP in patients with severe obstruction. Thus, a patient who is on CPAP of 5 cmH_2O and PS of 5 cmH_2O has an inspiratory pressure of 10 cmH_2O and end-expiratory pressure of 5 cmH_2O.
   b. If patient is comfortable and ABGs are acceptable, decrease PS by increments of 2–3 cmH_2O (as fast as every 1 hr for postoperative patients and possibly as slow as every other day for difficult-to-wean patients).

c. The **respiratory rate** is one of the best parameters to follow when PS is decreased; check ABG periodically or as needed.
d. Generally, a PS of 5 ± CPAP of 5 is an acceptable level for extubation, provided that other clinical factors (see **WEANS NOW** above) are acceptable.

Key References: Marino PL: The ICU Book, 2nd ed. Baltimore, Williams & Wilkins, 1998, pp 468–481; Yang KL, Tobin MJ: A prospective study of indexes predicting the outcome of trials of weaning from mechanical ventilation. N Engl J Med 324:1445–1450, 1991.

Troubleshooting During Weaning

I. **Definitions**
1. **AaO_2:** alveolar-arterial P_{O_2} gradient, calculated as follows: FiO_2 (Patm-P_{H_2O}) – ($PaCO_2$/0.8) – PaO_2
2. **PvO_2:** mixed venous PO_2, the partial pressure of oxygen measured from a sample of blood obtained from the right atrium.
3. **CaO_2:** oxygen content of arterial blood, calculated as 1.36 (Hb) × SaO_2, where Hb = hemoglobin in gm/dl.
4. **CvO_2:** oxygen content of mixed venous blood, calculated as 1.36 (Hb) × $S\bar{v}O_2$, where $S\bar{v}O_2$ is the mixed venous oxygen saturation.
5. **PI_{max}:** maximal inspiratory pressure (see Conventional Mechanical Ventilation).

II. **Tachypnea during weaning.** The major differential diagnoses are anxiety and muscle weakness or cardiopulmonary problems.
1. If V_T is decreased, measure PI_{max}. A low PI_{max} usually signifies muscle weakness.
2. If V_T is not decreased but AaO_2 is increased, a cardiopulmonary disorder is suggested.
3. IF V_T is not decreased, AaO_2 has not changed, but $PaCO_2$ has increased, measure PI_{max} to distinguish between neuromuscular disease (low PI_{max}) and central nervous system (CNS) disorder (normal PI_{max}).
4. If V_T is not decreased, AaO_2 has not changed, and $PaCO_2$ is low, consider sedation for anxiety.

III. **Hypoxemia during weaning**

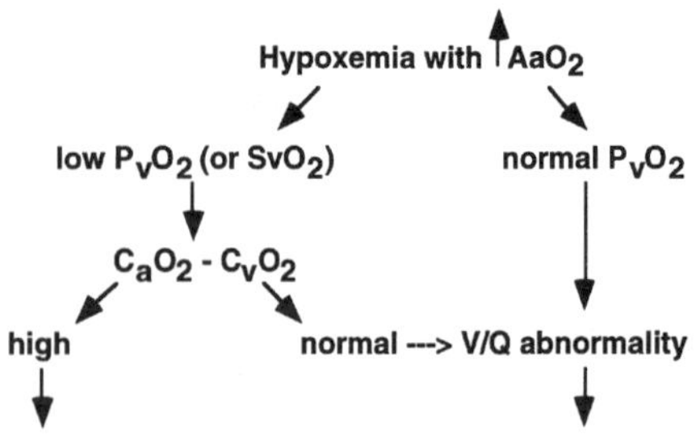

1. If **AaO_2 is normal or unchanged**, hypoxemia is more likely due to alveolar hypoventilation. Measure PI_{max} to distinguish between neuromuscular disorder (low PI_{max}) and CNS disorder (normal PI_{max}).
2. If **AaO_2 is increased, PvO_2 is low**, and **(CaO_2 – CvO_2) is high**, peripheral O_2 uptake is increased relative to delivery (e.g., due to low cardiac output [CO]

and/or high oxygen consumption $\dot{V}O_2$). The important point is that low CO or increased peripheral consumption may be causes of hypoxemia.

3. If **AaO_2 is increased** and the **PvO_2** and the **$CaO_2 - CvO_2$ are normal** (i.e., if PvO_2 is low, it is due to a low CaO_2, which also lowers CvO_2), $\dot{V}/Q$ is abnormal because of high dead-space ventilation or high shunt fraction. Thus the problem is in the lungs.

IV. **Hypercarbia during weaning**

1. If AaO_2 is increased, a cardiopulmonary disorder is suggested.
2. If AaO_2 is not increased and PI_{max} is decreased, respiratory muscle weakness is suggested.
3. If AaO_2 is not increased, PI_{max} is not decreased, and $\dot{V}CO_2$ is increased, hypermetabolism, lactic acidosis, or another cause of increased work of breathing is suggested.
4. If AaO_2 is not increased, PI_{max} is not decreased, and $\dot{V}CO_2$ is not increased, central hypoventilation or muscle fatigue is likely.

Adapted from: Marino PL: The ICU Book,. 2nd ed. Baltimore, Williams & Wilkins, 1998, pp 468–481.

Ventilating Severely Obstructed Patients

I. The current tendency is to ventilate patients with lower lung volumes and lower airway pressures and to accept higher $PaCO_2$ values as long as pH and mental status are acceptable (permissive hypercapnia). Hyperinflation increases the risk of pneumothorax and hypotension. **Strategies to prevent hyperinflation** include:

1. Increase expiratory time by decreasing $\dot{V}_E$ (minute ventilation), inspiratory time, and RR, increasing $\dot{V}insp$ (inspiratory flow rate), sedating the patient if needed, and using low-compliance tubing, square wave during inspiration, and lower V_T.
2. Aggressive **treatment of the airflow obstruction**.

II. Hypotension due to hyperinflation is due to the decreased venous return ← increased P_{RA} (right atrial pressure) ← increased Palveolus (alveolar pressure). Patients with emphysema have high lung compliance and therefore Palveolus caused by obstruction. Auto-PEEP is transmitted easily to the pleural space, compressing the great veins in the thorax and impeding venous return and cardiac output.

III. $\dot{V}_E > 12.5$ L/min increases risk of hyperinflation. Decreasing the $\dot{V}_E$ does **not** necessarily lead to increased $PaCO_2$ because the decreased hyperinflation may decrease dead space ventilation by improving perfusion to the ventilated lung units. Consider the intravenous administration of $NaHCO_3$ when pH < 7.20 if the patient has no evidence of heart failure and the acidosis is respiratory in nature.

IV. **Inspiratory time:expiratory time (I:E) ratio.** Although a low ratio is generally desirable in the obstructed patient (i.e, increased expiratory time), it can be misleading, as illustrated by the following example:

Patient 1: V_T = 1000 ml, RR = 15/min, $\dot{V}insp$ = 60 L/min (or 1 L/sec). Thus I = 1 sec, E = 3 sec.

Patient 2: If V_T and $\dot{V}insp$ remain the same but RR = 12/min (or 5 sec/breath), I = 1 sec, E = 4 sec.

Patient 3: If V_T and RR of 15/min remain unchanged but $\dot{V}insp$ = 120 L/min (or 2 L/sec), I = 0.5 sec, E = 3.5 sec.

Therefore, although the I:E ratio in patient 3 (1:7) is lower than in patient 2 (1:4), the absolute expiratory time is longer (and better) in patient 2 (4 sec vs. 3.5 sec).

V. **Auto-PEEP (intrinsic PEEP)** is the positive pressure that occurs at end-expiration when airway obstruction and inadequate expiratory time prevent complete gas emptying. It can reduce cardiac filling, increase work of breathing, and may cause barotrauma. Auto-PEEP may not be detected unless there is an expiratory hold, which allows equilibration of $P_{alveolus}$ with $P_{airway\ opening}$. In addition, auto-PEEP cannot be measured accurately if the patient has active respiratory muscle contractions.
   1. Auto-PEEP may occur without hyperinflation when expiratory muscle contraction is vigorous.
   2. Auto-PEEP may underestimate the degree of hyperinflation in asthmatics if airways are completely closed off from the alveoli.
   3. Auto-PEEP is treated by measures to prolong expiratory time (see above).

VI. **Peak airway pressure (Ppk) and plateau pressure (Pplat).** No convincing data indicate that Ppk correlates with barotrauma. Patients with asthma can tolerate Ppk of 70–90 cmH_2O as long as Pplat is < 30 cmH_2O. Decreasing the $\dot{V}insp$ to try to limit Ppk may only worsen hyperinflation. In contrast to Ppk, Pplat is a marker of hyperinflation; thus, it is often recommended that Pplat be kept at < 30 cmH_2O.

VII. **Recommended ventilator settings in asthmatics:** V_T (8–10 ml/kg), $\dot{V}insp$ (100 L/min), square wave. **In COPD:** V_T (7–8 ml/kg), $\dot{V}insp \approx (5 \times \dot{V}_E)$; keep $PaCO_2$ at or above baseline.

VIII. **Weaning in COPD**
   1. **Rest respiratory muscles:** increased sensitivity of trigger to –1 to –2 cmH_2O if on ACV, add PS if on SIMV, and treat auto-PEEP.
   2. **Improve respiratory muscle strength:** exercise during the day by decreasing SIMV rate and pressure support, or increasing T-piece time and rest on ventilator at night; correct potassium, calcium, magnesium, phosphorus, nutrition; search for myopathic effects of hypothyroidism, corticosteroids, aminoglycosides, and delayed effects of paralytics.
   3. **Decrease load on the respiratory system** by correcting factors that increase Ppk or Pplat (normal Ppk – Pplat ≤ 10 cmH_2O); e.g., aggressive bronchodilator therapy to decrease both hyperinflation and auto-PEEP.

IX. **Herpetic tracheobronchitis:** should be considered in both immunocompromised and immunocompetent (usually elderly) patients with new-onset wheezing unresponsive to conventional therapy. Severe bronchospasm and airway obstruction may lead to respiratory failure. Bronchoscopy may reveal erythema, ulceration, and a fibrinopurulent exudate that may cause luminal obstruction. Cytology of bronchial wash may show acute inflammatory cells with intranuclear inclusions. This disorder may cause difficulty in weaning.

Key References: Corbridge TC, Hall JB: Techniques for ventilating patients with obstructive pulmonary disease. J Crit Illness 9:1027–1036, 1994; Pepe PE, Marini JJ: Occult positive end-expiratory pressure in mechanically ventilated patients with airflow obstruction: The auto-PEEP effect. Am Rev Respir Dis 126:166–170, 1982.

Treatment of Severe Exacerbations of Chronic Obstructive Pulmonary Disease (COPD)

I. **Increase β_2-agonist dosage:** 6–8 puffs every ½–2 hr via metered-dose inhaler (MDI) with spacer, **inhalant solution** unit dose every ½–2 hr, or **terbutaline SQ**, 0.5 mg every 4–8 hr.

II. **Increase ipratropium dosage:** 6–8 puffs every 3–4 hr via **MDI** or **inhalant solution** 0.5 mg every 4–8 hr.

III. **Aminophylline** to maintain serum level at ~ 10–12 μg/ml (55–65 μmol/L). **Initial dose:** 2.5–5 mg/kg ideal body weight (IBW) load over 30 min. **Maintenance:** 0.5 mg/kg/hr (use 0.2–0.4 mg/kg/hr for patients with heart failure or liver disease or the elderly).

IV. **Methylprednisolone**, 50–100 mg IV initially, then every 6–8 hr; taper as soon as possible.

V. **Antibiotic** in patients with evidence of a bacterial infection such as purulent sputum and fever, with or without infiltrate. Acute bacterial exacerbation of COPD is not uncommon, especially in smokers. Besides *Streptococcus pneumoniae*, other organisms to consider include *Hemophilus influenzae* and *Moraxella catarrhalis*. Appropriate empiric antibiotic regimens include trimethoprim-sulfamethoxazole, doxycycline, second- or third-generation cephalosporin, or β-lactamase-resistant penicillin (e.g., amoxacillin-clavulanic acid).

VI. **Mucolytic agent** if sputum is highly viscous. N-acetylcysteine (NAC, Mucomyst) may be given by nebulization. The typical dose is 3–5 ml of a 20% solution via a nebulizer 3–4 times/day. Because NAC may be associated with bronchoconstriction, it should be combined with the inhaled β-agonist.

VII. **Recommended initial O_2 settings** to achieve $PaO_2 > 60$ mmHg

PaO_2 (room air, mmHg)	FiO_2 (%)	Nasal cannula (L/min)
50	24%	1
45	28%	2
40	32%	3
35	35%	4

VIII. **Sympathomimetic bronchodilator dosages after stabilization***

Drug	MDI dose	MDI puffs per PUFF	Standard doses of **inhalant** solutions (varies with manufacturer)
Epinephrine	0.16 mg	2–4 every 4–6 hr	0.25–0.5 ml (1.25–2.5 mg)
Metaproterenol (Alupent)	0.65 mg	1–2 every 3–4 hr	0.2–0.3 ml (10–15 mg) or 2–5 ml (10 mg) or 2–5 ml (15 mg)
Albuterol (Proventil)	0.09 mg	1–2 every 4–6 hr	0.5 ml (2.5 mg) or 3 ml (2.5 mg)
Terbutaline	0.20 mg	2 every 4–6 hr	0.25–0.5 ml (0.25–0.5 mg)
Salmeterol (Serevent)	0.02 mg	2 every 12 hr	

* Adapted from ATS Board of Directors: Standards for the diagnosis and care of patients with chronic obstructive pulmonary disease. Am J Respir Crit Care Med 152:S77–S120, 1995.

IX. Measures to mobilize secretions such as chest physiotherapy (percussion, postural drainage) may cause a transient fall in FEV_1. In general, consider the role of chest physiotherapy limited to patients with > 25 ml sputum/day or lobar atelectasis from mucus plugging. Intermittent positive pressure breathing (IPPB), positive expiratory pressure (PEP), and bland aerosol therapy are of no proven benefit.

Key Reference: ATS Board of Directors: Standards for the diagnosis and care of patients with chronic obstructive pulmonary disease. Am J Respir Crit Care Med 152:S77–S120, 1995.

Treatment of Status Asthmaticus

I. Consider other causes of dyspnea and wheeze such as pulmonary embolus, upper airway obstruction, and heart failure. Prevention of status asthmaticus cannot be overstressed. In the words of Tom Petty, M.D., "the best treatment of status asthmaticus is to treat it three days before it occurs."

II. Sequential (or even continuous) inhalation of aerosolized β-agonists is the treatment of choice:
Albuterol, 5 mg/ml: 2.5–5 mg (0.5 ml of 0.5% solution) every ½–2 hr via nebulizer. MDI: 6–8 puffs every ½–2 hr, or **metaproterenol**, 50 mg/ml: 0.3 ml (15 mg) in 3 ml normal saline (NS) every ½–2 hr. MDI (0.65 mg/puff): 2–3 puffs every ½–2 hr, or **racemic epinephrine**, 2.25% solution: 0.3–1 ml via nebulizer. For patients who have excessive tremor or tachycardia from the β_2 agonist, the stereoisomer of albuterol known as **levalbuterol** (Xopenex), 0.63 mg per dose via nebulizer, may be given instead of albuterol to reduce the side effects.

III. **Methylprednisolone**, 0.5–1.0 mg/kg IV every 6 hr; larger doses (125 mg every 6 hr) may result in more rapid improvement but have not been shown to improve outcome.

IV. **Oxygen:** mitigates against paradoxical bronchodilator-induced hypoxemia and reverses hypoxic pulmonary vasoconstriction (i.e., it may help prevent the transient $\dot{V}/Q$ mismatching following bronchodilator therapy).

V. **Ipratropium bromide**, 0.5 mg via nebulizer hourly or 4–10 puffs via MDI with spacer every 20 min × 3 doses, may be given but is not considered a first-line agent. However, patients with bronchospasm precipitated by β-blockers may particularly benefit from ipratropium bromide.

VI. **Aminophylline** (contains 80% theophylline by weight); not routinely used because it is not likely to have additional bronchodilatory effects over β_2-agonists and corticosteroids. Theophylline may have other benefits, such as increased diaphragmatic contractility and improved mucociliary clearance.
Loading dose: 5 mg/kg IBW IV over 20 min in patients not receiving theophylline
Maintenance infusion: **0.4 mg/kg/hr**
Check serum levels within 6 hr of loading dose and maintain theophylline level at ~ 10–12 μg/ml (55–65 μmol/L).

VII. **Antibiotics** for clinical evidence of bacterial tracheobronchitis or pneumonia.

VIII. **Heliox** may be tried in recalcitrant cases, although it is not considered standard therapy. Start with 80% helium, 20% oxygen mixture. If PaO_2 is too low, you may try a helium:oxygen ratio of 70:30 or 60:40. To maximize the reduction in its density, the FiO_2 should be < 40%.
Reference: Gluck EH, Onorato DJ, Castriotta R: Helium-oxygen mixtures in intubated patients with status asthmaticus and respiratory acidosis. Chest 98:693–698, 1990.

IX. **Magnesium sulfate: 1 gm in 50 ml normal saline IV over 20 min** may be tried in recalcitrant cases, although its use is not generally accepted. You may repeat in 20 min for a total dose of 2 gm.

X. **Criteria for endotracheal intubation and mechanical ventilation.** Many studies have shown that acute respiratory acidosis, although concerning, does not necessarily indicate the need for endotracheal intubation because many patients respond favorably to aggressive bronchodilator and corticosteroid treatment. Some generally accepted indications for intubation include:
1. Cardiac or respiratory arrest
2. Significant alterations in mental status

3. Progressive exhaustion and worsening respiratory acidosis or hypoxemia despite aggressive medical management.

Once intubation is achieved, sedation and avoidance of overventilation prevent excessive gas trapping and auto-PEEP.

Key References: Corbridge TC, Hall JB: The assessment and management of adults with status asthmaticus. Am J Respir Crit Care Med 151:1296–1316, 1995; Leby BD, Kitch B, Fanta CH: Medical and ventilatory management of status asthmaticus. Intens Care Med 24:105–117, 1998.

Pearls for Life-threatening Asthma

I. Signs of severe obstruction include change in mental status, diminished breath sounds, and upright position, but **respiratory failure may be imminent even in the absence of these signs**. Some patients perceive minimal dyspnea despite severe obstruction, especially in subacute cases. Lactic acidosis usually indicates severe obstruction.

II. Although many recommendations for therapy are based on peak expiratory flow rate or FEV_1, measurement of peak flow or FEV_1 in the acute setting may transiently worsen symptoms. Cardiopulmonary arrest has been reported after such maneuvers.

III. **Hypercapnia**, although always indicative of life-threatening exacerbations, does not predict the need for endotracheal intubation. The great majority of patients with hypercapnia (even those with initial $PaCO_2 > 55–60$ mmHg) can be successfully treated without mechanical ventilation. There is the potential for worsening of airway obstruction immediately after intubation because of stimulation of irritant receptors in the trachea.

IV. Addition of ipratropium to a β_2-agonist may be beneficial in some patients. Inhaled ipratropium is **contraindicated in patients with a hypersensitivity to soya lecithin, soybean, or peanuts.**

V. Corticosteroids reduce inflammation, upregulate β_2 receptors, decrease microvascular permeability, and may decrease mucus production.

VI. **Mechanical ventilation pearls**

1. The two major complications associated with positive pressure ventilation are **systemic hypotension** and **barotrauma**.
2. The peak airway pressure (Ppk) is **not** considered a predictor of hypotension or barotrauma.
3. **Dynamic hyperinflation (DHI)** is a reflection of the volume at end-inspiration (V_{EI}) and the amount of trapped gas or volume at end-expiration (V_{EE}): $V_{EI} - V_T = V_{EE}$. Thus, both V_{EI} and V_{EE} are indicators of the severity of DHI. Practically, the minute ventilation ($\dot{V}_E$) is the critical determinant of DHI. The peak inspiratory flow ($\dot{V}$insp) is proportional to 1/DHI. The higher the $\dot{V}$insp, the lesser the V_{EE} and DHI due to longer expiratory time; this may result in a higher Ppk, but the Pplat is lower. However, **decreasing the minute ventilation is of far greater value in decreasing DHI than increasing the $\dot{V}$insp.** Thus, **DHI is determined by three variables:**
   a. **Severity of air flow limitation**
   b. **Tidal volume**
   c. **Expiratory time**, which may be prolonged to decrease DHI by decreasing RR, higher $\dot{V}$insp, square wave, and low-compliance tubing.
4. Auto-PEEP seems to be an accurate gauge of DHI. If auto-PEEP is high, it is suggestive of DHI. However, some patients have negligible auto-PEEP and yet have significant DHI because many airways may close completely during

expiration, preventing accurate measurement of end-expiratory P_{alv}. In contrast, the trapped gas is reflected by an increase in Pplat. Therefore, **Pplat is preferred over auto-PEEP in assessing DHI.**

VII. **Sedation and paralysis**

1. Use short-acting benzodiazepines such as midazolam. Low doses (1–3 mg every 4 hr) of morphine usually do not cause histamine release.
2. The combination of neuromuscular-blocking agents **(NMBA) and corticosteroids may cause a profound myopathy**. NMBAs also suppress the cough reflex. Assess the degree of blockade with the **train-of-four** neuromuscular junction method: 1 twitch in response to 4 repetitive stimuli is best.

VIII. **Permissive hypercapnia**

1. Generally well tolerated; may be potentially harmful in patients with cerebral edema.
2. Consider slow infusion of $NaHCO_3$ for persistent pH < 7.2. Given rapidly, $NaHCO_3$ causes a significant increase in CO_2 production and may aggravate intracellular acidosis.
3. Tromethamine or Tris buffer—unlike $NaHCO_3$—reduces $PaCO_2$ during the buffering process: ml 0.3M tromethamine = desired increase in $NaHCO_3$ (mEq/L) × BW (kg)
   Tromethamine should not be given to patients with renal insufficiency because elimination of acid requires excretion of H+-tromethamine complex in the urine.

IX. **Unconventional therapy**

1. **Droperidol:** a butyrophenone derivative similar to haloperidol; 0.22 mg/kg IV over 10 min has been used successfully as an adjunct to mechanical ventilation when asthma has been unresponsive to conventional therapy. Possible side effects include hypotension and extrapyramidal reactions.
2. **General anesthesia:** use in patients with both severe DHI and hypercapnia refractory to therapy so that correction of one worsens the other.
   a. **Isoflurane** is preferred over halothane because it is a potent bronchodilator and is less arrhythmogenic.
   b. **Ketamine**, a potent bronchodilator, has been used as a continuous infusion at 5–10 μg/kg/min in attempts to avoid mechanical ventilation. Ketamine may increase cerebral blood flow (with an increase in intracranial pressure) and is also a myocardial stimulant due to increased sympathetic activity.
3. **Venous-venous bypass with ECMO and CO_2 removal (ECO_2R)** has been used to facilitate bronchoscopy for extensive mucus plugging.

Key Reference: Leatherman J: Life-threatening asthma. Clin Chest Med 15:453–479, 1994.

Managing Patients with Adult Respiratory Distress Syndrome (ARDS)

I. **Clinical definition of ARDS:** bilateral alveolar infiltrates with hypoxemia ($PaO_2/FiO_2 \leq 200$ regardless of PEEP), pulmonary arterial wedge pressure (PAWP) ≤ 18 mmHg, or no clinical evidence of increased left atrial pressure. Acute lung injury (ALI) is defined similarly except that the $PaO_2/FiO_2 \leq 300$ mmHg. ARDS may mimic pneumonia with fever, leukocytosis, and pulmonary infiltrates. Most patients who die of ARDS do so within the first 2 weeks of the illness. Infiltrates that persist after 7–10 days suggest inflammation and fibrosis or nosocomial pneumonia.

II. **Major causes:** sepsis, aspiration of gastric contents, diffuse pulmonary infection (bacterial, viral, fungal, *Pneumocystis carinii*), major trauma, acute pancreatitis, neurogenic, inhalational (oxygen, smoke, NO_2), near-drowning, incompatible or massive blood transfusion, drugs (heroin, cocaine, aspirin, chemotherapeutics), and reperfusion injury (after lung transplant or cardiopulmonary bypass).

III. **Ventilatory strategies**

1. **Lower tidal volume (V_T).** Lower V_T (6 ml/kg of predicted body weight) has been shown to improve mortality and ventilator-free days in the first month of mechanical ventilation for ARDS or ALI. The mean plateau pressure in the low V_T group was 25 ± 6 cm H_2O; for the "traditional" V_T group (~ 12 ml/kg), it was 33 ± 8 cm H_2O.

   Reference: The Acute Respiratory Distress Syndrome Network: Ventilation with lower tidal volumes as compared with traditional tidal volumes for ALI and the ARDS. N Engl J Med 342:1301–1308, 2000.

2. **PEEP.** Theoretically, PEEP increases lung volume at end expiration, thereby increasing functional residual capacity (FRC). Prophylactic PEEP does not prevent ARDS in susceptible people. It may prevent microatelectasis by preventing alveolar collapse during exhalation. Use of PEEP in improving oxygenation should be increased by increments of 3–5 cm (maximum = 15 cm), and its effects should be evaluated clinically (blood pressure, urine output, lung compliance) or hemodynamically (maximization of oxygen delivery [$\dot{D}O_2$] at an acceptable FiO_2).

   Reference: Pepe PE, Hudson LD, Carrico CJ: Early application of positive end-expiratory pressure in patients at risk for the adult respiratory distress syndrome. N Engl J Med 311:281–286, 1984.

2. **Permissive hypercapnia.** The rationale is to limit high airway pressures and overdistention of the alveoli. The most direct way to implement this form of lung protective strategy is to set the V_T at 4–8 ml/kg. Tracheal gas insufflation (TGI) at a rate of 2–14 L/min via a catheter above the carina may lower $PaCO_2$ by decreasing the dead space, although no clinical studies have demonstrated its efficacy in this setting. Complications associated with permissive hypercapnia include acidosis, hyperkalemia, increased cerebral blood flow, seizures, coma, and arrhythmias. Thus, it is not advisable to use permissive hypercapnia in patients with increased intracranial pressure.
3. **Inverse-ratio ventilation (IRV).** The rational for IRV (increased inspiratory time) is that the sustained inspiratory pressure, while maintaining Ppk at an acceptable level, may have an incremental effect on nonfunctioning atelectatic lung regions (recruiting alveoli). IRV may be applied to either volume-controlled (by decreasing peak flow sufficiently to prolong inspiratory time) or pressure-controlled ventilation (by inverting the I:E ratio). When used in ARDS, IRV results in lower Ppk and PEEP requirements, although mean P_{aw} rises. Its use often requires heavy sedation with or without paralytics because it is an uncomfortable mode of ventilation.
4. The following unconventional modes of oxygenating the patient are unproven and in fact have not been shown to improve survival in patients with ARDS.
   a. **High-frequency ventilation** (V_T 1–5 ml/kg at 60–3600 cycles/min, expiration is passive). Theoretical advantages include enhanced alveolar gas kinetics, less barotrauma, and maintenance of alveolar volume and better recruitment due to higher mean P_{aw}. Studies of HFV in patients with ARDS show no survival advantages.
   b. **Extracorporeal membrane oxygenation and/or extracorporeal CO_2 removal** have not been shown to affect survival in ARDS.

IV. **Positioning.** Consider lateral decubitus or prone positioning in patients who persistently require high FiO_2. Proposed mechanisms for improved PaO_2 include increased functional residual capacity, more efficient diaphragmatic motion, better postural drainage of secretions, and improved $\dot{V}/Q$ matching. Getting the patient to the prone position should not be taken lightly. It requires meticulous attention and coordination on the part of the respiratory therapists, nursing staff, and physicians to prevent inadvertent extubation and decannulation of various lines and tubes.

V. **Fluid management** is a controversial topic. There are theoretical benefits to maintaining the lowest PAWP possible that does not reduce cardiac output, tissue perfusion (monitored by capillary refill time and lactate levels), or urine output.

VI. **Oxygen delivery and consumption.** Present data suggest a benefit from normalization but not maximization of $\dot{D}O_2$.

VII. **Corticosteroids** generally are not recommended within the first week after the onset of ARDS and should not be routinely used even in the later stages of ARDS because only one small controlled trial has been done. However, in this trial, and in anecdotal and small case series, glucocorticoids (methylprednisolone 2 mg/kg load, then 2 mg/kg/day from days 1–14, 1 mg/kg/day from days 15–21, 0.5 mg/kg/day from days 22–28, 0.25 mg/kg/day from days 29–30, and 0.125 mg/kg/day from days 31–32) have been shown to be helpful during the fibroproliferative phase of ARDS (≈ 7–14 days after onset). Consider bronchoalveolar lavage, protected brush specimen, or possibly an open lung biopsy to rule out infection before initiating corticosteroids. One recommended regimen consists of a 1–2 week trial of methylprednisolone, 2–3 mg/kg/day (or prednisone, 2–4 mg/kg/day) beginning 7–14 days after the onset of ARDS in patients who are difficult to oxygenate or ventilate and in whom uncontrollable systemic infections are not an issue.

VIII. **Inhaled nitric oxide (NO).** In small case series, NO has been shown to reduce pulmonary artery pressures and intrapulmonary shunting with an increase in PaO_2/FiO_2 ratio. Inhaled NO selectively vasodilates the pulmonary vessels that have good ventilation, thus improving $\dot{V}/Q$ matching. In the study by Rossaint et al., 7 patients were treated with continuous inhalation of NO (5–20 parts per million) for 3–53 days.

IX. **Continuous renal replacement therapy (CRRT)** may be of benefit in ARDS to reduce extravascular lung water. In addition, CRRT-induced hypothermia may reduce CO_2 production, and its alkali effect of bicarbonate in the replacement solution may facilitate permissive hypercapnia.

X. **Amiodarone pulmonary toxicity:** occurs in 5–15% of treated patients with a 5–10% mortality rate. Chronic toxicity is characterized by an insidious progression of dyspnea, cough, weight loss, and pulmonary infiltrates that include diffuse interstitial and alveolar infiltrates and localized lobar, nodular, masslike, or cavitary lesions. Histopathology is nonspecific with fibrosis, hemorrhage, and organizing pneumonia. Bronchoalveolar lavage may show foamy macrophages laden with phospholipid inclusion bodies (present even in patients without pulmonary toxicity). **Acute toxicity may mimic a bacterial pneumonia with adult respiratory distress syndrome**. Even in the absence of preoperative manifestations of pulmonary toxicity, **patients treated with amiodarone are at increased risk for acute respiratory failure after surgical procedures**, possibly because of oxidant injury triggered by the high FiO_2.

Key References: Carmichael LC, Wheeler AP: Current practices in mechanical ventilation in ARDS. Contemp Intern Med 8:53–65, 1996; Fein AM, Calalang-Colucci MG: Acute lung injury and acute respiratory distress syndrome in sepsis and septic shock. Crit Care Clin 16:289–317, 2000; Kollef MH, Schuster DP: The acute respiratory distress syndrome. N Engl J Med 332:27–37, 1995; Meduri GU, Headley AS, Golden E, et al: Effort of prolonged methylprednisolone therapy in unresolving acute respiratory distress syndrome. JAMA 280:159–165, 1998; Rossaint R, Falke KJ, Lopez F, et al: Inhaled nitric oxide for the adult respiratory distress syndrome. N Engl J Med 328:399–405, 1993; Schetz M: Non-renal indications for continuous renal replacement therapy. Kidney Int 56(Suppl): S88–S94, 1999.

Diffuse Alveolar Hemorrhage

I. Diffuse alveolar hemorrhage (DAH) is a group of disorders in which the majority of the small pulmonary vessels are the source of bleeding. Approximately one-third of patients do not have hemoptysis. Underlying histology include bland DAH, capillaritis, and unique histologies such as lymphangioleiomyomatosis and pulmonary veno-occlusive disease.

II. **DAH with pulmonary capillaritis**

Isolated pauciimmune necrotizing pulmonary capillaritis	Henoch-Schönlein purpura
Wegener's granulomatosis	Goodpasture's syndrome*
Systemic necrotizing vasculitis (microscopic polyangiitis)	Pauci-immune glomerulonephritis
Mixed cryoglobulinemia	Immune-complex-associated glomerulonephritis
Behcet's syndrome	Collagen-vascular disease (polymyositis, rheumatoid arthritis, mixed-connective tissue disease, scleroderma)

III. **DAH without capillaritis**

Idiopathic pulmonary hemosiderosis	Trimellitic anhydride
Systemic lupus erythematosus*	Mitral stenosis
Goodpasture's syndrome*	Coagulation disorders
Diffuse alveolar damage—e.g., after cytotoxic drug preconditioning therapy for bone marrow transplantation	Pulmonary veno-occlusive disease
Penicillamine—bland hemorrhage; uncommon; occurs after 1 yr of therapy	Pulmonary capillary hemangiomatosis
	Lymphangioleiomyomatosis—due to rupture of postcapillary venules, which are infiltrated by smooth muscles
	Tuberous sclerosis

* Capillaritis may or may not be persent.

IV. **Laboratory tests recommended**: urinalysis, ANCA, ANA, RF, dsDNA, anti-phospholipid antibody, complement, cryoglobulin, coagulation studies.

V. **Immunohistochemistry**
1. Linear immunofluorescence: Goodpasture's syndrome
2. Granular immunofluorescence: systemic lupus erythematosus, Henoch-Schönlein purpura, cryoglobulinemia, other connective tissue diseases
3. Pauci-immune: Wegener's granulomatosis, microscopic polyangiitis, isolated rapidly progressive glomerulonephritis.

VI. **Treatment** for DAH + capillaritis: anti-inflammatory therapy, including corticosteroids, cyclophosphamide, intravenous immunoglobulin (IVIG), and plasmapheresis, depending on the underlying etiology.

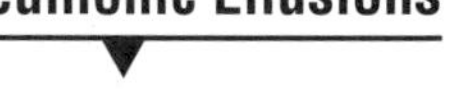

Parapneumonic Effusions

I. **Transudative vs. exudative pleural effusions.** Transudates are due to alterations in the hydrostatic and oncotic forces that control fluid formation and resorption; they are not due to intrinsic pleural pathology. Exudates are due to primary pleural pathology, usually inflammation of the pleura or obstruction of lymphatic drainage. Exudative effusions meet at least one of the following criteria, whereas transudative effusions meet none (pf = pleural fluid):
1. Protein (pf)/protein (serum) > 0.5
2. Lactate dehydrogenase (LDH) (pf)/LDH (serum) > 0.6
3. LDH (pf) > ⅔ of the upper normal limit for serum LDH

II. **Indications for tube thoracostomy in parapneumonic effusion**

1. Gross pus
2. Organisms present on Gram stain
3. Glucose < 50 mg/dl (2.8 mmol/L)
4. ph < 7.00 or at least 0.15 units < arterial pH
5. Consider if LDH > 100 IU/L

In borderline cases, serial thoracenteses at 12–24 hr intervals may indicate the need for tube thoracostomy if LDH is increasing or pH and glucose are decreasing.

III. **Thrombolytics** may be tried in patients with loculated effusions: **streptokinase**, 250,000 U, or **urokinase**, 100,000 U, in 30–60 ml of normal saline intrapleurally via chest tube each day as needed for up to 10–14 days. Clamp chest tube for 1.5–2 hr before draining.

IV. **Algorithm for empyema**

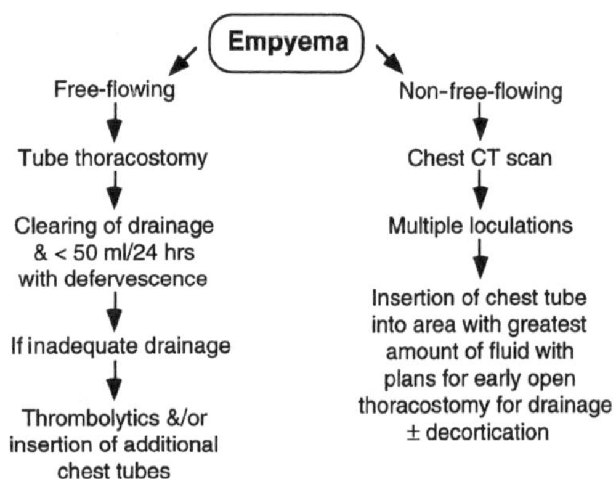

Key Reference: Light RW: Pleural diseases. Dis Mon 38:265–331, 1992.

Diagnostic Strategies in Pulmonary Embolism

I. **Algorithm for diagnosing pulmonary embolism (PE).**

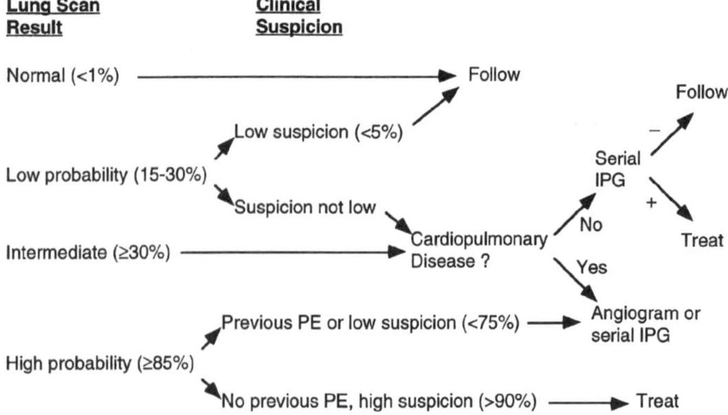

Adapted from Kelly MA, Carson JL, Palevsky HI, Schwartz JS: Diagnosing pulmonary embolism: New facts and strategies. Ann Intern Med 114:300–306, 1991.

There is a certain amount of uncertainty in the diagnosis of PE. The probability that a patient has PE correlates with clinical suspicion plus the degree of abnormality on the ventilation-perfusion ($\dot{V}/Q$) lung scan (see table).

II. **Probability of PE (%) based on $\dot{V}/Q$ scan and clinical suspicion in 887 patients**

	Clinical Suspicion			
Scan Category	**High**	**Moderate**	**Low**	**All Clinical Probabilities**
High	96 (28/29)	88	56 (5/9)	87 (103/118)
Intermediate	66	28	16	30
Low	40	16	4	14 (40/296)
Normal/near normal	0 (0/5)	6	2 (1/61)	4 (5/128)
All categories	68	30	9	28

Adapted from PIOPED Investigators: Value of the ventilation/perfusion scan in acute pulmonary embolism. JAMA 263:2753–2759, 1990.

Anticoagulation with Heparin

I. For treatment of pulmonary embolus, it is crucial that the level of anticoagulation with heparin be obtained quickly. Numerous studies have shown that therapeutic anticoagulation is often delayed unnecessarily. Most cases of pulmonary embolism can be treated with heparin alone without thrombolytics. See next section for patients who are candidates for thrombolysis.

II. The following is one recommended protocol for **unfractionated heparin:**

1. Give **bolus of heparin, 5000 U IV, then 31,000 U/24 hr** (1,300 U/hr) infusion.
2. **Check activated partial thromboplastin time (APTT) 6 hr after the bolus injection** and use the following protocol:

APTT (sec)	Repeat bolus dose (units)	Stop infusion (min)	Change rate of infusion. [heparin] = 40 U/ml	Next APTT test
< 50	5000	0	+3 ml/hr +2880 U/24 hr	6 hr
50–59	0	0	+3 ml/hr +2880 U/24 hr	6 hr
60–85	0	0	0	Next morning
86–95	0	0	–2 ml/hr –1920 U/24 hr	Next morning
96–120	0	30	–2 ml/hr –1920 U/24 hr	6hr
> 120	0	60	–4 ml/hr –3840 U/24 hr	6 hr

III. **Low–molecular-weight heparins (LMWH)** have several advantages over unfractionated heparin, including longer half-lives, administration of a fixed dose without laboratory monitoring, potential lower incidence of bleeding, and perhaps greater efficacy in preventing recurrences. Unfractionated heparin–antithrombin II complex can bind to factors IXa, Xa, and thrombin and inactivate all three. In contrast, LMWH–antithrombin III complex can inactivate only factor Xa.

Dose of LMWH:

LMWH	Deep vein thrombosis prophylaxis	Acute DVT
Ardeparin	50 units/kg 2 times/day	—
Dalteparin	2500 IU SQ 2 times/day	120 IU/kg/day SQ or 2 times/day
Danaparoid		750 units/kg BID
Enoxaparin	30 mg SQ 2 times/day	1 mg/kg SQ 2 times/day
Nadroparin		225 units/kg BID
Reviparin		100 units/kg BID
Tinzaparin		175 units/kg QD

IV. **Management of heparin-induced thrombocytopenia** (see Hematology section)
1. Discontinue heparin.
2. If there is no evidence of extension of preexisting thrombus and warfarin has been initiated (and international normalized ratio [INR] is in therapeutic range for at least 24 hr), continue warfarin.
3. If there is extension of preexisting venous thrombosis (or a large thrombus), insert inferior vena cava filter and continue warfarin.
4. If there is a new arterial thrombus, a **rapid-acting anticoagulant** should be used:
   a. **Ancrod**, 1–2 U/kg IV over 6 hr, with the dose adjusted to maintain a fibrinogen level of 0.3–0.8 gm/L.
   b. **Danaparoid sodium**, 2000 U SQ every 12 hr or 2500 U IV bolus followed by 400 U/hr IV infusion for 4 hr, 300 U/hr for 4 hr, and a maintenance infusion of 200 U/hr.
   c. **Hirudin**, 0.4 mg/kg IV bolus, followed by 0.15 mg/kg/hr IV infusion.
   d. **Refludan**, 0.4 mg/kg IV bolus, followed by 0.15 mg/kg/hr IV infusion.

Key References: Ginsberg JS: Management of venous thromboembolism. N Engl J Med 335: 1816–1828, 1996; Hirsh J: Heparin. N Engl J Med 324:1565–1574, 1991.

Administration of Protamine Sulfate

I. Protamine consists of low–molecular-weight cationic proteins that act as a heparin antagonist by complexing with heparin to form a stable salt.

II. **Major indication:** heparin-associated bleeding that requires rapid reversal of anticoagulation. Most bleeding complications may be controlled without using protamine, which may itself cause a life-threatening allergic reaction.

III. **Dose requirement of protamine** decreases as time has elapsed after the last dose of heparin. If heparin was given by bolus, see the table below for dosing protamine. **If heparin was given by IV infusion, give 25–50 mg protamine by slow IV infusion after stopping infusion of heparin.**

Time since IV heparin bolus given	Dose of protamine (mg)/100 U heparin
Few minutes	1–1.5 mg
30–60 min	0.5–0.75 mg
≥ 2 hr	0.25–0.375 mg

IV. **Method of administering protamine:** Must be given **very slowly by IV injection at a concentration of about 10 mg/ml over 1–3 min**. No more than 50 mg of protamine should be given in an 10-min period.

V. **Adverse effects**
1. Rapid injection may cause acute hypotension, bradycardia, pulmonary hypertension, dyspnea, and flushing.

2. **Hypersensitivity reactions:** urticaria, angioedema, anaphylaxis (especially in patients with allergy to fish because protamine is isolated from the sperm or mature testes of salmon). Patients who have previously been treated with protamine, who use protamine containing insulin (NPH, neutral protamine Hagedorn), and men with vasectomies may be at increased risk for subsequent hypersensitivity reactions to protamine.

Key Reference: Freed M, Grines C: Essentials of Cardiovascular Medicine. Birmingham, MI, Physicians' Press, 1994, p 247.

Thrombolytic Therapy in Venous Thromboembolism

I. Although patients with refractory hypotension or profound hypoxemia are currently considered candidates for thrombolytic therapy, some data suggest that patients with only right ventricular hypokinesis also may benefit by (1) staving off long-term right ventricular (RV) dysfunction and pulmonary hypertension and (2) decreasing the recurrence rate of pulmonary emboli (PE), but the use of thrombolytics in this latter group remains controversial.

II. **Thrombolytic Regimens:**

Agent	Standard Regimen	Bolus	Comments
Streptokinase	250,000 IU over 30 min, then 100,000 IU/hr for 24-72 hr		
Urokinase	4400 IU/kg over 10 min, then 4400 IU/kg/hr for 12–24 hr		
rTissue Plasminogen Activator	100 mg IV over 2 hr	0.6 mg/kg over 2 min or 50 mg over 10 min	Bolus regimen not FDA-approved

III. **Practical decision tree**
1. Hemodynamic compromise + high clinical suspicion + high-probability lung scan—angiogram may not be necessary before thrombolysis.
2. In patients with medium or large PE who are normotensive, an echocardiogram showing RV dilatation or dysfunction may help decide whether to use thrombolytics.

IV. **Contraindications to thrombolytics**
1. Major internal bleeding in the previous 6 months
2. Intracranial or intraspinal disease (head trauma within 6 weeks or hemorrhagic stroke within 2 months)
3. Operation or biopsy in the preceding 10 days
4. Hypertension > 200 systolic or 110 diastolic pressure
5. Infective endocarditis
6. Pericarditis
7. Bleeding disorder
8. Although advanced age is not an absolute contraindication, elderly patients have a higher risk of intracranial hemorrhage.
9. Prolonged or traumatic cardiopulmonary resuscitation

V. **Significant hemorrhage** varies greatly (6–30%) but with more recent trials, the incidence of major hemorrhage is ≈ 5–10% and of fatal hemorrhage, ≈ 1–2%.

VI. **Practical issues in massive PE:** (the primary cause of death is RV dysfunction due to increased afterload)

1. In extremely unstable patients, echocardiography may support the diagnosis of PE.
2. Fluids required for hypotension may potentially increase afterload and worsen RV dysfunction.
3. For hemodynamic instability, norepinephrine with or without dobutamine is a good option for blood pressure support, inotropy, and decreased pulmonary afterload.
4. Techniques to consider other than IV thrombolysis in patients with hemodynamically significant PE but contraindications to thrombolysis: suction-cup catheter embolectomy, intraembolic (low-dose) thrombolytic infusion, surgical embolectomy.
5. Consider inferior vena cava (IVC) filter (see next section).

Key Reference: Goldhaber SZ: Thrombolytic therapy in venous thromboembolism. Clin Chest Med 16:307–320, 1995.

Inferior Vena Cava (IVC) Filters

I. It is important to remember that even with adequate anticoagulation, recurrent or primary pulmonary emboli (PE) may still occur, with an incidence as high as 19% in anticoagulated patients with cancer. Most inferior vena cava (IVC) filters are placed via the right internal jugular approach. The filter is typically placed below the renal veins and above the bifurcation of the iliac veins. If it is necessary to place a filter above the renal veins because of IVC thrombosis, the Greenfield filter type should be used because it can remain patent to blood flow despite trapping clots.

II. **Standard indications for IVC filters**

1. **Contraindications to anticoagulation** in patients at high risk for proximal vein thrombosis and PE.
2. **Complications of anticoagulation**, such as bleeding, thrombocytopenia
3. Recurrence of PE despite adequate anticoagulation
4. Large, free-floating vena caval thrombus
5. Chronic thromboembolic pulmonary hypertension
6. Surgical pulmonary embolectomy or pulmonary endarterectomy

III. **Expanded indications**

1. Prophylaxis in surgical patients at high risk for PE: major trauma; pelvic, lower extremity, or hip orthopedic surgery; urologic surgery.
2. Primary treatment in patients at high risk for complications of PE or anticoagulation (obviously does not apply to all patients): elderly or pregnant patients, patients with cancer or advanced COPD.

IV. **Types of IVC filters**

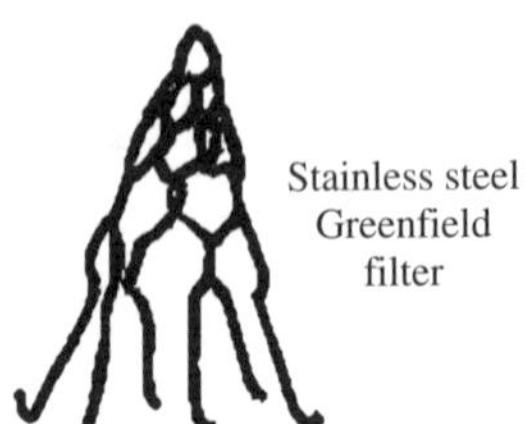

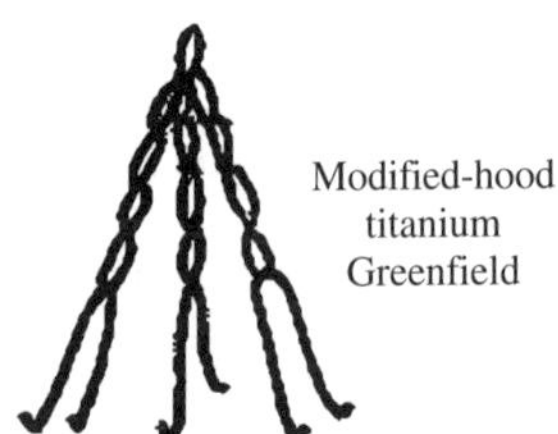

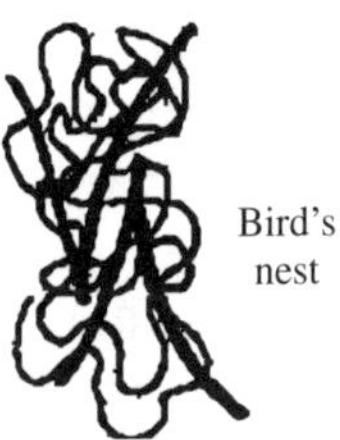

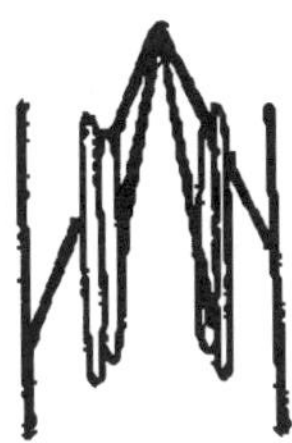
Lehmann-Girofflier-Metais

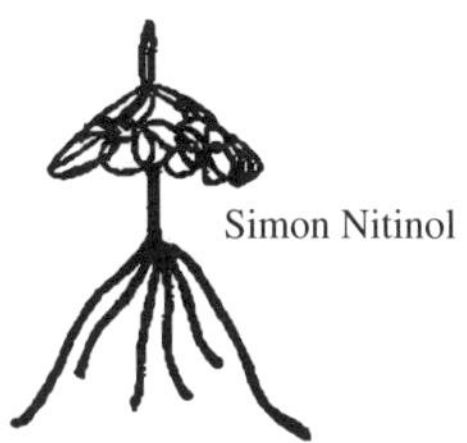
Simon Nitinol

V. **Comparison of the different types of IVC filters**

IVC Filter Type	Advantages	Disadvantages
Greenfield-stainless steel	Resistant to dislodgement from magnetic resonance field strengths	Significant artifact with MRI
Greenfield-titanium	Small cross-sectional profile, allowing percutaneous insertion; no artifacts on MRI studies	
Bird's nest	Can be anchored well, even in large vessels; can be inserted percutaneously through small (14-F) sheath	Significant artifact with MRI
Lehmann-Girofflier-Metais	No significant artifact on MRI	
Simon Nitinol	Can be inserted through a small sheath (9-F), allowing placement through antecubital or external jugular vein; Creates only minor artifact with MRI.	

VI. **Complications of IVC filters**

1. **Migration.** Limited migration is not uncommon and usually of no significance. Long-distance migration of the filter during or after placement may cause cardiac arrest. **Thus, it is extremely important to know whether a patient has an IVC filter before inserting a central venous catheter (especially a femoral line) because the guidewire may be snared and trapped by the IVC filter.**
2. **Massive caval occlusion** may lead not only to edema and lower extremity stasis but also to proliferation of the clot superior to the filter, creating more pulmonary emboli. For these reasons, it is generally recommended that **anticoagulation be continued indefinitely after IVC filter placement** if there is no contraindication.
3. **Insertion site deep venous thrombosis** may occur even with smaller catheters; if looked for, the incidence varies from 6% up to 28% although clinically significant DVT is much less common.
4. **Malpositioning.** Tilting of the IVC filter decreases its filtering efficiency.

Key References: Hyers TM, Hull RD, Weg, JG: Antithrombotic therapy for venous thromboembolic disease. Chest 108:335S–351S, 1995; Schilz R, Wirth JA: Does your patient need an inferior vena cava filter? J Respir Dis 17:1022–1030, 1996; Schilz R, Wirth JA: IVC filters: Update on evolving indications. J Respir Dis 18:30–44, 1997.

Airway Management in Burn Patients

I. **Carbon monoxide poisoning** (see Carbon Monoxide Poisoning in Toxicology Section) accounts for ≈ 50% of all burn deaths. Other medical issues to consider in a fire-burned patient are **cyanide poisoning** (see Cyanide Poisoning in Toxicology Section) and **lactic acidosis**.

II. **Upper airway injury** (edema) is usually due to thermal insult. **Lower airway injury** is primarily due to a chemical injury: (1) oxides of sulfur/nitrogen that combine with lung water to yield corrosive acids and alkalis and (2) products of polyvinylchlorides (e.g., cyanide). Noncardiogenic pulmonary edema may develop 6–72 hr after exposure in approximately 25% of patients with smoke inhalation; therefore, any patient with evidence of upper airway burns or edema, hypoxemia, bronchoconstriction, crackles, abnormal chest radiograph, or tracheobronchitis should be observed for 24–48 hr. Other lower respiratory tract manifestations associated with smoke inhalation include atelectasis (due to mucus secretion and plugging) and infectious pneumonia (complication of parenchymal injury or inflammation).

III. **Setting and signs associated with an increased risk of mucosal damage at the laryngeal level and thus increased risk of upper airway obstruction**
1. Fire in an enclosed space
2. Facial and neck burns
3. Singed nasal hairs
4. Sooty sputum and bronchorrhea
5. Hoarseness, rales, wheezes

IV. A normal flow-volume curve has a high specificity with a 94% posttest probability that intubation will not be required. However, **physiologic dysfunction** may be detected by spirometry before detectable anatomic abnormalities. Pain, anxiety, narcotics, and facial burns complicate and impose practical limitations on flow-volume curves. Abnormal spirometry results indicative of airway injury include:
1. Decreases in spirometry and expiratory flow rates
2. Sawtoothing of expiratory flows (see figure below)
3. Pattern consistent with upper airway obstruction

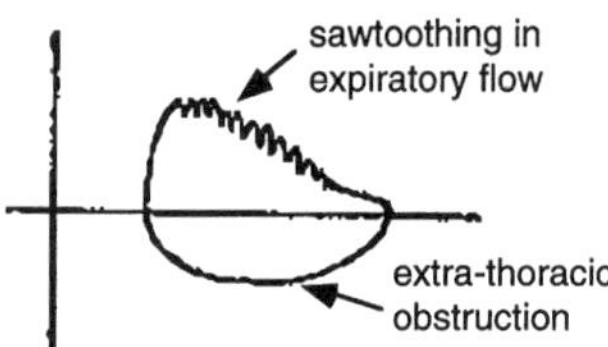

V. **Indications for prophylactic intubation.** One caveat to remember is that critical upper airway edema may develop in hospital because of supination of patient plus administration of large amounts of intravenous fluids.
1. Patients with abnormal spirometry
2. Patients with multiple risk factors for upper airway obstruction (see III above).

Key Reference: Haponik EF, Munster AM, Wise RA, et al: Upper airway function in burn patients. Am Rev Respir Dis 129:251–257, 1984.

Miscellaneous Upper Airway Obstruction

I. **Achalasia-induced upper airway obstruction:** postprandial megaesophagus may develop in achalasia due to increased upper esophageal sphincter tone after food is swallowed (acts as a one-way valve), poor peristalsis, and increased lower esophageal sphincter tone, thus trapping the food in the esophagus. The expanding esophagus causes the upper airway obstruction by compressing the trachea at the thoracic inlet. Cervical venous congestion, a compressible bulge in the neck (representing the esophagus), and respiratory distress are clues to the diagnosis. **In patients with adequate respiratory reserve, decompress the esophagus with a nasogastric tube. With respiratory failure, do tracheal intubation first with a small (≤ 7) tube, and then decompress the esophagus.**

II. **Bilateral vocal cord paralysis:** the cords are adducted in midline. During exhalation, the cords passively abduct, pushed aside by the positive airway pressure. During **inspiration** the cords **abut**, acting as one-way valves and **obstructing** the airways. Because of the neutral position of the cords at midline, the voice may be relatively preserved. For severe inspiratory stridor and respiratory failure requiring intubation, note function of the cords during tube placement. Long-term treatment options include (1) tracheotomy tube and (2) arytenoidectomy with lateralization of a vocal cord. Although bilateral vocal cord paralysis may simulate aspirated foreign body or upper airway tumor, these conditions have a component of expiratory stridor.

Key Reference: Dominguez P, et al: Acute upper airway obstruction in achalasia. Am J Gastrol 82:362–364, 1987.

Management of Massive Hemoptysis

I. Definition is arbitrary, but usually massive hemoptysis is bleeding > 100–600 ml in 24 hr. The rate of bleeding is inversely related to the prognosis. It is important to differentiate **hemoptysis** (bright red, sputum, frothy) from **hematemesis** (darker, food particles, acidic).

II. **Major causes:** aspergilloma, bronchial adenoma, bronchiectasis, bronchogenic carcinoma (central tumors, such as squamous cell carcinoma, eroding into a central pulmonary artery), broncholithiasis (due to tuberculosis or histoplasmosis), cystic fibrosis, Goodpasture's syndrome, lung abscess, pulmonary embolism, systemic lupus erythematosis, tuberculosis (Rasmussen's aneurysm in a cavity), endobronchial metastases (colon, breast, melanoma), trauma, Osler-Weber-Rendu syndrome, Kaposi's sarcoma, mitral stenosis, diffuse alveolar hemorrhage, and cryptogenic (~ 8–15%).

III. **Pathophysiology.** Massive hemoptysis generally involves bleeding from the high-pressure bronchial arteries or from the pulmonary circulation that has been pathologically exposed to the bronchial circulation via enlarged bronchopulmonary anastomoses.

IV. **Diagnosis**

1. The history, physical examination, and chest x-ray may be inaccurate in determining the hemithorax that is bleeding; thus, bronchoscopy is the most valuable diagnostic procedure in massive hemoptysis. An infiltrate on chest x-ray indicates either an airway or parenchymal source, whereas a clear chest x-ray indicates an airway source. In general, the earlier the bronchoscopy is performed, the more accurate the localization of bleeding: ~ 91% are localized < 24 hr after onset of bleed, ~ 34–50% < 48 hr, and ~ 11% > 48 hr.
2. **Arteriography** is particularly helpful when the bleeding source is peripheral to the bronchoscope's area of visualization.
3. **Pulmonary angiography** is indicated with suspicion of Rasmussen's aneurysm, arteriovenous malformation (AVM), or pulmonary artery aneurysm.

V. **Management**

1. **Control the airway.** Death is usually due to asphyxiation rather than exsanguination. Correct any coagulopathy with fresh frozen plasma and vitamin K.

Lower head of the bed to drain blood from the airway, and position patient with the **affected side down**. Coughing should be suppressed slightly.

2. If endotracheal intubation is required, try to **intubate the nonaffected side selectively.** If the bleeding is from the right lung, an endotracheal tube (ETT) can be placed in the left lung as a temporary measure. Because of the high proximal take-off of the right upper lobe bronchus, it is often not feasible to insert an ETT into the right mainstem bronchus in the case of a left lung bleed. Insert a double-lumen ETT in the case of a left lung bleed.
3. **Tamponade with the balloon of a pulmonary artery catheter or a Fogarty balloon** (may remain inflated for 24–48 hr) guided outside the bronchoscope channel. A manometer should be attached to the balloon port via a 3-way stopcock, and the inflation pressure should be < 40 mmHg to avoid mucosal necrosis.
4. **Embolization therapy** with Gelfoam following bronchial arteriography is palliative. Major complications include (1) spinal cord ischemia and (2) retrograde flow of emboli material resulting in a stroke or bowel ischemia.
5. Obtain **early surgical consultation.**

Key Reference: Thompson AB, Teschler H, Rennard SI: Pathogenesis, evaluation, and therapy for massive hemoptysis. Clin Chest Med 13:69–82, 1992.

Dyspnea in Peripartum Patients

I. The **differential diagnoses** include amniotic, air, or thrombotic embolism; aspiration of gastric contents; sepsis; preeclampsia with pulmonary edema; cardiac dysfunction (peripartum cardiomyopathy, idiopathic hypertrophic subaortic stenosis, diastolic dysfunction of obesity, and mitral valve disease); and tocolytic-related pulmonary edema.

II. **Amniotic fluid embolism (AFE).** The traditional risk factors of tumultuous labor, uterine stimulants, and/or large baby are **not** present in most patients. In a large study, risk factors for AFE are **advanced maternal age, multiparity, premature placental separation, fetal death, and meconium staining of amniotic fluid.** Endocervical vein lacerations or lower uterine tears during normal labor (or tears from a cesarean, ruptured uterus, or retained placenta) may be sites of entry. **Signs and symptoms** (during and up to 48 hr after delivery) include dyspnea, cardiorespiratory collapse, seizure, and hemorrhage from coagulopathy. The maternal mortality rate is 80–100%. Although it seems that hemodynamic compromise results from pulmonary vascular obstruction with right ventricular failure due to pulmonary hypertension, recent observation suggests that primary LV dysfunction is the major factor. Pulmonary artery catheterization, therefore, may show evidence of **pulmonary hypertension and left ventricular failure.** Thus, **diuresis and inotropic agents** are the treatment of choice rather than vasodilators and volume replacement. Presence of squamous cells in the maternal circulation is a **nonspecific** finding and **not** pathognomonic for AFE. These cells are also found in pregnant patients without AFE and even in nonpregnant patients (probably due to epidermal contamination during catheter placement). A promising method is the finding of elevated zinc coproporphyrin (a characteristic component of meconium) in maternal plasma.

III. **Tocolytic-induced pulmonary edema (ritodrine, salbutamol, terbutaline, isoxsuprine)** occurs most often during treatment (30–72 hr into therapy) with IV (or oral) β-agonist therapy. Pulmonary artery catheter studies are conflicting in regard to cardiogenic or noncardiogenic origin. Varying degrees of heart failure, pulmonary vasoconstriction, capillary leak syndrome, volume overload, and/or reduced oncotic pressure may play a role. Treatment is supportive and recovery relatively rapid after discontinuation of the tocolytic. (β-agonists may increase sodium/water retention, renin, and antidiuretic hormone.)

IV. **Volume overload.** Sodium/water retention is augmented by pregnancy, oxytocin, and iatrogenesis (IV fluids or hypertonic saline to induce abortion).

V. **Peripartum cardiomyopathy** typically presents with congestive heart failure (CHF) and embolic phenomena in the last trimester or early months postpartum; it may be unmasked by tocolytics.

VI. **Therapeutic considerations**

1. Hyperemia in pregnancy may increase **risk of endotracheal intubation trauma.**
2. Alkalosis, dopamine, dobutamine, or norepinephrine may decrease uterine blood flow.
3. For **hypotension, elevate the right hip** to move the gravid uterus off the IVC; Trendelenberg position may decrease venous return by IVC compression; for refractory hypotension, β-adrenergics such as **ephedrine or metaraminol** may be the best choice.

Key Reference: Phelan JP: Pulmonary edema in obstetrics. Obstet Gynecol Clin North Am 18:319–331, 1991.

Venous Air Embolism

I. **Venous air emboli** are marked by the sudden occurrence of unexplained cardiopulmonary dysfunction during or soon after a surgical procedure. Neurologic dysfunction may occur with a paradoxical embolus through a patent foramen ovale or, more likely, through microvascular intrapulmonary shunts. Some degree of asymptomatic air emboli occurs in up to 40% of patients undergoing **cesarean section or craniotomy in the upright position. Positive pressure ventilation and central line placement** are other settings. Air embolism also may occur through a skin tract that persists after catheter removal.

II. **Diagnosis** may be made by auscultation of the "mill-wheel" murmur, aspiration of air via a central line, air-fluid level in the pulmonary artery, or Doppler echocardiography. Nonspecific signs include elevated right heart pressures, wheezing or rales due to pulmonary edema, systemic embolization to the central nervous system or heart, and localized livedo reticularis.

III. **Treatment**

1. Extreme **left** lateral decubitus position with the chest dependent and head down
2. Aspiration of air via an existing central line
3. 100% O_2
4. Hyperbaric chamber
5. Discontinuation of nitrous oxide anesthesia, which is 20 times more soluble than oxygen or nitrogen and diffuses rapidly into and thus enlarges the air bubbles.

Systemic Air Embolism

I. **Systemic gas embolism** may be a manifestation of barotrauma during mechanical ventilation. The triad of signs and symptoms includes **cerebral manifestations** (often infarction), **myocardial infarction** (often right coronary artery or inferior wall myocardial infarct), and **livedo reticularis localized to the shoulder or anterior chest**.

II. **Predisposing factors** include adult respiratory distress syndrome, especially in the presence of necrotizing pneumonia or parenchymal cysts, which facilitates air entry into the pulmonary veins. **Emboli can be arterial (via the pulmonary veins) or venous.**

III. **Diagnosis** is made by exclusion in the setting of other signs of barotrauma.

Key Reference: Marini JJ, Culver BH: Systemic gas embolism complicating mechanical ventilation in the adult respiratory distress syndrome. Ann Intern Med 110:699–703, 1989.

Fat Embolism Syndrome

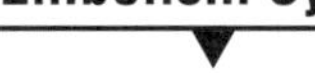

I. The classic presentation of fat embolism syndrome (FES) is a triad of **neurologic dysfunction, petechial rash, and respiratory insufficiency** after a long bone fracture. The definition is arbitrary and clinical because in up to 90% of patients with long bone or pelvic fractures and in all patients during insertion of a prosthesis in total hip replacement, fat globules are released into the venous circulation.

II. **Causes: fractures** (especially of pelvis and long bones of lower extremities), nontraumatic orthopedic procedures, soft tissue injuries, burns, osteomyelitis, diabetes mellitus, pancreatitis, sickle-cell anemia, alcoholic liver disease, lipid infusion, bone marrow harvesting and transplant, liposuction, bone tumor lysis, and cyclosporin A solvent.

III. **Features**

1. **Timing.** Massive embolization may result in acute pulmonary obstruction and right heart failure. Typically there is a delay of symptoms 24–72 hr (as late as 2 weeks after injury) after a fracture due to the release of fatty acids (from neutral fat) that results in tissue injury.
2. **Neurologic.** Intrapulmonary shunts result in microvascular fat occlusion in the CNS. Pathologically, there is diffuse petechial hemorrhage in the white matter, ischemic lesions, and intravascular fat globules. Signs and symptoms include confusion, stupor, focal neurologic deficits, seizures, and coma. The caveat is that even severe cases with cerebral edema and decorticate posturing may recover.
3. **Dermatologic. Petechiae** (present in only 20–50% of cases) typically occur over the head, neck, anterior thorax, and axillae. They represent fat globules lodged in dermal capillaries with extravasation of red blood cells.
4. **Respiratory.** Intrapulmonary shunts increase as the pulmonary artery pressure increases. Respiratory insufficiency is due to (1) initial microvessel occlusion by fat globules and (2) subsequent hydrolysis by lipase to toxic free fatty acids, resulting in lung injury characterized pathologically by intravascular clot, hemorrhagic interstitial and alveolar edema, and inflammation.
5. **Arterial embolization.** Fat globules shunted to the arterial circulation result in central retinal artery occlusion and renal fat emboli with lipiduria. **Coagulation abnormalities** occur mimicking disseminated intravascular coagulation (DIC).

IV. **Diagnosis** rests on the clinical triad. Amazingly, numerous studies have shown that laboratory tests for fat (in the serum, sputum, urine, and even bronchoalveolar lavage [BAL]) lack sensitivity and specificity (e.g., BAL is associated with a high false-positive rate in patients with pneumonia and patients with fractures but without clinical FES).

V. **Treatment.** The prophylactic use of corticosteroids may decrease the incidence and severity of FES. The difficulty is in identifying the $< 5\%$ of patients who develop clinically significant FES. It may be tried in patients who have developed early microvascular obstruction to stave off development of the later signs of acute lung injury. In one study the dose of methylprednisolone used was 30 mg/kg initially, then 4 hr later. Early immobilization and operative correction may decrease the incidence of FES.

Key Reference: King MB, Harmon KR: Unusual forms of pulmonary embolism. Clin Chest Med 15:561–580, 1994.

Tumor Embolism

I. The diagnosis of **tumor embolism (TE)** is made ante mortem in only about 6% of cases, even in patients with known cancer. Therefore, the diagnosis is often missed. TE may be the ultimate source of lymphangitic carcinomatosis. It is associated with many different solid tumors, but the most common are **liver, breast, renal, and stomach cancers**. **Intravascular lymphomatosis** is a special case of TE in which a B-cell lymphoma is confined to small blood vessels (angioendotheliomatosis). Many such patients have cutaneous violaceous plaques or nodules and central nervous system disease (dementia, focal deficits, seizures).

II. **Clinical manifestations and timing**
   1. The course and presentations are typically subacute with dyspnea over days to weeks, with or without chest pain, cough, and hemoptysis.
   2. Because of the subacute nature, **pulmonary hypertension** is often present.
   3. **Large fragments of TE** presenting acutely with hemodynamic and respiratory compromise are rare but reported with chondrosarcoma, renal cell carcinoma, right atrial myxoma, and Wilms' tumor.
   4. Death usually results from right heart failure.

III. **Ventilation-perfusion scan** may show peripheral subsegmental defects, often with a mottled appearance, similar to fat embolism and persistent pulmonary hypertension.

IV. **Cytology of blood aspirated through a wedged pulmonary artery catheter** may make the diagnosis (false positives may occur with misidentification of pulmonary megakaryocytes).

Key Reference: King MB, Harmon KR: Unusual forms of pulmonary embolism. Clin Chest Med 15:561–580, 1994.

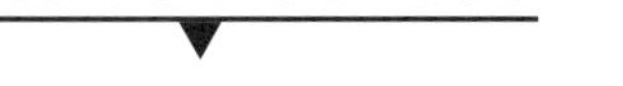

Tracheoinnominate Fistula

I. **Tracheoinnominate fistula (TIF)** results when the tip of the tracheotomy tube erodes into the innominate artery where it crosses the anterolateral surface of the trachea at the level of the upper sternum.

II. **Diagnosis**
   1. Bleeding may occur days to months after surgery.
   2. **Fifty percent of all life-threatening tracheal bleeding more than 48 hr after tracheotomy results from TIF.**
   3. Ideally, patients should be examined in the operating room because tube manipulation may result in massive hemorrhage.

III. **Treatment**
   1. **Temporizing measures**
      a. Overinflation of the cuff to tamponade the artery

   b. Endotracheal tube passed through the stoma with cuff placement adjacent to the fistula
   c. Finger insertion through a suprasternal notch incision with compression of the artery against the sternum.
2. **Definitive therapy is resection of the necrotic section of artery through a median sternotomy.**

IV. **Prevention**: avoiding low tracheotomies, using a tube of correct length that does not place the tip at the level of the innominate artery, and securing the ventilator hoses to avoid excessive tube movement.

Post-pneumonectomy Complications

I. **Bronchopleural fistula (BPF)**
1. Frequency of BPF is ~ 1.5 to 4.5% after pneumonectomy. Most BPFs occur within 2–4 weeks after surgery. Nearly all cases of BPF are associated with post-pneumonectomy empyema.
2. **Risk factors**
   a. Right-sided pneumonectomy due to a short right mainstem
   b. Current radiation or chemotherapy
   c. Age > 60 years
   d. Impaired wound healing (diabetes mellitus, corticosteroids, malnutrition)
   e. Residual tumor
   f. Surgeon's level of experience
3. **Clinical manifestations**
   a. Fever
   b. Cough with purulent sputum
   c. Hemoptysis
4. **Diagnosis**
   a. Chest radiograph
   b. V/Q scan shows aerosolized isotope in the post-pneumonectomy pleural space.
5. **Treatment**
   a. Antibiotics
   b. Drainage of space
   c. Temporary closure of tissue glue
   d. Permanent closure with muscle flap

II. **Post-pneumonectomy space (PPS)** may result from a bronchopleural fistula. The fluid in the PPS does not organize after surgery; rather, it persists or is reabsorbed even years after surgery. If the fluid does not get reabsorbed, the PPS becomes very small and the heart and great vessels may shift and rotate significantly, often lying against the lateral and posterior portions of the chest wall. Thus a "blind" thoracentesis may be quite hazardous with the risk of puncture of the heart or great vessels; worse yet, tube thoracostomy of the heart or aorta will be catastrophic.
1. **Clinical features**: Presentation may be insidious without localizing findings. Infection may develop decades after surgery.
2. **Diagnosis**: If infection of the PPS is suspected, sonography (or CT scan) of the chest should be obtained to guide a diagnostic thoracentesis and, if positive, to guide placement of a chest tube.

III. **Post-pneumonectomy empyema**
1. Differences between "early" vs "late" post-pneumonectomy empyema

	Early	Late
Onset	10–14 days	> 3 months
Incidence	60%	40%
Etiologies	Bronchopleural fistula Direct contamination Esophagopleural fistula	Bronchopleural fistula Esophagopleural fistula Blood dissemination
Symptoms	Fever, productive cough	Flu-like illness

2. Mostly due to *Staphylococcus aureus* or *Pseudomonos aeruginosa*
3. Overall mortality rate is ~ 25%.
4. Treatment consists of drainage and irrigation of the space, correction of any underlying fistula, and antibiotics.

IV. **Post-pneumonectomy pulmonary edema**

1. **Risk factors** include right-sided pneumonectomy (the right lung represents about 55% of lung mass and lymphatic capacity), carinal resection, transfusion of blood products perioperatively, amiodarone treatment perioperatively, iatrogenic fluid overload, long duration of surgery, high airway pressures during surgery, and pleural drainage with an underwater seal system. After pneumonectomy, the mean pulmonary artery pressure increases, resulting in a greater difference between pressures in the arterial and venous ends of the capillary, a greater net filtration force, and capillary leak. Excessive fluid administration exacerbates this process, which most often occurs 24–48 hr postoperatively. Although less common, pulmonary edema also may occur after a lobectomy.
2. **Criteria for diagnosis**
   a. Respiratory distress 24–96 hrs after surgery
   b. Pulmonary edema by chest radiograph
   c. Rule out cardiac dysfunction
   d. Rule out other causes of acute respiratory distress syndrome (e.g., sepsis, aspiration, hospital-acquired pneumonia)
3. **Mortality rate is > 80%**. At autopsy, the histopathology is consistent with diffuse alveolar damage.
4. **Treatment** is mainly supportive. Keep total fluid balance to ≤ 20 ml /kg in the first 24 hr after surgery. Optimize strategies to minimize ventilator-associated lung injury. Preventive measures include **meticulous fluid balance, positioning patient with the remaining lung up, and pain control to limit catecholamine release**.

V. **Pulmonary artery stump hemorrhage**

1. Uncommon complication of a BPF
2. Results from inflammation of BPF with erosion into the pulmonary artery stump.

VI. **Chylothorax**

1. Usually seen in patients who have undergone extensive lymph node resection
2. Rapid filling of space in the immediate post-operative period may be due to either hemorrhage or chylothorax
3. **Treatment**
   a. Asymptomatic: bowel rest
   b. Symptomatic: requires surgery because "tension in the space" results in increased central venous pressure.

VII. **Pulmonary embolus**

1. Thrombi can form in the pulmonary artery stump and embolize to the contralateral lung
2. Thrombi formation is more common after right sided procedures
3. Most are incidental findings and probably do not need to be treated.

VIII. **Right to left intracardiac shunt through a patent foramen ovale (PFO)** occurs with rotation of the heart and a mediastinal shift that results in preferential flow through the PFO.

IX. **Cardiac torsion** (also known as herniation or volvulus)
   1. Occurs only when the pericardium is opened during lung resection
   2. The heart moves through the defect in the pericardium and into the vacated pleural space.
   3. Right pneumonectomy-associated torsion → obstruction of aorta and/or superior vena cava. Left pneumonectomy-associated torsion → strangulation of the myocardium.
   4. Torsion is typically seen within 24 hr after surgery. It is rare after 72 hr postoperatively.
   5. Hypotension is a cardinal feature of cardiac herniation.

Thoracic Trauma

I. **Airway obstruction.** In trauma, airway obstruction may result from direct injury to the larynx and soft tissues and bony structures of the face or from edema of the upper airways. The possibility of cervical spine injury may make securing an airway more difficult. If time permits, a lateral cervical spine film should be obtained in patients with head or neck trauma before securing an airway, although a negative film does not rule out cervical fracture. If the patient is spontaneously breathing but an airway is required emergently, nasotracheal intubation may be attempted. For apneic patients, orotracheal intubation with inline cervical immobilization should be performed. For patients in whom intubation is not technically possible but who are airway compromised, needle cricothyroidotomy followed by surgical cricothyroidotomy or the latter alone should be performed (see Transtracheal Ventilation in Procedures Section).

II. **Tension pneumothorax** is a clinical diagnosis and should not be made radiographically. It is characterized by respiratory distress, tachycardia, hypotension, contralateral tracheal deviation, unilateral absence of breath sounds, neck vein distension, and cyanosis. Tension pneumothorax may be confused with cardiac tamponade, but the former is more common. Differentiation may be made by a hyperresonant percussion over the ipsilateral chest. Management involves placement of a chest tube.

III. **Open pneumothorax** (sucking chest wound). Because air tends to follow the path of least resistance through the large chest-wall defect, effective ventilation is impaired, leading to hypoxia. Management includes closing the defect with a sterile occlusive dressing, large enough to overlap the wound's edges and taped securely on three sides. Definitive surgical closure of the defect is usually required.

IV. **Massive hemothorax** is defined as rapid accumulation of > 1500 ml of blood in the chest cavity. It is most commonly caused by penetrating wounds but may result from blunt trauma. Management includes placement of a large-bore chest tube (38-French); early thoracotomy is usually required if 1500 ml or more is immediately evacuated or rate of blood loss is ≥ 200 ml/hr.

V. **Flail chest** occurs when a segment of the chest wall does not have bony continuity with the rest of the thoracic cage. It usually results from multiple rib fractures, causing a paradoxic motion of the chest wall due to loss of the structural integrity of the rib cage combined with the now unopposed influence of the negative intrapleural pressure during inspiration. The severity of the chest wall injury does

not correlate with the degree of respiratory dysfunction. Rather, respiratory failure most commonly occurs in patients with severe lung contusions, development of adult respiratory distress syndrome, or underlying respiratory compromise (e.g., emphysema). Thus **the decision to ventilate the patient mechanically is determined by the presence of respiratory failure and not by the presence of the flail chest itself, no matter how severe**. Bronchial hygiene is best managed with aggressive analgesia (intercostal nerve blocks, epidural anesthesia) and timing respiratory therapy and coughing exercises to periods of maximal pain control. Administer IV fluids judiciously because the injured lung is sensitive to edema formation.

VI. **Cardiac tamponade** consists of the classic triad of elevated venous pressure, hypotension, and muffled heart sounds. It may occur with both blunt and penetrating injuries. Pericardiocentesis may not be diagnostic or therapeutic because the blood in the pericardial sac is clotted.

VII. **Pulmonary contusion with or without flail chest.** Respiratory failure may be subtle and may develop subacutely. The contusion, manifested radiographically within 1–6 hr after trauma as ill-defined alveolar infiltrates, is due to hemorrhage and edema. Although hemoptysis and hypoxemia may occur, most patients who have chest contusion without flail chest do well.

VIII. **Myocardial contusion** may be established by symptoms of chest pain in the appropriate setting with EKG abnormalities (premature ventricular contractions, sinus tachycardia, atrial fibrillation, right bundle-branch block, and ST segment changes), two-dimensional echocardiography, and cardiac muscle enzyme elevations.

IX. **Traumatic aortic rupture** usually occurs in the setting of car collision or fall from great height (deceleration injuries). Angiography should be performed liberally because the findings of chest films are unreliable. Radiographic signs that may be suggestive include widened mediastinum, fractures of the first and second ribs, obliteration of the aortic knob, deviation of the trachea to the right, presence of a pleural cap, elevation and rightward shift of the right mainstem bronchus, depression of the left mainstem bronchus, obliteration of the space between the pulmonary artery and aorta, and deviation of the esophagus (and nasogastric tube) to the right.

X. **Traumatic diaphragmatic rupture.** If laceration of the left diaphragm is suspected, a nasogastric tube should be inserted; a diaphragmatic rupture is likely if the tube appears in the thoracic cavity. Right diaphragmatic rupture is more difficult to diagnose because the liver obliterates the defect on the right; the only finding may be an elevated right hemidiaphragm.

XI. **Laryngeal fracture** is suggested by hoarseness, subcutaneous emphysema, palpable fracture, and crepitus.

XII. **Tracheal injury.** Airway obstruction and associated injuries in the neck and upper chest areas are the major concerns.

XIII. **Bronchial injury** is an unusual but underappreciated and often fatal complication of thoracic trauma. Most cases involve blunt trauma to the anterior part of the chest and occur within 1 inch distal to the carina. The first three ribs are often fractured. Frequently the patient presents with hemoptysis, subcutaneous emphysema, bilateral pneumothoraces, or tension pneumothorax with a mediastinal shift. In addition, obstructive bronchus and atelectasis may occur when the fracture end is displaced. Findings suggestive of bronchial injury in a trauma patient include (1) pneumothorax associated with a **persistent large air leak** after tube thoracotomy, (2) **pneumothorax and pneumomediastinum in the absence of pleural effusion,** and (3) **pneumomediastinum in a trauma patient not on mechanical ventilation.**

XIV. **Esophageal trauma** is most commonly due to penetrating injury. Blunt trauma causes include forceful expulsion of gastric contents into the esophagus from a severe blow to the upper abdomen. Consider esophageal trauma in any patient who has a left pneumothorax or hemothorax without rib fracture, who received a severe blow to the lower sternum or epigastrium, who is in pain or shock out of proportion to the apparent injury, and who has particulate matter in the chest tube.

XV. **Pulmonary lacerations** may develop with severe blunt chest trauma or from broken rib ends. Lacerations that extend to the pleural surface may result in bronchopleural fistula and hemopneumothorax. Hemorrhage within a parenchymal laceration may appear as a spherical hematoma. Traumatic pneumatoceles may form rather quickly or days after the trauma because the elastic lung recoils from the site of rupture. Pneumatoceles may take 4–6 months for complete radiographic resolution.

XVI. **Blunt chest trauma:** may result in (1) **pulmonary contusion**, which is characterized by a patchy or homogeneous infiltrate at region of maximal trauma (or a contrecoup effect) that is apparent within 1 hr in 70% of patients and invariably within 6 hr of the trauma (a new infiltrate occurring after 6 hr suggests another diagnosis), or (2) **pulmonary lacerations**, which may remain intrapulmonary, presenting as a **hematoma** (spherical infiltrate) or **traumatic pneumatocele** (lung contracts from the laceration immediately or days after trauma), or may extend through the pleural surface, presenting with a **bronchopleural fistula** and **hemopneumothorax**.

Key Reference: Committee on Trauma: Advanced Trauma Life Support. Chicago, American College of Surgeons, 1988.

Radiology

Monitoring and Troubleshooting Catheters, Wires, and Tubes

I. **Endotracheal tubes (ETT)**
   1. With the neck in neutral position, the ETT tip should be 4–6 cm above the carina.
   2. Early radiographic signs of tracheal rupture:
      a. Orientation of the distal portion of the ETT to the right relative to the tracheal lumen in association with an overdistended balloon cuff
      b. Migration of the balloon cuff toward the tip of the ETT
      c. Pneumomediastinum and subcutaneous emphysema

II. **Thoracostomy tubes**
   1. Subcutaneous placement of a chest tube results in no visualization of the non-radiopaque tube edge because it is silhouetted by subcutaneous tissue.
   2. After removal of a chest tube, a residual pleural or parenchymal line from the tube tract is often noted and may be confused with a pneumothorax.

III. **Central venous catheters**
   1. For accurate central venous pressure readings, the tip of the catheter should be past the last venous valves, usually distal to the anterior first rib.
   2. Keep the catheter tip above the right atrium to lessen the risk of arrhythmia and right atrial perforation from the catheter itself or from hypertonic solutions infused through the catheter.

IV. **Pulmonary artery catheters**
   1. When the catheter is positioned too far distally or the balloon is overinflated, pulmonary infarction, embolism, hemorrhage, pulmonary artery rupture with a bronchial tree fistula, or pseudoaneurysm may occur.
   2. In the nonwedged position, the tip of the catheter should be located in the right or left central pulmonary artery.

V. **Transvenous pacemakers**
   1. Best positioned in the right ventricular apex.
   2. Cardiac perforation (eventually occurs in ≈ 5–7% of placements after migration) can be detected when the tip extends beyond the expected border of the myocardium or into the epicardial fat pad or when the cardiac shadow rapidly enlarges.

VI. **Intraaortic balloon pump**
   1. The catheter tip should be just distal to the left subclavian artery so as not to occlude the aortic arch vessels.
   2. Aortic dissection is a known complication.

Key Reference: Swensen SJ, Peters SG, LeRoy AJ, et al: Radiology in the intensive-care unit. Mayo Clin Proc 66:396–410, 1991.

Cardiopulmonary Disorders

I. **Distinguishing pulmonary abscess from empyema**
   1. Typically an **abscess has air-fluid level widths that are equal** on both frontal and lateral chest radiographs because abscesses are more likely to be spherical.

2. Pleural fluid collections tend to have a more vertical orientation. The inner wall margins are smooth in an empyema, whereas **abscess walls are shaggy**. In addition, empyema has an air-fluid level that extends to the chest wall.
3. On computed tomography, the **walls of an empyema are uniform in thickness**, and when the empyema occupies > 10% of a hemithorax, lung compression and distortion are common (lung compression is rarely caused by an abscess).
4. Angle of contact with the chest wall: acute in abscess, obtuse in empyema.
5. Lobar boundaries are preserved by abscess, crossed by empyema.
6. Bronchial vessels are displaced by empyema, obliterated by abscess.

II. **Atelectasis**

1. Common in the left lower lobe after cardiac surgery, in part because of paralysis and paresis of the phrenic nerve related to stretch or cold-induced injury.
2. Absence of air bronchogram in a region of persistent atelectasis is suggestive of mucoid impaction. Therapeutic bronchoscopy may help.

III. **Pulmonary embolism and infarction**

1. Nonspecific chest x-ray findings: elevated hemidiaphragm, subsegmental atelectasis, patchy infiltrates (due to associated edema, hemorrhage, or infarction), effusions, oligemia (Westermark's sign), Hampton's hump (wedge-shaped peripheral opacity).

IV. **Pleural effusions**

1. In a recumbent position, the effusion layers posterosuperiorly, resulting in a hazy opacity that increases in density in a cephalocaudad direction.
2. Radiographic detection of **pleural effusions**
   a. < 75 cc—no radiographic changes
   b. > 75 cc—blunting of posterior diaphragmatic sulcus on lateral chest x-ray
   c. > 175 cc—blunting of lateral costophrenic angle on posteroanterior chest x-ray
3. Five clues to the presence of a **subpulmonic effusion**
   a. Elevation of ipsilateral diaphragm
   b. Lateral displacement of apex of diaphragm
   c. Medial flattening of diaphragm
   d. Nonvisualization of lower lobe vessels behind the diaphragm
   e. Increased distance between the diaphragm and stomach bubble

V. **Postpneumonectomy**

1. The fluid level in the hemithorax should rise slowly.
2. A rapid accumulation of fluid is consistent with a pulmonary hemorrhage.
3. A decrease in fluid level is consistent with a bronchopleural fistula.

VI. **Effects of positive end-expiratory pressure (PEEP)**

May result in better aerated lungs, decreased heart size, and a narrower vascular pedicle radiographically.

VII. **Pneumothorax (PTX)**

1. Most PTXs demonstrated radiographically in recumbent patients are situated in an anteromedial or subpulmonic location. Increased lucency over the diaphragm, cardiac apex, or fat pad or a deepened diaphragmatic sulcus may be the only clue.
2. A simple PTX appears as a thin dense **line**, bordered by aerated lung on one side and pleural air on the other. In a supine patient with a hydropneumothorax, the pleural space does not appear as black because of the pleural fluid.
3. A skin-fold appears as an **edge**, not a line, with bronchovascular markings visible distal to the edge.
4. **Pneumomediastinum.** On frontal views, mediastinal air deflects the pleura laterally along the left heart border, creating a lucent stripe of air medially bounded by a lateral, vertical pleural line. A continuous diaphragm sign (central

portions of the diaphragm are visualized behind the heart) and air lucencies around the aorta, vena cava, or trachea may be seen. On the lateral view, air within the mediastinal tissue planes and surrounding the cardiac shadow may be seen.

5. **Estimating the size of pneumothorax**
   1. Measure the maximal apical interpleural distance in cm (1).
   2. Measure the interpleural distance ¼ the distance from the apex in cm (2).
   3. Measure the interpleural distance ¾ the distance from the apex in cm (3).
   4. Average the 3 interpleural distances in cm.

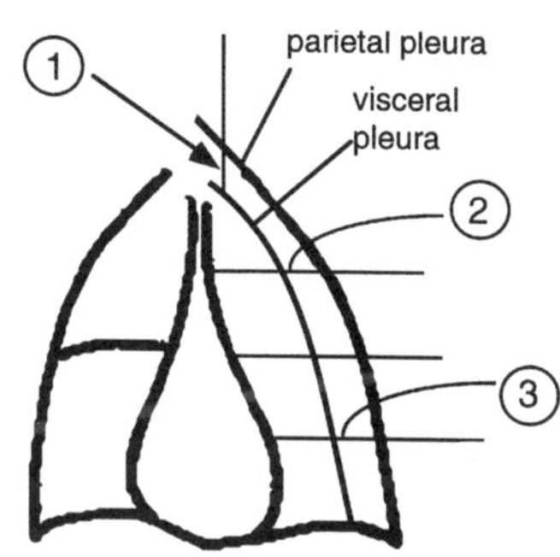

Percentage pneumothorax	Average interpleural distance (cm)
5	< 0.5
10	0.5
25	2.25
50	5.0

Key Reference: Swensen SJ, Peters SG, LeRoy AJ, et al: Radiology in the intensive-care unit. Mayo Clin Proc 66:396–410, 1991.

Radiographic Recognition of Barotrauma

I. Although a number of retrospective studies have clearly shown an association between high peak airway pressure (Ppk) and barotrauma, a cause-and-effect relationship has not been demonstrated.

II. A more predictive variable for the occurrence of barotrauma is the degree of **lung distention**, which correlates with the **transalveolar pressure** in experimental animal studies. In humans, this pressure correlates best with the **plateau or static airway pressure (Pplat).** The critical or toxic Pplat is ~ 35 cmH_2O.

III. **Radiographic signs of barotrauma (includes pneumothorax, interstitial emphysema, and pneumomediastinum).** Barotrauma is indicated by a number of radiographic signs, including visible pleural line *(A)*, deep sulcus sign *(B)*, hyperlucency localized to the upper abdomen *(C)*, inverted diaphragm *(D)*, air-fluid level *(E)*, mediastinal shift *(F)*, subpleural air cyst *(G)*, interstitial emphysema *(H)*, complete diaphragm *(I)*, and pneumomediastinum *(J)*.

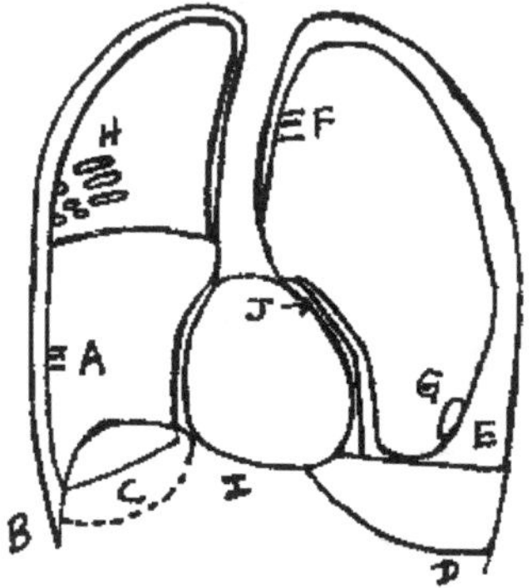

Key Reference: Marini JJ, Wheeler AP: Critical Care Medicine: The Essentials. Baltimore, Williams & Wilkins, 1989, p 265.

Radiographic Recognition of Atelectasis

I. Atelectasis is not uncommon in patients who are intubated, sedated, comatose, or in pain because secretions are not cleared normally. Atelectasis may be segmental, lobar, or involve the whole lung. Air bronchograms may be seen in atelectasis and usually indicate that the atelectasis is peripheral rather than the result of a central obstruction. Some patients have multiple areas of scattered atelectasis that simulate patchy alveolar infiltrates of widespread pneumonia.

1. **Primary signs of atelectasis:** opacification (indicating airlessness) and shift of an interlobar fissure, hilum, or main bronchus.
2. **Secondary signs:** shift of hemidiaphragm, heart, or mediastinal structures; crowded vessels, rib cage size discrepancy, and compensatory hyperaeration in the uninvolved parts of the lung are other signs of atelectasis. Hilar displacement is the best sign of lobar collapse; remember that the left hilum is higher than the right in 97% of normal people.

II. **Normal fissure positions**

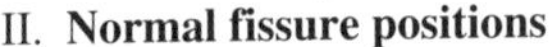

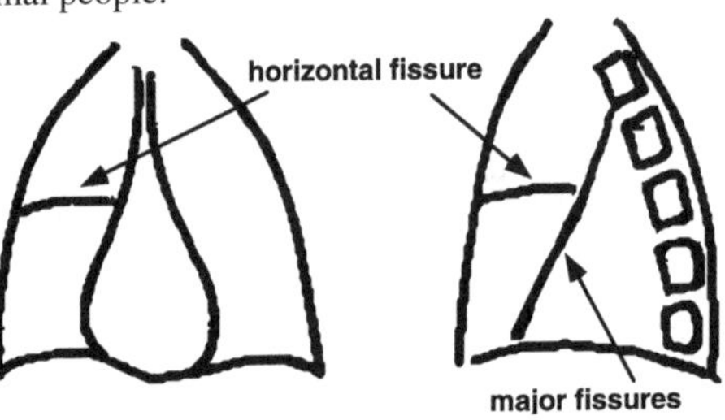

III. **Left upper lobe collapse:** collapses anteriorly and superiorly

1. Opacification of the left upper chest
2. Partial loss of the left heart border

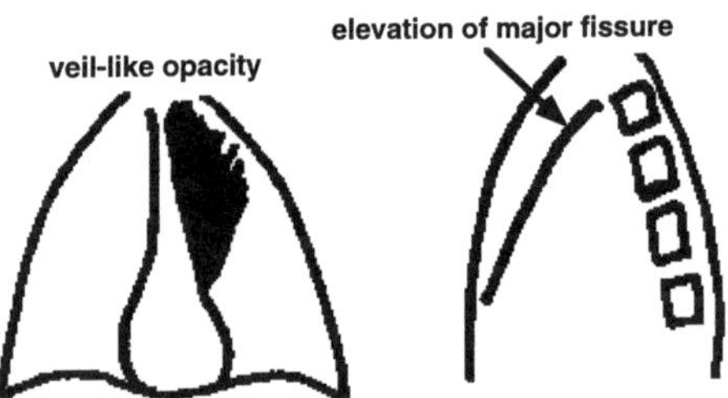

IV. **Right upper lobe collapse:** Collapses superiorly and medially

1. Opacification of the right upper medial chest
2. Elevation of the minor fissure
3. Reverse S sign of Golden represents the elevated minor fissure

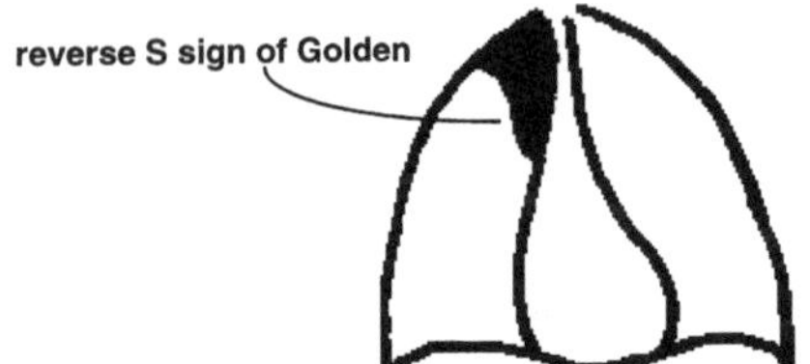

V. **Right middle lobe collapse**
1. Minimal loss of the right heart border
2. On lateral view, the linear band or wedge-shaped triangle of the right middle lobe is sandwiched between the depressed minor fissure and the elevated major fissure.

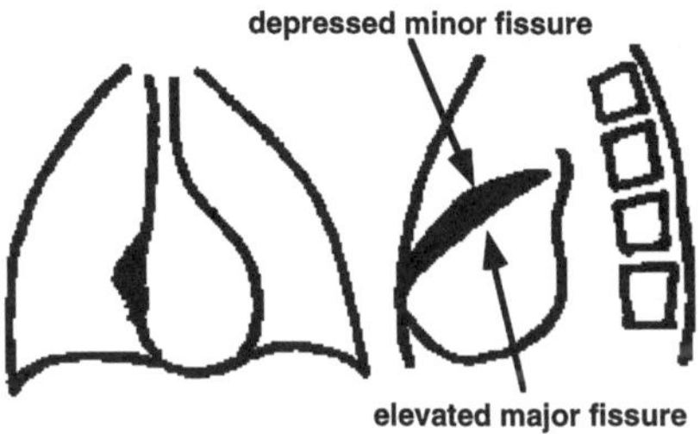

VI. **Right upper and middle lobe collapse**
1. Opacification along the medial aspect of the right chest
2. Absence of much of the right heart border
3. Smaller right lung
4. On lateral view, elevation of the major fissure

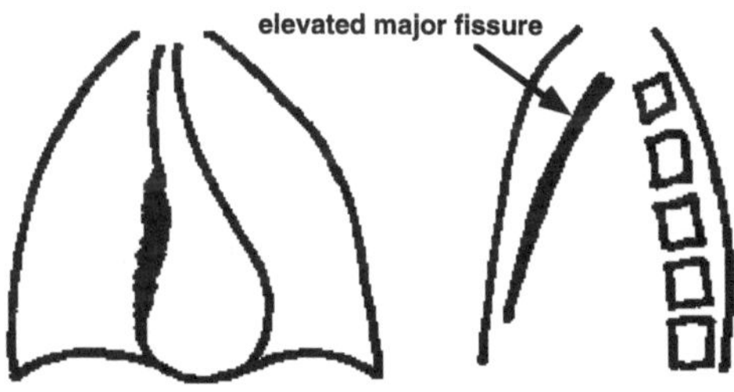

VII. **Lower lobe collapse:** both lower lobes collapse in a posterior medial and inferior direction. The shifted major fissure is most often seen on the frontal radiograph.
1. **Left lower lobe collapse**
   a. Retrocardiac density
   b. Lack of visualization of the descending aorta and left hemidiaphragm
   c. Shift of mediastinum to the left

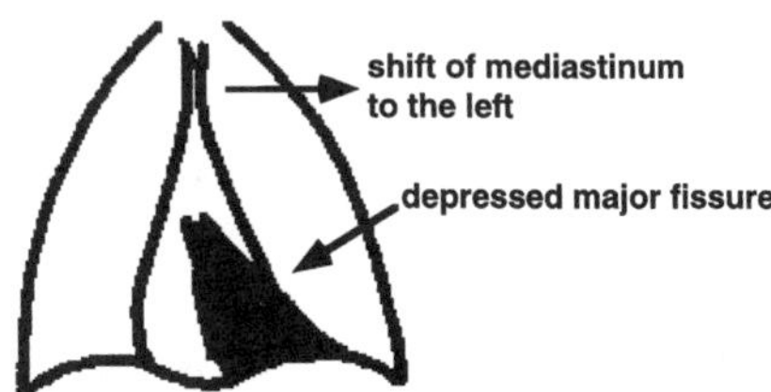

2. **Right lower lobe collapse**
   a. Lack of visualization of the right hemidiaphragm
   b. Shift of mediastinum to the right

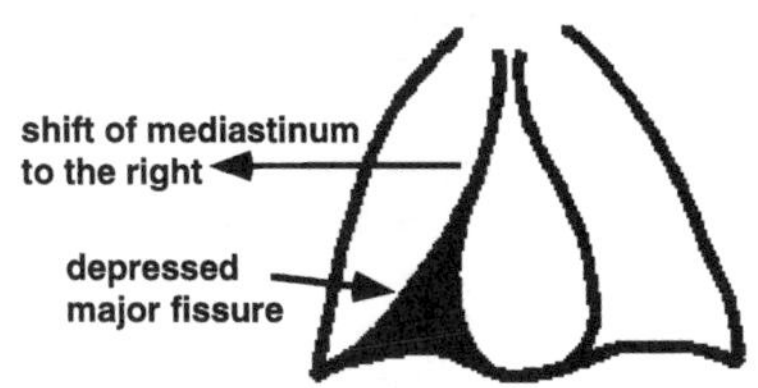

Key Reference: Freundlich IM, Bragg DG: A Radiologic Approach to Diseases of the Chest. Baltimore, Williams & Wilkins, 1992.

Intravenous Contrast Media Reactions

I. Intravenous contrast agents are low-molecular-weight iodinated compounds that are highly hyperosmolar. Two main types of reactions may occur in patients receiving these agents: **chemotoxic and anaphylactoid**.

II. **Chemotoxic reactions** include (1) interactions with the hypothalamus causing fever, nausea, increased vagal tone leading to bradycardia and bronchospasm, and seizures; (2) alteration of cardiac conduction and decreased contractility leading to arrhythmias; and (3) renal toxicity due to renovascular constriction, osmotic diuresis, and direct tubular toxicity. Chemotoxic effects are mainly related to the high osmolality of the agents and include initial plasma expansion with subsequent osmotic diuresis and volume depletion.

III. **Risk factors for anaphylactoid reactions** (risk is less with lower-osmolality, nonionic compounds):
   1. Age 30–40 years
   2. History of atopy or asthma
   3. Previous reaction
   4. Current use of beta blockers
   5. Significant cardiovascular disease
   6. Cerebral or coronary angiography

III. **Prophylaxis regimen**
   1. **Prednisone**, 50 mg, 13 hr, 7 hr, and 1 hr before radiocontrast procedure.
   2. **For emergent radiocontrast procedure**, give hydrocortisone, 200 mg IV immediately and 4 hr after the procedure. Also give diphenhydramine, 50 mg orally or IM 1 hr before the procedure.
   3. **Use nonionic contrast media**

IV. **Treatment** of anaphylactoid reactions includes beta agonists, diphenhydramine, epinephrine, corticosteroids, fluids, and H_2 blockers.

Key Reference: Crnkovich DJ, Carlson RW: Anaphylaxis: An organized approach to management and prevention. J Crit Illness 8:332–346, 1993.

Prevention of Radiographic Contrast Agent-induced Renal Insufficiency

I. Intravenous radiographic contrast agents can precipitate acute renal failure. **Risk factors include**:
   1. Preexisting renal dysfunction, especially diabetic nephropathy.
   2. Dehydration
   3. States of reduced effective arterial volume such as congestive heart failure and cirrhosis.
   4. Concomitant administration of drugs that interfere with the regulation of renal perfusion (e.g., angiotensin-converting enzyme inhibitors).
   5. Higher volume of contrast agent given.

II. **Preventive measures**
   1. Use of **low-osmolality, nonionic radiocontrast agent**
   2. **Saline hydration**
   3. **N-acetylcysteine**, 600 mg orally twice daily on the day before and on the day of administration of the contrast agent.

Key Reference: Tepel M, et al: Prevention of radiographic contrast-agent-induced reductions in renal function by acetylcysteine. N Engl J Med 343:180–184, 2000.

Acid–Base Disorders

Acid–Base Pearls

I. **Bedside interpretation**

Disorder	Rule of thumb of compensatory findings
Metabolic acidosis	$PaCO_2$ decreases by 1–1.5 times the decrease in $[HCO_3]$ or the last 2 digits in pH ≈ $PaCO_2$
Metabolic alkalosis	$PaCO_2$ increases by 0.25–1.0 times the increase in $[HCO_3]$
Acute respiratory acidosis	$[HCO_3]$ increases 1 mmol/L for each 10 mmHg increase in $PaCO_2$ or 10 mmHg increase in $PaCO_2$ → decrease in pH of 0.08 units
Chronic respiratory acidosis	$[HCO_3]$ increases by 4 mmol/L for each 10 mmHg increase in $PaCO_2$
Acute respiratory alkalosis	$[HCO_3]$ decreases 1–3 mmol/L for each 10 mmHg decrease in $PaCO_2$ but usually not to < 18 mmol/L
Chronic respiratory alkalosis	$[HCO_3]$ decreases 2–5 mmol/L for each 10 mmHg decrease in $PaCO_2$ but usually not to < 14 mmol/L.

II. **The serum anion gap (AG)** is the difference between the unmeasured anions (UA) and unmeasured cations (UC) in the serum and is equivalent to [Na] – [Cl] – $[HCO_3]$. Normal AG is 3–11 mEq/L.

1. Factors that may cause a decrease in the AG are hypoalbuminemia, abnormal paraproteinemias (which have a net positive charge), hyponatremia, and increases in measured cations (potassium [K], magnesium [Mg], calcium [Ca]) as well as unmeasured cations (NH_4^+ and other ammonium compounds, as occur in chronic renal failure).
2. A 50% reduction in serum albumin decreases the AG by 5–6. Therefore, an AG of 12 should be corrected to 17–18; this may uncover an increased AG acidosis.

III. **Urinary AG = urinary UA – urinary UC = $[U_{Na}] + [U_K] - [U_{Cl}]$** is a useful parameter in patients with non-AG acidosis to determine renal or gastrointestinal loss of HCO_3.

Urine AG	Urine pH	Diagnosis
Negative	< 5.5	Normal
Positive	> 5.5	Type 1 renal tubular acidosis (RTA)
Negative	< 5.5	Diarrhea

NH_4 is the major UC. When urine acidification is deranged (RTA), the urinary NH_4 (UC) is decreased, and the urinary AG is increased and becomes more positive.

IV. **General clues to the presence of a mixed disorder** (see Differential Diagnosis of Metabolic Acidosis and Alkalosis):

1. Normal pH (with the exception of respiratory alkalosis)
2. pCO_2 and HCO_3 deviating in opposite directions
3. pH change in the opposite direction for a known primary disorder

Key Reference: Dunagan WC, Ridner ML (eds): Manual of Medical Therapeutics, 26th ed. Boston, Little, Brown, 1989, p 66 (table in Section I.)

Differential Diagnosis of Metabolic Acidosis and Alkalosis

I. **Normal AG metabolic acidosis** (determine the urinary AG = $U_{Na} + U_K - U_{Cl}$) Positive urinary AG → renal loss; negative urinary AG → gastrointestinal (GI) loss.
   1. Potassium usually decreases with:
      GI losses (diarrhea, ureterosigmoidostomy, pancreatic fistula)
      Type I and II RTA
      Acetazolamide
      Post-ATN diuretic phase
      Excessive chloride administration for diabetic ketoacidosis (DKA)
      Mild renal insufficiency
      Volume infusion with chloride containing fluids or oral $CaCl_2$
      Toluene toxicity
   2. Potassium is normal or increases with:
      Type IV RTA
      Spironolactone, triamterene, amiloride
      Hyperparathyroidism
      Mild renal insufficiency
      Ingestion of acids with Cl (NH_4Cl, arginine HCl, HCl)

II. **High AG metabolic acidosis** ("klumpies")
   Ketoacidosis (diabetic, alcoholic, starvation)
   Lactic acidosis
   Uremia
   Methanol, ethanol
   Paraldehyde, propylene glycol
   Isoniazid, iron
   Ethylene glycol, toluene
   Salicylate

III. **Metabolic alkalosis** (unclassified: milk-alkali syndrome) may be subdivided into chloride-responsive (U_{Cl} < 10 mmol/L) or chloride-resistant alkalosis (U_{Cl} > 20 mmol/L).

Chloride-responsive (volume-depleted)	Chloride-resistant (mineralocorticoid excess)
Vomiting	Hyperaldosteronism
Nasogastric suction	Bartter's syndrome
Diuretic use (U_{Cl} > 10 mmol/L)	Cushing's syndrome
Contraction alkalosis	Malignant hypertension
Villous adenoma	Exogenous steroids
Rapid correction of chronic respiratory acidosis	English licorice (glycyrrhizic acid)
Zollinger-Ellison syndrome	Liddle syndrome
	Hypercalcemia
	Potassium depletion

   Treatment: K and NaCl solutions. Chloride may be the most important ion to replace.

IV. **Mixed acid–base disorders**
   1. pH < 7.35 indicates primary acidosis; pH > 7.45 indicates primary alkalosis.
   2. Metabolic acidosis and respiratory acidosis (e.g., cardiopulmonary arrest, severe congestive heart failure).
   3. Metabolic acidosis and respiratory alkalosis (salicylate intoxication)—both P_{CO_2} and HCO_3 are low, but the P_{CO_2} is lower than predicted.

4. Metabolic acidosis and metabolic alkalosis (renal failure with vomiting, ketoacidosis with vomiting, critically ill patients with gastric suction)—increased anion gap with normal or high HCO_3 is suggestive.
5. Metabolic alkalosis and respiratory acidosis (chronic obstructive pulmonary disease with vomiting, adult respiratory distress syndrome with gastric suction)—characterized by high HCO_3 and high $PaCO_2$ but increase in HCO_3 greater than predicted.
6. Metabolic alkalosis and respiratory alkalosis (inappropriate mechanical hyperventilation with gastric suction or diuretic use, pregnancy with vomiting).
7. Triple acid–base disorder (e.g., alcoholic with ketosis, vomiting, and tachypnea due to sepsis or liver disease; see Practical Approach to Acid-Base Disorders below).

Lactic Acidosis

I. **Definition:** [lactate] > 4 mmol/L (normal = ~ 1 mmol/L) + metabolic acidosis.

II. **Causes**

1. **Type A**
   a. **Tissue hypoxia** (shock, decreased cardiac output, hypoxemia, carbon monoxide poisoning, severe anemia, hemorrhage, methemoglobinemia)
   b. **Increased oxygen demand** (vigorous exercise, seizures, sepsis)
   c. Both a and b are associated with **elevated NADH/NAD ratio** (ratio of reduced to oxidized nicotinamide adenine dinucleotide). This ratio directly correlates with the amount of pyruvate metabolized to lactate because tissue hypoxic states, which result in low oxidized NAD levels and high NADH/NAD ratio in the mitochondria, increase lactate production.
2. **Type B**
   a. **Liver disease**
   b. **Diabetes mellitus, hypoglycemia**
   c. **Malignancy** (lymphoma, leukemia, small cell carcinoma)
   d. **Renal failure**
   e. **Alkalosis**
      - Elevates lactate because the key glycolytic enzyme phosphofructokinase [PFK] is pH-sensitive.
      - Acidosis inhibits and alkalosis stimulates glycolysis by inhibiting and stimulating PFK, respectively.
      - **Caveat:** sodium bicarbonate or hypocapnia may increase lactic acid production.
   f. **Drugs** (phenformin, metformin, ethanol, methanol, ethylene glycol, paraldehyde, cyanide, nitroprusside, isoniazid, epinephrine [pheochromocytoma])
   g. **Hereditary defects** (pyruvate decarboxylase [biotin] deficiency, mitochondrial disorders, glucose-6-phosphatase deficiency)
   h. **D-lactic acidosis**
      - Occurs in patients with small bowel dysfunction (e.g., short bowel syndromes) in which excess carbohydrate is metabolized by bacterial D(–)-lactic dehydrogenase, an enzyme lacking in humans.
      - Accompanied by neurologic syndrome consisting of confusion, ataxia, and slurred speech.
      - Because standard lactate determinations measure only L(+)-lactate, the lactate level in D(–)-lactic acidosis is "normal."

III. **Symptoms and signs:** hyperventilation, abdominal pain, mental status change.

IV. **Treatment**

1. **Treat underlying disorder** (e.g., sepsis, cardiogenic shock, or toxin exposure): fluid resuscitation with or without inotropic support.
2. **Sodium bicarbonate:** controversial because bicarbonate therapy has been shown to be deleterious in experimental models and patients; generally not recommended unless severe acidosis is refractory to fluid and inotropic resuscitation.
3. **Hemodialysis:** beneficial effects include removal of lactate and excessive fluid and delivery of bicarbonate.
4. **Dichloroacetate** (activator of pyruvate dehydrogenase) failed to show benefit in hemodynamics or survival in a prospective study. **Carbicarb** (contains sodium bicarbonate and carbonate) theoretically may alkalinize without raising $PaCO_2$. Neither is FDA-approved for treatment of lactic acidosis.

Key Reference: Stacpoole: Lactic acidosis. Endocrinol Metab Clin North Am 22:221–245, 1993.

Renal Tubular Acidosis (RTA)

Type	Associated Conditions	K	Urinary pH	Therapy
I (distal)	Autosomal dominant, systemic lupus erythematosus, sickle cell, hyperparathyroid hormone, medullary sponge kidney, amphotericin B, lithium, toluene, hypergammaglobulinemia states (cirrhosis, sarcoidosis, multiple myeloma)	Low to normal	> 5.5	Oral HCO_3, 1–2 mmol/kg/day
II (proximal)	Fanconi syndrome, acetazolamide, medullary cystic disease, multiple myeloma, nephrotic syndrome	Low to normal	< 5.5	Oral HCO_3, 10–25 mmol/kg/day
IV (distal)	Hyporeninemic hypoaldosteronism (diabetes, interstitial nephritis, obstructive uropathy), Addison's disease, heparin, K-sparing diuretics	High	< 5.5	Fludrocortisone 0.1–0.4 mg orally a day

HCO_3 deficit (mmol/L HCO_3) = weight (kg) × (24 – HCO_3) × 0.5

Practical Approach to Acid–Base Disorders

I. **Determine whether the data are internally consistent.**

1. $[H+] = 24\ PaCO_2/[HCO_3]$
2. For each 0.01 unit change in pH, [H+] will change inversely by 1 mmol/L, i.e., **$[H+] = 40 + (\Delta pH)(1\ mEq/L)/(0.01)$**
3. Example: 7.32/24/104; HCO_3 = 23
   a. [H+] = (24)(24)/23 = 24
   b. However, for pH of 7.40 → 7.32, [H+] = 40 + (0.08)(1 mEq/L)/0.01 = 48
   c. Thus, the data is not internally consistent because for the pH to be 7.32 with a pCO_2 of 24, the [H+] should be 48 and not 24 (i.e., the HCO_3 should be lower).

II. **Determine whether the patient is acidemic or alkalemic and diagnose the primary disorder** (see Acid–Base Pearls).

III. **Determine whether respiratory compensation is adequate for metabolic acidosis.**

$$pCO_2 = 1.5(HCO_3) + 8 \pm 2$$

IV. **Measure the urine AG in patients with hyperchloremic metabolic acidosis** (see Acid–Base Pearls).

V. **To sort out high AG acidosis mixed with other acid–base disorders, measure the ΔGap = ΔAG – ΔHCO_3**

$= (AG_{obs} - AG_{ULN}) - (HCO_{3LLN} - HCO_{3obs})$; $AG_{ULN} \approx 12$; $HCO_{3LLN} \approx 24$,

where ULN = upper limit of normal, LLN = lower limit of normal, obs = observed.

ΔGap ≈ 0: Simple high AG acidosis

ΔGap > 0: Mixed high AG metabolic acidosis + primary metabolic alkalosis
 Mixed high AG metabolic acidosis + chronic respiratory acidosis with metabolic compensation

ΔGap < 0: Mixed high AG metabolic acidosis + non-AG metabolic acidosis
 Mixed high AG metabolic acidosis + chronic respiratory alkalosis with compensatory non-AG metabolic acidosis
 Mixed high AG metabolic acidosis + low AG metabolic acidosis

VI. A **more rapid method** to determine the presence of a mixed disorder:

1. **If ΔAG + HCO_3 is normal** → high AG metabolic acidosis only.
2. **If ΔAG + HCO_3 > normal** → high AG metabolic acidosis + metabolic alkalosis.
3. **If ΔAG + HCO_3 < normal** → high AG metabolic acidosis + non-AG metabolic acidosis.

Key Reference: Narins RG, Emmett M: Simple and mixed acid–base disorder: A practical approach. Medicine 59:161–187, 1980.

Pearls on the Anion Gap (AG)

I. The AG has traditionally been used to assign a patient with metabolic acidosis to one of two diagnostic categories—high AG or normal AG acidosis—with a different set of diagnoses for each.

II. Because of electrical neutrality, the total cations must equal the total anions in the blood. Thus,

Na + K + **Ca + Mg** = HCO_3 + Cl + **PO_4 + SO_4 + protein + organic acids**

Na + **UC** = HCO_3 + Cl + **UA** (UC = unmeasured cation, UA = unmeasured anion)

UA – UC = AG = Na – HCO_3 – Cl

Therefore, increased AG may be due to an increase in UA, decreased in UC, or both, and acidosis is only one factor that may affect the AG.

III. Normal AG has gone from 12 ± 4 to 3–11 mmol/L; downward shift is mainly due to an upward shift in Cl value.

IV. One major caveat to the AG is that non-HCO_3 buffers may ameliorate the decrease in HCO_3 so that for each 1 mmol increase in AG, there is less than 1 mmol decrease in HCO_3. Therefore, with long duration of acidosis, increased intracellular buffering → less decrease in HCO_3 → decrease in the widened AG. **Thus, if the duration of the illness is prolonged, an AG acidosis may become a non-AG acidosis.**

V. The AG may also be altered by **non–acid–base disorders:**

1. **Hypoalbuminemia:** For every 1 gm/dL decrease in albumin, a 2.5–3 mmol/L decrease in AG occurs because albumin is the major component of UA. The

corollary is that a **high AG acidosis may masquerade as a normal AG acidosis in patients with low albumin.**

2. **Hypercalcemia** due to hyperparathyroidism causes a decrease in AG due to increased Ca + decreased PO_4. Hypercalcemia due to malignancy does not affect the AG because PO_4 is proportionately increased.
3. **Lithium:** small decrease in AG due to increased UC (Li^{2+})
4. **Carbenicillin:** increased UA → increased AG; **polymyxin:** increased UC → decreased AG.
5. **Hyperlipidemia** causes decrease in AG because of various factors, including interference with the colorimetric assay of Cl giving a falsely elevated Cl.
6. **Air exposure of blood sample:** increased CO_2 loss → decreased HCO_3 → overestimation of AG.
7. **Heparin** → decreased $PaCO_2$ → decreased HCO_3 → overestimation of AG.

VI. **AG in alkalosis:** High AG does not necessarily imply acidosis. It may be increased in metabolic alkalosis because of (1) associated volume contraction leading to hyperproteinemia, (2) release of protons from proteins, which yields higher % of UAs, and (3) induction of glycolysis, which yields hyperlactatemia. Respiratory alkalosis also may increase lactate production, with lactate levels reaching 11.1–16.6 mmol/L with severe hyperventilation ($pCO_2 < 20$) because of increased activity of phosphofructokinase, a key enzyme in the glycolysis pathway.

VII. **AG in special circumstances of metabolic acidosis**

1. **AG and methanol:** In patients with both ethanol and methanol ingestion, ethanol inhibits methanol metabolism; thus, neither acidosis nor a high AG may be seen.
2. **AG in hyperlactatemia:** Moderate elevation of AG up to 24 mmol/L is not associated with an identifiable organic acid in 35% of cases (false positive); the increase in AG may be related to alterations in UCs, protein, or PO_4. Conversely, the presence of a readily identifiable excess of an organic acid is not always accompanied by a high AG. In one study, an increase in blood lactate in acidotic patients was associated with a normal AG in 32/45 patients. Thus, the serum AG lacks sensitivity and specificity in lactic acidosis. **Mild-to-moderate lactic acidosis should be included in the differential diagnosis of normal AG acidosis.**
3. **AG in diarrhea:** Although most patients have a normal AG acidosis, volume depletion (→ lactic acidosis), hemoconcentration (→ hyperproteinemia), or prerenal azotemia (→ hyper-PO_4) tends to increase the AG.
4. **AG in uremia:** Decreased glomerular filtration rate tends to increase AG by retention of UAs, whereas tubular dysfunction leads to hyperchloremic acidosis (renal tubular acidosis). However, in a study of 70 consecutive patients with end-stage renal disease, an elevated AG was present in only 20%.
5. **AG in nonketotic hyperosmolar coma (NKHC):** In two studies of NKHC, the AG averaged 34 mmol/L and 22 mmol/L with neither lactic acidosis nor ketoacidosis as an explanation for the high AG. The AG was present with or without acidosis. Postulated mechanisms include:
   a. Hyperosmolality releasing intracellular protons, phosphate, and organic acid anions
   b. Beta-hydroxybutyric acidosis not detectable on routine testing
   c. Mild hyperlactatemia
   d. Acute renal insufficiency

Key Reference: Salem MM, Mujais SK: Gaps in the anion gap. Arch Intern Med 152:1625–1629, 1992.

Special Circumstances of Acid–Base Disorders

I. **Severe (metabolic) alkalemia in patients with renal failure**

1. A potential scenario is a patient with cirrhosis on nasogastric suction who develops renal failure. The alkalosis, caused by the nasogastric suction, requires treatment because of increased hepatic encephalopathy and associated arrhythmia. The renal failure complicates the treatment of alkalemia with NaCl.
2. **Treatment:** HCl infusion into a central vein at 0.1 M at 100–125 ml/hr. **Do not exceed** 0.2 mmol/kg/hr or 140 ml/hr. Monitor pH of blood.
3. **Cautions:**
   a. Serum potassium may rise slightly because of exchange of H+ with intracellular K+.
   b. Extravasation of HCl results in severe skin necrosis; HCl should be administered through a central venous catheter.

II. **Severe (respiratory) alkalosis**

1. A potential scenario is a patient who overbreathes a ventilator because of anoxic brain injury resulting in severe respiratory alkalosis. Problems of alkalosis include central nervous system complications (anxiety, confusion, tremors, myoclonus, seizures, coma), atrial and ventricular tachyarrhythmias, and depressed myocardial function with a decrease in systemic vascular resistance resulting in hypotension.
2. **Treatment**
   a. Avoid superimposed metabolic alkalosis by correcting hypokalemia, volume depletion, and avoiding nasogastric suction.
   b. Consider intermittent mandatory ventilation, although it is often not effective in patients with central nervous system insult.
   c. Muscle paralysis may be required for rapid correction of the alkalosis.

Key Reference: Knutsen OH: New method for administration of HCl in metabolic alkalosis. Lancet 1:953–956, 1983.

Acid–Base Problems

(see Practical Approach to Acid–Base Disorders)

I. **Hint:** Determine Δgap in patients with high AG metabolic acidosis to assess for mixed disorder.

II. **Hint:** If the ΔAG + HCO3 is ≈ normal, no metabolic alkalosis disorder coexists with the AG metabolic acidosis.

III. **Example 1:** A 68-year-old woman with 70 pack-year smoking history and chronic analgesic abuse admitted with severe bronchitis. Na, 140; K, 5.0; Cl, 102; HCO_3, 15; blood urea nitrogen (BUN), 86, creatinine (Cr), 10.1; pH, 7.1, pCO_2, 50, pO_2, 51.
Answer: The patient has a low HCO_3 and a high pCO_2, both of which may contribute to her acidosis. The AG is 23 and the ΔAG = 23–12 = 11. Because ΔAG + HCO_3 = 11 + 15 is relatively normal, no other metabolic process is present other than the high AG metabolic acidosis. Thus, the patient has a high AG metabolic acidosis + respiratory acidosis.

IV. **Example 2:** A 64-year-old woman with a psychiatric disorder and cardiac arrest. Na, 141;K, 6; Cl, 105; HCO_3, 8; pH, 6.99; pCO_2, 34; pO_2, 60. Hint: Is the respiratory compensation adequate?

Answer: AG = 28. She therefore has a high AG metabolic acidosis. $\Delta AG = 28 - 12 = 16$ and $\Delta AG + HCO_3 = 24$ (normal). Therefore, there is no other metabolic problem. Expected $pCO_2 = 1.5\ (HCO_3) + 8 \pm 2 = 1.5(8) + 8 \pm 2 = 20 \pm 2$. Therefore, the patient is not adequately compensated and has respiratory acidosis in addition to high AG metabolic acidosis.

V. **Example 3:** A 47-year-old woman with systemic lupus erythematosus and chronic renal insufficiency with fever and chills and LLQ pain. Na, 136; K, 5.5; Cl, 106; HCO_3, 8; pH, 7.44; pCO_2 12; pO_2, 108; BUN, 124; Cr, 6.8.
Answer: AG = 22. $\Delta AG = 22 - 12 = 10$. $\Delta AG + HCO_3 = 18 \neq$ normal. Thus, there is another metabolic process. $\Delta gap = \Delta AG - \Delta HCO_3 = 10 - (24 - 8) = -6$. Because the Δgap is negative, it is either a high AG metabolic acidosis + non-AG metabolic acidosis or a high AG metabolic acidosis + chronic respiratory alkalosis with metabolic compensation. Because the patient is acutely ill, it is more likely the former. The expected respiratory compensation is $pCO_2 = 1.5(8) + 8 \pm 2 = 20 \pm 2$. Therefore, she also has primary respiratory alkalosis.

VI. **Example 4:** A 64-year-old woman with chronic obstructive pulmonary disease and watery diarrhea for 3 days. Na, 136; K, 3.3; Cl, 105; HCO_3, 19; pH, 7.09; pCO_2, 65; pO_2, 48.
Answer: Non-AG metabolic acidosis (AG = 12) + respiratory acidosis.

VII. **Example 5:** A 58-year-old man with vomiting for several days, loss of consciousness, and labored breathing. Na, 127; K, 3.1; Cl, 75; HCO_3, 2; pH, 6.7; pCO_2, 12; pO_2, 108.
Answer: AG = 50. $\Delta AG = 50 - 12 = 38$. $\Delta AG + HCO_3 = 38 + 2 = 40$. Thus there is another metabolic process. The $\Delta gap = 38 - (24 - 2) = +16$. Thus the patient has a high AG metabolic acidosis + 1° metabolic alkalosis.

Analgesia, Sedation, Paralysis

Analgesia and Sedation

I. **General statements**

1. Opioids are poor amnestic agents.
2. The histamine releasing effects of narcotics are more likely to be seen with meperidine and morphine but are usually minimal except with large IV doses.
3. All narcotics are hepatically metabolized and renally excreted.
4. Agitation from pain/dyspnea → opioids; anxiety → benzodiazepines; delirium → haloperidol ± benzodiazepines.
5. Proper ventilatory support necessary when using these agents.
6. Continuous sedation of patients who require mechanical ventilation is a common practice in many intensive care units. However, this practice may be associated prolonged sedation and prolonged duration of mechanical ventilation. It has been shown that daily discontinuation of sedative infusions shortens the duration of mechanical ventilation and reduces the length of ICU stay. Alternatively, sedation given as an "as needed" basis may help prevent over-sedation of patients and reduce the cost of these expensive agents.

   Reference: Kress JP, Pohlman AS, O'Connor MF, Hall JB: Daily interuption of sedative infusions in critically ill patients undergoing mechanical ventilation. N Engl J Med 342:1471–1477, 2000.

II. **Choice of sedatives and analgesics**: in general, a large number of trials have been published comparing midazolam with propofol. Both are comparable in sedation and although propofol may result in a faster time to extubation, it is also more problematic with hypotension than midazolam.

Sedative	Dose for agitation	Metabolism Half-life (hr)	Comments
Lorazepam (Ativan)	0.5–10 mg every 2–4 hr as needed *or* **Load:** 0.5–2 mg IV every 15 min as needed. **Infusion:** 1 mg/hr, increase by 1 mg/hr	No active metabolite (16 hr)	Best amnestic potency
Midazolam (Versed)	1 or more loading doses of 0.03 mg/kg (~ 1–2 mg), then 0.5 mg/hr, increase by ~ 1 mg/hr as needed	Liver, active metabolites (2 hr)	Half-life is long with prolonged infusion
Diazepam (Valium)	**Load:** 5–10 mg IV every 15 min to effect. **Maintenance:** 5–20 mg every 2–4 hr, then every 8–12 hr after 2–4 days	Liver, active metabolites (24 hr)	Hypotensive
Haloperidol (Haldol)	**Load:** 1–5 mg IV every 20 min to calming effect **Maintenance:** ¼ loading dose every 6 hr for 24–48 hr, then decrease by 25–50%/day If > 40 mg/day, add	Liver, active metabolites; (20–24 hr)	Hypotension due to α-blockade; synergistic with lorazepam; discontinue if QTc > 0.48. For acute dystonia: benztropine, 1–2 mg IV every 12 hr

(Table continued on next page.)

Sedative	Dose for agitation	Metabolism Half-life (hr)	Comments
Haloperidol (Haldol) *(cont.)*	lorazepam, 1–4 mg/hr **Note:** IV adminstration is not FDA approved		as needed. For other extrapyramidal syndromes: diphenhydramine, 25–50 mg IV every 6 hr as needed
Propofol (Diprivan)	5–50 μg/kg/min (start at 5, increase by 5 every 5 min)	Liver to inactive metabolites (3–6 hr)	No dose adjustment for chronic liver or renal failure; potential seizure with prolonged use; potential acidosis with increased creatine phosphokinase (CPK) large doses
Fentanyl	**Load:** 50–100 μg IV every 5 min to effect. **Maintenance:** ¼ loading dose/hr, increase as needed to 500 μg/hr	Liver metabolized, urine excretion (2–6 hr)	Minimal hemodynamic effect, high lipid solubility, chest wall rigidity, seizures
Morphine	**Load:** 2–10 mg IV every 15 min to effect. **Maintenance:** ⅕ loading dose/hr, increase to 100 mg/hr	Liver, active metabolites; (1–3 hr)	Slow infusion lessens histamine release, decrease maintenance dose for hepatic and renal dysfunction
Thiopental	**Load:** 3–4 mg/kg IV **Infusion:** none	Liver (3–8 hr)	Used for intubation; hypotension in hypovolemic patients.
Etomidate	**Load:** 0.3 mg/kg or 20 mg IV over 30–60 sec	Rapid onset ≈ 1 min Duration ≈ 3–5 min Liver (1 hr, 15 min)	Useful for endotracheal intubation
Ketamine	**Load:** 0.5–1 mg/kg IV **Infusion:** none	Should be used with a benzodiazepine to prevent hallucinations; liver, active metabolites (2–3 hr)	Tachycardia and increased blood pressure may occur; avoid with head trauma (can increase ICP). Useful for intubating hypotensive patients.

QTc = Q-T interval corrected for heart rate, ICP = intracranial pressure.

III. Antidotes for sedatives

Agent	Dose	Comments
Naloxone (Narcan)	0.4–2 mg every 2 min; up to 10 mg	Repeat dosing every 1–2 hr as narcotics have a longer half-life than naloxone.
Flumazenil (Mazicon)	0.2–0.5 mg IV every 30 sec to desired effect or total of 3 mg (peak: 6–10 min)	Antidote to benzodiazepines. Avoid in situations in which seizures are likely.

Key References: Hansen-Flaschen J: Sedation of mechanically ventilated patients. Pulmon Crit Care Unit 10:1–10, 1995; Ostermann ME, Keenan SP, Seiferling RA, Sibbald WJ: Sedation in the intensive care unit: A systematic review. JAMA 283: 1451–1459, 2000; Shapiro BA,Warren J, Egol AB, et al: Practice parameters for intravenous analgesia and sedation for adult patients in the intensive care unit: An executive summary. Crit Care Med 23:1596–1600, 1995; Wheeler AP: Sedation, analgesia, and paralysis in the intensive care unit. Chest 104: 566–577, 1993.

Neuromuscular Paralytic Agents or Blockers

I. **Indications in the ICU:** muscle relaxation to facilitate endotracheal intubation, tetanus, cardiovascular or metabolic instability due to intractable convulsive activity, facilitation of mechanical ventilation (e.g., modes of ventilation with prolonged expiratory time, permissive hypercapnia, or high levels of positive end-expiratory pressure, all of which may be difficult). The important caveat, which cannot be overemphasized, is that sedation alone should be tried first. If neuromuscular blockers (NMBs) are required, adequate sedation must be maintained.

II. **Complications:** inadequate sedation (increased blood pressure, increased heart rate, diaphoresis, and lacrimation may be the only clues), concealment of physical signs and prevention of communication, decubitus ulcers, nerve compression syndromes, corneal erosions, muscle atrophy, deep vein thrombosis, prolonged paralysis after discontinuation, malignant hyperthermia, **myopathy** with corticosteroids, and cord compression with unstable cervical spine.

1. Conditions and drugs that reduce or **antagonize** the effectiveness of paralytics: burns, edema, methylxanthines, phenytoin, lithium, corticosteroids, carbamazepine.
2. Factors that **potentiate** neuromuscular blockade: respiratory acidosis, metabolic alkalosis, hypokalemia, hyponatremia, hypocalcemia, hypermagnesemia, beta blockers, calcium channel blockers, cyclosporine, aminoglycosides, tetracycline, clindamycin, quinidine, and procainamide.
3. Patients with neuromuscular disease (e.g., myasthenia gravis, Guillain-Barré syndrome, amyotrophic lateral sclerosis) and denervation hypersensitivity may be prone to develop hyperkalemic effects of paralytics, especially with succinylcholine.

III. **Neuromuscular agents**

Agent	Loading Dose	Maintenance	Metabolism	Comments
Succinylcholine (Anectine)	0.5–1.5 mg/kg	—	By pseudo-cholinesterase Onset: 1 min Duration: ~ 10 min	Contraindicated in neuroleptic malignant syndrome, malignant hyperthermia, hyperkalemia, crush or brain injuries, and neuromuscular disorders
Atracurium (Tracrium)	0.4–0.5 mg/kg	2–15 μg/kg/min 0.4–1 mg/kg/hr	Onset: 2 min; Duration: 30 min	Undergoes plasma (Hoffman) degradation
Cisatracurium (Nimbex)	0.15–0.2 mg/kg	3 μg/kg/min	Onset: 2–3 min Duration: 30 min	Undergoes plasma (Hoffman) degradation
Vecuronium (Norcuron)	0.06–0.1 mg/kg	0.08–0.1 mg/kg/hr	Liver, kidney Half-life: 60–100 min Onset: 2 min Duration: 40 min	Avoid in renal insufficiency due to accumulation of active metabolite, 3-desacetyl-vercuronium
Pancuronium (Pavulon)	0.06–0.15 mg/kg	0.01–0.05 mg/kg/hr	Onset: 2–3 min Duration: 60–120 min Kidney > liver	Vagolytic effect causes tachycardia

(Table continued on next page.)

Agent	Loading Dose	Maintenance	Metabolism	Comments
Rocuronium (Zemuron)	0.5 mg/kg over 5 sec	—	Onset: 1 min; Duration: ~ 30 min Liver	Use when succinylcholine is contraindicated
Doxacurium (Nuromax)	0.01–0.05 mg/kg	0.005–0.01 mg/kg every 30–45 min as needed as boluses	Kidney > liver Onset: 5 min Duration: 80–100 min	Dose of 0.025 mg/kg may last over 2 hr with hepatic or renal failure
Rapacuronium (Raplon)	1.5 mg/kg	—	Onset: 90 sec Duration: ~15 min	Continous infusion not recommended Used for intubation

IV. **Conditions associated with succinylcholine-induced hyperkalemia**

1. Upper motor neuron lesion
2. Lower motor neuron lesion
3. Muscle denervation
4. Trauma, severe tissue damage
5. Muscle immobilization and atrophy
6. Thermal burns
7. Muscular dystrophy
8. Clostridial infections
9. Severe prolong infections (?)
10. Anterior horn cell disease (?)
11. Diffuse CNS insult (head injury, aneurysmal rupture, encephalitis) (?)

V. Both aminosteroid NMBs (e.g., pancuronium, vecuronium) and benzylisoquinolinium (nonsteroidal) neuromuscular blockers (e.g., atracurium, doxacurium) may cause profound myopathy (especially in use with corticosteroids), although it appears to be more common with the aminosteroid NMBs.

Key Reference: Hansen-Flaschen J, Cowen J, Raps EC: Neuromuscular blockade in the intensive care unit: More than we bargained for. Am Rev Respir Dis 147:234–236, 1993.

Neuromuscular-Blocking Drugs in Particular Settings

I. **Elderly patients:** Effects of many NMBs may be prolonged due to age-related decrease in renal and hepatic dysfunction. The plasma clearance of **atracurium** appears unaffected.

II. **Cardiac disorders:** Because the vagolytic effect of pancuronium causes tachycardia, it should be avoided in patients with ischemic heart disease or congestive heart failure. Most other NMBs are devoid of vagolytic effect.

III. **Renal disease:** Because ~ 10% of the dose of **atracurium** is renally excreted, it is a preferred NMB in patients with renal insufficiency. Avoid doxacurium and pipecuronium in patients with renal failure.

IV. **Hepatic disease: atracurium** clearance in cirrhotics approximates clearance in noncirrhotics.

V. **Neuromuscular disorders:** Avoid succinylcholine because of risk of severe hyperkalemia or malignant hyperthermia syndrome. Patients with myotonic dystrophy may have severe contractures with succinylcholine, preventing intubation. If short-term paralysis is absolutely required, consider reduced doses of atracurium, vecuronium, or rocuronium. Patients with myasthenia gravis may have increased resistance to succinylcholine but increased sensitivity to the nondepolarizing NMBs.

VI. **Burn injury:** Avoid succinylcholine because a massive efflux of potassium may be released from damaged muscles.

VII. **Reduced plasma cholinesterase activity:** Effects of succinylcholine may be prolonged. Patients who may have reduced cholinesterase activity include those with pregnancy, hepatic disease, renal disease, cancer, collagen vascular disease, hypothyroidism, or genetic predisposition.

VIII. **Increased intracranial pressure:** Both etomidate and succinylcholine are generally contraindicated. Alternative agents should be tried.

Key Reference: Hunter JM: New neuromuscular blocking drugs. N Engl J Med 332:1691–1699, 1995.

Infectious Diseases

Bronchoalveolar Lavage for Diagnosing Pulmonary Infections

I. **Significance of microorganisms isolated from bronchoalveolar lavage (BAL)** (American Thoracic Society criteria)

1. **Diagnostic of infection:** *Pneumocystis carinii*; *Toxoplasma gondii; Strongyloides, Legionella, Coccidioides*, and *Histoplasma* spp.; *Mycobacterium tuberculosis*, influenza; respiratory syncytial virus
2. **Possible cause of infection:** herpes simplex virus, cytomegalovirus (CMV), bacteria, *Aspergillus* and *Candida* sp., cryptococci, atypical mycobacteria
3. **Cytomegalic cell due to CMV**
   Enlarged cell: may be macrophages, endothelial cells, or bronchiolar mucosal cells

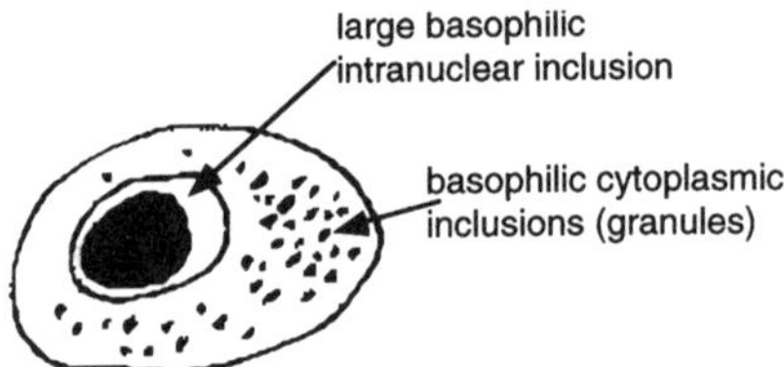

4. ***Pneumocystis carinii***
   a. Cysts: 5–6 μm in diameter. Stained with methenamine silver and toluidine blue O stains.
   b. Sporozoite: an intracytoplasmic cell (up to 8 may be in an intact cyst) and stains with Giemsa or Wright stains.
   c. Trophozoites: an excysted sporozoite that changes into a cyst after attaching to a cell surface and stains with Giemsa or Wright stains.

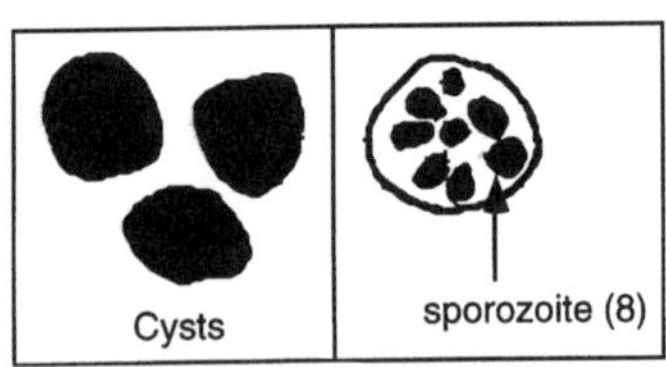

5. ***Toxoplasma gondii.*** Pseudocysts (or oocysts, not shown) are ingested in meats. Tachyzoites infect liver cells. Infected macrophages distribute tachyzoites throughout the body. The sexual cycle (oocysts) occurs only in cats.

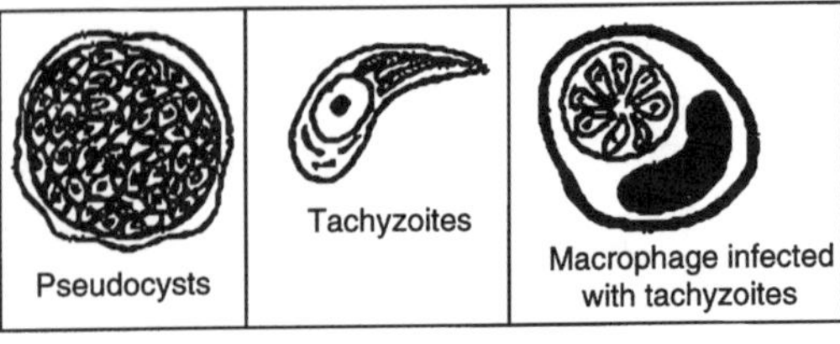

6. ***Coccidioides immitis.*** Direct examination of the sputum (or BAL) after 10% KOH digestion or after staining with Papanicolaou stain (the latter method may be better) may reveal the diagnostic spherule. The spherule may be confused with pollen grains.

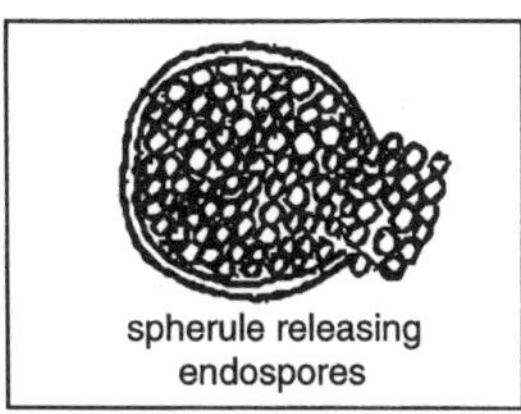

7. ***Histoplasma capsulatum.*** Intracellular *Histoplasma* organisms packed in a macrophage can be seen by H&E. During fixation, the protoplasm retracts from the rigid cell wall, giving an artificial appearance of a capsule. Unlike intracellular histoplasma, *Histoplasma* organisms in necrotic and granulomatous tissue require special fungal stains such as Gomori methenamine silver (GMS). *Histoplasma* organisms exist mainly as a yeast form in the host, although hyphal forms also may be seen.

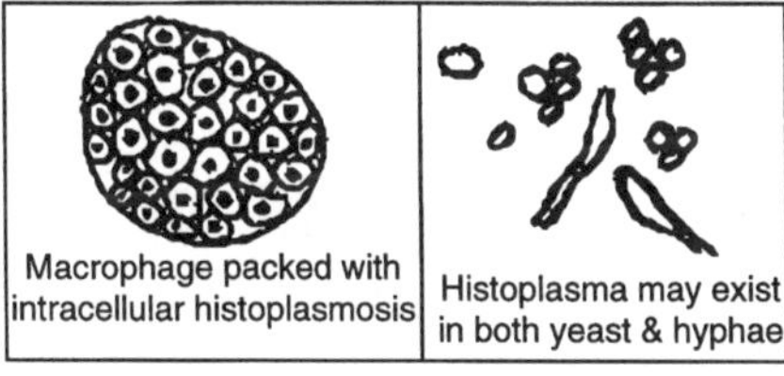

Macrophage packed with
intracellular histoplasmosis
Histoplasma may exist
in both yeast & hyphae

II. **Immunocompromised patients**
   1. **AIDS.** BAL is usually sufficient when sent for culture, cytology, and acid-fast staining. Exceptions that may require a biopsy are patients with coccidioidomycosis, lymphocytic interstitial pneumonitis (LIP), or CMV pneumonia as culture from BAL is nonspecific and thus biopsy is needed to show tissue invasion.
   2. **Non-AIDS.** BAL and transbronchial biopsy are usually sufficient. A notable exception is *Aspergillus* sp., which is frequently missed even on open lung biopsy. In cardiac transplant patients, CMV may be missed even on biopsy.

III. **Immunocompetent patients (bacterial pneumonia)**
   1. **Protected specimen brush**
      a. **Technique.** Avoid injecting lidocaine through the bronchoscope channel, because this approach contaminates the lung with upper respiratory flora. Use nebulized lidocaine instead. When at the appropriate segmental orifice, advance the catheter ~ 3 cm, then advance the inner cannula, and lastly brush. Rotate gently, retract the brush into the inner cannula, the inner cannula into the outer cannula, and remove from the scope. Wipe the outer and then the inner cannula with 70% ethanol before advancing the brush. Cut brush off into exactly 1 ml of sterile nonbacteriostatic saline. Send immediately for quantitative and semiquantitative cultures; the latter is not subjected to serial dilutions.
      b. **Interpretation.** Cutoff is 10^3 CFU/ml. Sensitivity is 59–100%; specificity is 86–100%. If the patient is taking antibiotics, accuracy drops.

IV. **Accuracy of BAL and infectious diseases**

Parameter	Definition	Results of BAL
Diagnostic yield	No. of positive BALs/total no. of BALs	40–95% (variable) (higher in HIV series)
Sensitivity	No. of positive BALs/no. of positive cases	55–88%
Specificity*	No. of negative BALs/no. of negative cases	22–53%

* Overdiagnosis of infection (false positives) may be a problem.

V. **Sensitivities of BAL in diagnosing various infections**
1. Pneumocystosis—> 90% in the AIDS population
2. Tuberculosis—90–100% in both HIV-positive and HIV-negative patients
3. Fungal
4. Bacteria—the protected catheter method (using an inflatable balloon at the end of the catheter to isolate the lavage tip from the proximal airways) may be more accurate to diagnose nosocomial/ventilator-associated pneumonia. The threshold reported as diagnostic of pneumonia has varied from 10^3–10^5 CFU/ml. It is unclear whether this threshold should apply to the sum of all bacteria recovered or only to individual isolates.
5. CMV—a diagnosis of exclusion, but four tests may be used on the BAL sample:
   a. Conventional: difficult to distinguish asymptomatic infection from pneumonitis
   b. Centrifugation culture: (shell vial) followed by immunofluorescence staining with monoclonal antibodies
   c. Examination of lavage cells for the presence of cytopathogenic effects
   d. Use of DNA probes for CMV

Key References: Pisani RJ, Wright AJ: Clinical utility of bronchoalveolar lavage in immunocompromised hosts. Mayo Clin Proc 67:221–227, 1992; Shellito J: Bronchoalveolar lavage: A tool for diagnosing pulmonary infections. Mediguide to Pulmonary Infectious Diseases. Miles Inc., 1994, pp 1–6.

Fever

I. Fever in the ICU may be **infectious or noninfectious, nosocomial or community-acquired**, and its underlying cause may range from **benign to lethal**.

II. Fever is considered to be **produced by the following mechanism for gram-negative bacterial infections:** lipopolysaccharide → increased production of endogenous pyrogen (interleukin 1 and 6, tumor necrosis factor alpha) → increased prostaglandin E_2 production by endothelial cells in the anterior hypothalamus → increased cyclic adenosine monophosphate → reset of the hypothalamic thermoregulatory center → increased internal heat production (e.g., shivering) and decreased peripheral heat loss.

III. **Noninfectious causes**
1. **Malignancy**
2. **Intracranial hemorrhages**
3. **Seizures**
4. **Myocardial infarction**
5. **Pericarditis**
6. **Alcohol withdrawal**
7. **Hemorrhage** (gastrointestinal, occult, hematoma, retroperitoneal)
8. **Deep venous thrombosis–pulmonary embolism**
9. **Ischemic bowel**
10. **Cholecystitis**
11. **Thrombotic thrombocytopenic purpura**

12. **Adrenal insufficiency**
13. **Malignant hyperthermia**
14. **Hyperthyroidism**
15. **Atelectasis**
16. **Transfusion**
17. Subcutaneous and **intramusuclar injections of medications**
18. **Postoperative fever:** noninfectious causes are more likely to occur within the first 2 days after surgery and to have a shorter duration than infectious causes.

IV. **Infectious causes**

1. The three most common causes: **urinary tract infections** (especially with indwelling catheters), **pneumonia** (major risk is mechanical ventilation > 24 hr), and **septicemia**.
2. **Nosocomial sinusitis:** risk factors are nasogastric and nasotracheal intubation. Orotracheal intubation may have the same risk. Most cases are due to gram-negative organisms.
3. **Intraabdominal infections:** occult abscesses, biliary source (e.g., cholecystitis with or without gallstones, cholangitis), diverticulitis, and pseudomembranous colitis.
4. **Catheter-associated septicemia**
5. **Miscellaneous:** endocarditis, encephalitis, meningitis, perinephric abscess, decubitus ulcers, and fasciitis.

Key Reference: Green RJ, Clarke DE, Fishman RS, et al: Investigating the causes of fever in critically ill patients. J Crit Illness 10:51–64, 1995.

Staphylococcal Toxic Shock Syndrome

I. Toxic shock syndrome (TSS) is associated with *Staphylococcus aureus* colonization and is due to the **toxin TSST-1**, especially in the menstrual cases of TSS. Staphylococcal enterotoxin B (SEB) and to a lesser extent SEA and SEC have been implicated as well. Blood cultures are usually negative.

II. **Menstruating women** (who have genital colonization of toxin-producing *S. aureus* and use highly absorbent tampons) and patients with surgical/nonsurgical **wound infections** are the two groups particularly at risk. Since removal of super-absorbent tampons from the market, the incidence of TSS has decreased although menstrual cases of staphylococcal TSS continue to occur.

III. **Clinical signs:** fever, sore throat (without exudate and culture-negative), myalgias, diffuse macular blanching **erythroderma** → desquamation of plantar and palmar skin, and culture-negative inflammatory arthritis.

IV. **Definition**

1. Temperature > 102°
2. Hypotension
3. Diffuse or palmar erythroderma due to maximal capillary dilatation → desquamation
4. Hyperemia of conjunctivae or mucous membrane of oropharynx or vagina
5. Multisystem dysfunction (3 or 4 of the following):
   a. Vomiting or diarrhea
   b. Altered mental status
   c. Renal insufficiency
   d. Hepatic insufficiency
   e. Decreased platelets
   f. Increased creatine phosphokinase (CPK)
   g. Cardiopulmonary dysfunction
   h. Low calcium or phosphate
6. No clinical or laboratory evidence of another illness

V. **Laboratory tests.** No diagnostic test; > 50% have elevated white blood cell count with left shift; blood cultures are negative; hypocalcemia and sterile pyuria are common.

VI. **Differential diagnosis.** Group A streptococcal infection, drug reaction, vasculitis (Kawasaki disease), meningococcemia, Rocky Mountain spotted fever.

VII. **Treatment.** Beta-lactamase-resistant penicillin or cephalosporin, removal of foreign body, drainage or irrigation of infected area in nonvaginal TSS, irrigation of the vaginal vault in menstrual-associated cases, and volume resuscitation. Addition of antibiotics such as clindamycin, erythromycin, rifampin, or fluoroquinolones that suppress TSST-1 synthesis has theoretical advantages. Use of pooled immunoglobulins may be helpful in recalcitrant cases by neutralizing TSST-1.

Key Reference: Stevens DL: The toxic shock syndromes. Infect Dis North Am 10:727–746, 1996.

Streptococcal Toxic Shock Syndrome

I. **Definition**: any group A streptococcal infection associated with the early onset of shock and organ failure.

II. **Case definitions**

1. **Isolation of group A streptococci** (GAS)
   a. From a sterile body site
   b. From a nonsterile body site
2. **Clinical signs of severity**
   a. **Hypotension** *and*
   b. **Clinical and laboratory abnormalities** (at least two of the following):
      - Renal insufficiency
      - Coagulopathy
      - Liver abnormalities
      - Acute respiratory distress syndrome
      - Extensive tissue necrosis (i.e., necrotizing fasciitis)
      - Erythematous rash
3. **Definite case** = 1a + 2 (a and b), **Probable case** = 1b + 2(a and b)

III. Comparison of staphylococcal vs streptococcal TSS

Feature	Staphylococcal	Streptococcal
Age	Mainly 15–35 years	Mainly 20–50 years
Sex	Greatest in women	Either
Severe pain	Rare	Common
Hypotension	100%	100%
Erythroderma rash	Very common	Less common
Renal failure	Common	Common
Bacteremia	Low	60%
Tissue necrosis	Rare	Common
Predisposition	Tampons, packing	Cuts, burns, bruises
Thrombocytopenia	Common	Common
Mortality rate	< 3%	30–70%

IV. **Treatment**

1. **Penicillin** is still effective against cutaneous infections although treatment failures have occurred.

2. More agressive Group A streptococcal infections (necrotizing fasciitis, empyema, burn wound sepsis, subcutaneous gangrene, and myositis) seem to respond less well to penicillin.
3. **Clindamycin** is efficacious for a number of reasons in addition to its antibiotic effect including suppression of bacterial toxin synthesis and facilitation of phagocytosis of *S. pyogenes* by inhibiting M-protein synthesis.
4. **Exploration and debridement** of suspected deep-seated *S. pyogenes* infection.
5. **Massive fluid resuscitation** may be required.
6. **Commercial iv γ-globulin** contains neutralizing antibodies and its use may result in dramatic improvement in the patient's condition.

Key Reference: Stevens DL: The toxic shock syndromes. Infect Dis North Am 10:727–746, 1996.

Clostridial Infections

	Tetanus	Botulism	Gas gangrene
General		Botulus: Latin for sausage	Responsible organism widespread in soil
Microbiology	*C. tetani* produces tetanospasmin toxin	*C. botulinum* produces powerful neurotoxin	*C. perfringens*
Epidemiology	Trauma, skin ulcers, burns, frost bites	Wound infection or eating foods containing preformed toxin	Incidence low, although > 30% of deep wounds are contaminated
Pathogenesis	Toxin inhibits inhibitory interneurons and thus causes increased motor and sympathetic activity	Neurotoxin binds to presynaptic membranes and prevents release of acetylcholine at peripheral cholinergic synapses (motor endplates)	Essential factor appears to be trauma, especially deep lacerated muscle wounds and devitalized tissues
Clinical	Median onset of tetany is 7 days: trismus dysphagia, risus sardonicus, rigid proximal muscles and abdomen, opisthotonus, respiratory muscle spasm and laryngospasm Severe autonomic instability: sympathetic overactivity and cardiac arrhythmias	Incubation of foodborne: ~ 18–36 hr. **Descending paralysis:** cranial nerve paralysis (diplopia, dysarthria, ptosis, decreased gag, blurred vision, dysphagia) → neck, arms, thorax, legs → respiratory failure. **Cholinergic blockade:** paralytic ileus, dry mouth, dilated pupils, and urinary retention. Sore throat, nausea, vomiting, abdominal pain. No significant fever.	Short incubation: < 24 hr–3 days. Sudden pain at wound site, local swelling, hemorhagic exudate (may or may not be frothy). Skin is tense, cool, white, and blue. Septic shock. Gas appears late.
Diagnosis	Clinical diagnosis: (+) culture is not specific; bacterium has terminal spore: resembles squash racquet	Toxin in serum, stool, or food	Gram stain of exudate reveals gram-positive rods with few inflammatory cells

(Table continued on next page.)

	Tetanus	Botulism	Gas gangrene
Treatment	Airway protection, wound debridement. Penicillin G, 10–12 million U/d, or metronidazole. Antitoxin: human tetanus Ig **(hTIG)**, 3000–6000 U IM in divided doses. Benzodiazepines, vecuronium for spasms and rigidity	Respiratory monitoring Test for hypersensitivity to horse serum → 2 vials Polyvalent antitoxin IV; repeat in 2–4 hr. Penicillin may prevent further production of toxin. Cathartics and enemas if no ileus	Penicillin G, 20 million U/day, *or* chloramphenicol 4 gm/day. Surgical debridement and resection with or without hyperbaric oxygen
Prevention	Primary series in adults: 4–8 weeks apart for 2 doses, then third dose 6–12 mo later. Booster: tetanus-diptheria toxoid every 10 yr	Antitoxin is from the **Centers for Disease Control.**. Days: (404) 639-375; Nights and weekends: (404) 639-2888	

Key References: Bleck TP: Tetanus: Pathophysiology, management and prophylaxis. Dis Month 37:551–603, 1991. Davis LE: Botulism toxin. West J Med 158:25–29, 1993.

Identification of Fungal Elements and Treatment Guidelines for Systemic (Disseminated) Disease

Fungus	Setting	Tissue forms	Treatment
Candida albicans	Neutropenic fever Line sepsis Prolonged broad-spectrum antibiotics	**Yeast** **Pseudohyphae** **Hyphae**	Amphotericin B, 0.5–1 mg/kg/day IV for total of 0.5–2 gm
Aspergillus fumigatus* or *flavus	Invasive aspergillosis (may mimic pulmonary infarct) in neutropenic fever, prolonged antibiotics, AIDS, old age, diabetes, renal and hepatic failure; necrotizing bronchitis in AIDS	**Septate hyphae** branching at 45° angles with conidiophores	Amphotericin B, 1–1.5 mg/kg/day IV for total of 2–4 gm
Histoplasma capsulatum	Progressive disseminated histoplasmosis (PDH): in AIDS, lymphoma, and immunosuppressive therapy (disorders with T-cell defects)	In soil and in culture media < 35°C, it grows as a mold with macro- and microconidia (the latter are infectious). In tissues, mainly in **yeast** forms but may grow as hyphal elements	Itraconazole, 200 mg orally twice daily *or* amphotericin B, 0.5–0.6 mg/kg/day IV
Coccidioides immitis	Primary pulmonary, chronic progressive pulmonary, miliary, disseminated (skin, bones, meninges); disseminated disease more common in Filipinos, blacks, AIDS, transplant patients, cancer patients, diabetics.	Mycelial morphology in saprobic state, but in tissues it exists as **endosporulating spherule**	Fluconazole, 400–800 mg/day orally *or* amphotericin B, 0.5 mg/kg/day IV (1–2.5 gm for pulmonary disease, 2.5–3 gm for disseminated disease)

(Table continued on next page.)

Fungus	Setting	Tissue forms	Treatment
Blastomyces dermatitidis	Acute infection may be asymptomatic or flulike; chronic blastomycosis may mimic malignancy	Mycelial form in nature, **yeast** form in tissues with broad-based buds ("daughter cells")	Itraconazole, 200 mg orally once or twice daily, *or* amphotericin B, 0.5–0.6 mg/kg/day IV
Sporothrix schenckii	AIDS Hematologic malignancies	As a mold at 25°C but as **yeast** in tissues	Amphotericin B, 0.5 mg/kg/day IV
Paracoccidioides brasiliensis	AIDS	Double-walled oval to round **yeast** cell with single or multiple buds	Itraconazole, 100–200 mg/day orally, *or* amphotericin B, 0.4–0.5 mg/kg/day IV
Mucorales (order) ***Mucor* sp.** ***Rhizopus* sp.** ***Absidia* sp.**	Diabetic ketoacidosis: **rhinocerebral forms.** Hematologic malignancies: **disseminated and pulmonary forms**	Hyphal invasion of blood vessels	Amphotericin B, 1–1.5 mg/kg/day IV
Cryptococcus neoformans	AIDS Transplantation Immunosuppressives	Small encapsulated **yeastlike** cells with narrow-based budding daughter cells	Amphotericin B, 0.3–0.7 mg/kg/day IV with or without flucytosine, 100 mg/kg/day orally

I. **Candidemia** may occur in the setting of endocarditis, septic thrombophlebitis, or disseminated candidiasis.

1. **Candidal endocarditis.** Risk factors include cardiac valve surgery, heroin addiction, and prolonged intravenous catheters. In candidal prosthetic valve endocarditis, blood cultures may be negative in ~26% of cases. In addiction-associated candidal endocarditis, *C. parapsilosis* is the leading candidal pathogen. In contrast, *C. albicans* is seen with contaminated heroin and causes mainly candidemia without endocarditis. Treatment of candidal endocarditis is with amphotericin, 0.6–0.8 mg/kg/day, and immediate surgery.
2. **Septic thrombophlebitis.** Associated with intravenous catheters that may occlude the great and peripheral veins. For diagnosing involvement of large veins (e.g., subclavian vein), helpful tests include radionuclide scan, venography, and magnetic resonance imaging. Patients should be treated with amphotericin for a total dose of 1.5–2 gm.
3. **Disseminated candidiasis.** At-risk individuals include patients with neutropenia, organ transplantation, abdominal surgery, burns, treatment with prolonged broad-spectrum antibiotics, cannulation with central venous catheters, and hyperalimentation. Microabscesses are present in multiple organs. Blood cultures may be negative in as many as 50% of cases. Blood culture yield may be increased by (1) subculturing, (2) multiple sets, (3) venting culture bottles, and (4) use of lysis-centrifugation tubes (isolator). The species most commonly involved in dissemination are *C. albicans, C. tropicalis*, and *C. glabrata*. There is no clear consensus about prophylaxis for disseminated candidiasis, but for patients with more than three risk factors for disseminated candiasis, ketoconazole, 200 mg/day, has been shown to to decrease the incidence of candidal sepsis. In at-risk patients, meticulous **physical examination is probably one of the best ways to diagnose disseminated candidiasis:**
   a. **Macronodular skin lesions**, 0.5–1 cm reddish pink with fungus seen on biopsy; lesions also may be ecthyma–gangrenosum-like.

b. **Myositis with myalgia:** the skin lesion is often over the myositis site.
c. **Endophthalmitis:** white, cotton or wool, chorioretinal foci of infection
d. **Hepatosplenomegaly**
e. Myocardial involvement may manifest as chest pain, arrhythmias, QRS changes mimicking myocardial ischemia, pronounced triphasic waves.
f. **Candiduria may indicate kidney infection**, such as perinephric abscess, papillary necrosis, emphysematous pyelonephritis, and hematuria. Pyuria may be notably absent in systemic neutropenia.

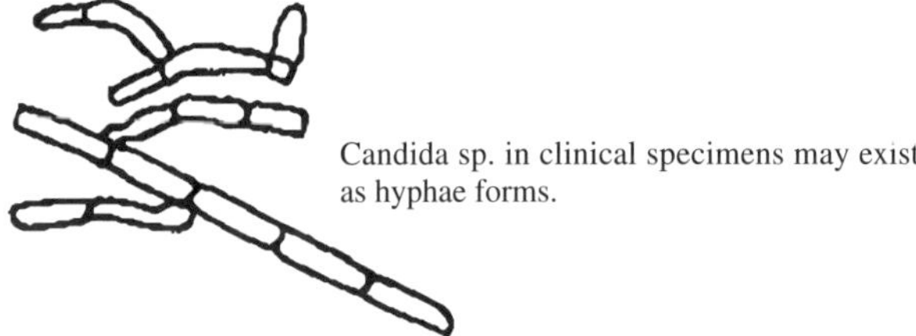
Candida sp. in clinical specimens may exist as hyphae forms.

II. **Invasive aspergillosis.** Most cases occur in severely immunocompromised patients, but it may occur in patients receiving low-dose corticosteroid therapy with no other major risk factor. In absolute neutropenia, the risk of invasive aspergillosis is ~ 1% per day during the first 3 weeks and increases to 4% per day thereafter. A focal infiltrate that does not improve with antibiotics, single or multiple wedge-shaped infiltrates, and nodules with or without cavitations are radiographic patterns suggestive of aspergillosis. Blood cultures are rarely positive despite the angioinvasive nature of *A. fumigatus*. The presence of aspergilli in bronchoalveolar lavage or bronchial washings in a patient with fever, pleuritic chest pain, and hemoptysis with pleural-based pulmonary infiltrates (or multiple nodules with or without cavitation or diffuse consolidation) is justification for beginning amphotericin B therapy.

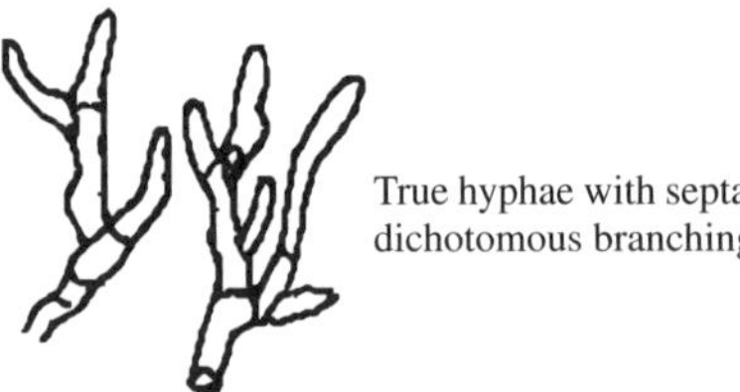
True hyphae with septate and dichotomous branching.

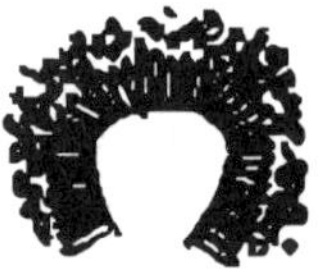
Asexual spores known as conidiophores.

III. **Rhinocerebral mucormycosis.** The acidosis in diabetic ketoacidosis is believed to be the major predisposing factor. The infection begins in the nasal passages and spreads into the paranasal sinuses, palate, and orbit. Meningitis and brain infarction may occur by extension through the cribriform plate or the apex of the orbit. Ischemic necrosis of cranial nerves II, III, IV, VI, and VII may occur. The cavernous sinus and internal carotids also may be invaded. There should be a high index of suspicion in the susceptible host with any of the following signs and symptoms: facial, ocular, or dental pain; epistaxis; facial numbness; cellulitis of the face; stroke syndromes. The presence of black pus draining from the eye and black eschar on the palatine or nasal mucosa are late findings.

1. **Diagnosis** requires the presence of tissue invasion by the fungus. A positive culture from a nasal wash alone is insufficient to make the diagnosis; similarly, the culture is positive in only 15% of invasive cases.

2. **Treatment** includes (1) correction of the acidosis or tapering of immunosuppressives, (2) amphotericin B, with the dose rapidly advanced to 1–1.5 mg/kg/day, and (3) tissue debridement.

IV. **Progressive disseminated histoplasmosis (PDH).** Patients at greatest risk are those with T-cell disorders, such as lymphoma, AIDS, and immunosuppressive therapies. Clinical manifestations include fever, hepatosplenomegaly, pancytopenia, disseminated intravascular coagulation, and chest radiograph that may reveal a miliary pattern. Adrenal insufficiency, meningitis, intracranial histoplasmoma, and aortic or mitral valve endocarditis are other disease manifestations of PDH. In diagnosing patients with PDH, blood cultures with the DuPont isolator should be obtained, but a bone marrow biopsy may be required. Buffy-coat examination for organisms and urine Histoplasma antigen are also useful for diagnosis.

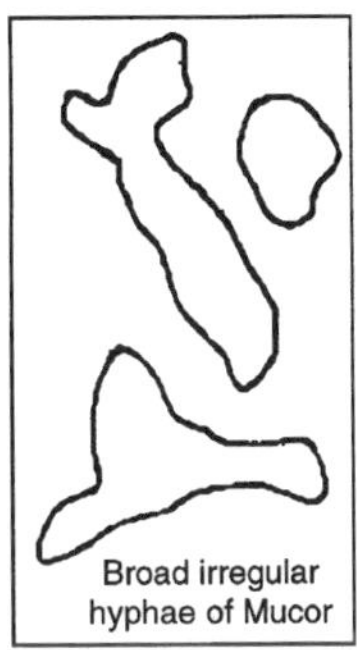
Broad irregular hyphae of Mucor

Key References: Gorbach SL, Bartlett JG, Blacklow NR: Infectious Diseases. Philadelphia, W.B. Saunders, 1992; Systemic fungal drugs. Med Lett 38:10–12, 1996.

Practical Approach to Administering Amphotericin B

I. **Major adverse effects:** fevers, chills, nausea, vomiting, hypokalemia, renal magnesium wasting, anemia, phlebitis, and nephrotoxicity.

II. **Pretreatment to control fevers and chills**
   1. **Acetaminophen**, 650 mg orally or rectally, and **diphenhydramine**, 25–50 mg orally or IV 30 min before amphotericin B dose.
   2. If fever develops despite premedication, consider adding **hydrocortisone, 25 mg,** to the amphotericin B infusion.

III. **Test dose** (may or may not be required): 1–2 mg IV

IV. **Dose escalation**
   1. Begin at 0.25 mg/kg; increase to 0.5 mg/kg on the second day.
   2. If a dose > 0.5 mg/kg is required, give full dose on the third day and thereafter.

V. **Infusion rate**
   1. Administer amphotericin B over 4 hr for the first 5–7 days.
   2. After 5–7 days, increase infusion rate to 45 min to 1 hr (unless renal disease, hyperkalemia, or myocardial disease is present).

VI. **Sodium supplementation**
   1. **Normal saline (NS)**, 250–500 ml 30 min before and 30 min after each amphotericin dose, has been recommended to prevent nephrotoxicity (in patients with no contraindication to sodium loading). 500 ml of NS is ~ 77 mmol of sodium.
   2. Alternatively, antibiotics that contain sodium (ticarcillin, ~ 156 mmol sodium per day's dose; carbenicillin, ~188 mmol/day; piperacillin, ~ 44 mmol/day; azlocillin, ~52 mmol/day; ceftazidime, ~14 mmol/day) may be given in place of or supplement normal saline if they are also indicated for bacterial infections.

VII. **Monitoring**
   1. Serum chemistries every other day
   2. Complete blood count twice weekly

3. Magnesium weekly
4. Total cumulative dose
5. Intravenous site for phlebitis

Key Reference: Bult J, Franklin CM: Using amphotericin B in the critically ill: A new look at an old drug. J Crit Illness 11:577–585, 1996.

Bacterial Meningitis

I. The incidence of bacterial meningitis is ~ 3 cases per 10^5 per year. The most common organisms have varied according to the population studied. Due to the widespread use of the *Hemophilus influenzae* type B vaccine in children, there has been a significant decline in the incidence of this organism.

II. The **signs and symptoms** include headache, fever, meningismus, with or without decreased cognition. Other manifestations include Kernig and Brudzinski signs, cranial nerve dysfunction (most commonly 3rd, 6th, and 8th), seizures, lateralizing deficits, and cerebral edema. With meningococcal meningitis, there is also a high incidence of bacteremia with characteristic rash: **macules** (which blanch on pressure) lead to a **petechial and purpuric rash**, especially on the lower extremities and trunk (sparing the face, palm, and soles), which may progress to **hemorrhagic bullae, large ecchymoses,** and **cutaneous gangrene**. There may be nonspecific signs and symptoms such as poor appetite and failure to thrive, especially in infants and the elderly. Papilledema is uncommon early in the course of bacterial meningitis. When present, papilledema suggests the possibility of venous sinus thrombosis, brain abscess, subdural empyema, or syphilitic meningitis.

III. **Differential diagnosis**: acute viral meningitis, nonsteroidal anti-inflammatory drug (NSAID)–induced meningitis, chemical meningitis due to craniopharyngiomas, carcinomatous meningitis, and parameningeal foci. In patients with lateralizing signs or papilledema and a suspicion of meningitis, blood cultures should be obtained and antibiotics begun *before* imaging studies are done.

IV. **Diagnosis**

1. **Cerebral spinal fluid pleocytosis** is typically > 1000/μl with neutrophilic predominance but many will have WBC < 1000/μl, and about 10% may present with lymphocyte predominance (more common in neonate and patients with *Listeria monocytogenes* meningitis).
2. **CSF glucopenia** (< 40 mg/dL [< 2.22 mmol/L], normal 45–65 mg/dl [2.5–3.6 mmol/L]), **CSF:blood glucose ratio** (< 0.4, normal = 0.6), and **protein** (> 150 mg/dl [> 1.5 gm/L], normal 20–45 mg/dl [0.2–0.45 gm/L]). One caveat is that the CSF glucose and protein are not independently sensitive or specific enough to establish or exclude the diagnosis of bacterial meningitis.
3. **Gram stain of CSF**: sensitivity is ~ 40–60%, depending on the observer, time spent reviewing the microscopy fields, slide preparation, and whether the patient has received antibiotics. Specificity is > 90%.
4. **CSF culture** sensitivity is 70–85% but falls below 50% in patients who received prior antibiotics.
5. **Latex agglutination**: should be considered in patients in whom CSF findings are consistent with bacterial meningitis but Gram stain is negative. Antigen tests are available for *H. influenzae* type B, *S. pneumoniae*, *N. meningitides*, *E.coli* K1, and group B streptococci (*S. agalactiae*). The specificity is high, but the sensitivity varies from 50% to 100%; therefore, a negative test does not rule out meningitis.

V. Empiric treatment

Patient Characteristics	Probable organisms	Drug of choice	Alternatives
Age < 18 yr	*Neisseria meningitidis* *Haemophilus influenzae* *Streptococcus pneumoniae*	Cefotaxime, 2 gm every 6 hr; *or* Ceftriaxone, 2 gm every 12 hr	
Age 18–50 yr	*Streptococcus pneumoniae* *Neisseria meningitidis*	Cefotaxime, 2 gm every 6 hr; *or* Ceftriaxone, 2 gm every 12 hr	Ampicillin, 2 gm IV every 4 hr Penicillin G, 4 million units every 4 hr Chloramphenicol, 1–1.5 gm every 6 hr Meropenem 1 gm every 8 hr
Age > 50 yr	*Streptococcus pneumoniae* Gram-negative bacilli *Listeria monocytogenes*	Ampicillin, 2 gm IV every 4 hr *plus either* Cefotaxime, 2 gm every 4 or 6 hr, *or* Ceftriaxone, 2 gm every 12 hr	Cefotaxime, 2 gm every 6 hr *plus* Trimethoprim-sulfamethoxazole, 10–20 mg/kg/day TMP in 6–8 hr dosing Meropenem, 1 gm every 8 hr
Impaired cellular immunity	Gram-negative bacilli *Listeria monocytogenes* *S. pneumoniae*	Ampicillin, 2 gm IV every 4 hr *plus* Ceftazidime, 50–100 mg/kg IV every 8 hr up to 2 gm every 8 hr	
Head trauma, neurosurgery, or cerebrospinal fluid shunt	Gram-negative bacilli *Streptococcus pneumoniae* Staphylococcal species	Vancomycin, 15 mg/kg IV every 6 hr up to 2 gm/day *plus* Ceftazidime, 50–100 mg/kg IV every 8 hr up to 2 gm every 8 hr	

VI. Suggested duration of therapy

1. 7 days for *H. influenzae* or *N. meningitidis*
2. 10–14 days for *S. pneumoniae*
3. 14–21 days for *L. monocytogenes* or group B streptococci
4. 21 days for gram-negative bacilli (other than *H. influenzae*)

VII. Special issues in bacterial meningitis

1. For household contacts, children and personnel in day care centers, or medical personnel after cardiopulmonary resuscitation of patients with meningococcal meningitis, **rifampin prophylaxis** should be given: adults, 600 mg every 12 hr × 4 doses; children, 10 mg/kg every 12 hr × 4 doses.
2. *S. pneumoniae* resistant to penicillin and cephalosporins must be considered and thus susceptibility testing should be performed promptly.
3. ***Listeria* sp.** appears to affect individuals with the following risk factors: pregnancy, organ transplantation, cirrhosis, hemodialysis, steroid therapy, chemotherapy, malignancies, and alcoholism. *Listeria* sepsis and peritonitis may occur.

4. The beneficial role of corticosteroids (decreased audiologic and neurologic sequelae) is more evident in children with bacterial meningitis who are > 2 mo old and infected with *H. influenzae*. The use of corticosteroids is much less clear in adults with bacterial meningitis; thus, it is generally **not** recommended. However, adults most likely to benefit from corticosteroids are those with (1) high bacterial concentration in the cerebrospinal fluid and (2) increased intracranial pressure. The dose of **dexamethasone is 0.15 mg/kg (~ 10 mg for a 70-kg person) IV every 6 hr for 4 days, given at the same time as antibiotics.**

Key References: Quagliarello VJ, Scheld WM: Treatment of bacterial meningitis. N Engl J Med 336:708–716, 1997; Segreti J, Harris AA: Acute bacterial meningitis. Infect Dis Clin North Am 10:797–809, 1996.

Spontaneous Bacterial Peritonitis

I. Spontaneous bacterial peritonitis (SBP) may occur in patients with ascites from any cause, although alcoholic cirrhosis is the most common underlying cause. The pathogenesis is due to impaired host defense in the cirrhotic liver plus invasion of ascites by gut organisms via portal blood.

II. **Microbiology:** *Escherichia coli* > streptococci (pneumococci and enterococci) > *Klebsiella* sp. > other aerobic gram-negative bacilli > anaerobic or microaerophilic bacteria (~10% of cases are polymicrobial). Anaerobes are infrequent (ascitic fluid has high PO_2).

III. **Clinical manifestations:** fever, abdominal tenderness, hepatorenal failure, and worsening hepatic encephalopathy. Patients, however, may have little or no abdominal symptoms. Septicemia may occur early because of shunting of portal blood into the systemic circulation.

IV. **Ascitic fluid characteristics**
1. Gram stain positive in 30–40% of cases (low yield because of low organism concentration)
2. Protein < 1 gm/dl (< 10 gm/L)
3. Glucose (peritoneal fluid) ~ glucose (serum)
4. **Absolute neutrophil count > 250 cells/µl (2.5 × 10^9/L)** is the best indicator of infection in patients with a negative Gram stain + signs and symptoms consistent with SBP. Neutrophil count of > 500 cells/µl (5.0 × 10^9/L) indicates SBP even in patients without signs or symptoms.
5. pH, lactate, and ascitic-blood pH gradients are **not** particularly useful because they do not become abnormal until neutrophil count is > 250 cells/µl.
6. Higher sensitivity of peritoneal fluid culture if 10 ml of ascitic fluid is directly inoculated into a blood culture bottle. Positive blood cultures in ~40% of patients.

V. **Empiric treatment regimens** (in an area with a high rate of extended-spectrum β-lactamase [ESBL], consider a fluoroquinolone or carbapenem).
1. Cefotaxime 2 gm every 6 hr or ceftriaxone 2 gm every 12 hr

   or
2. Ticarcillin-clavulanate, 3.1 gm IV every 4–6 hr

   or
3. Piperacillin-tazobactam, 3.375 gm IV every 6 hr or 4.5 gm IV every 8 hr

   or
4. Ampicillin-sulbactam, 1.5–3 gm IV every 6 hr

   or
5. Cefoxitin, 1 gm IV to 2 gm IV every 4 hr

VI. Role of albumin: among patients with SBP, ~1/3 develop irreversible renal insufficiency, a sensitive predictor of death. In a multicenter, randomized, controlled trial of cefotaxime vs. cefotaxime + albumin in SBP patients, the addition of albumin significantly reduced the rates of renal failure and mortality.

Key References: Gilbert JA, Kamath PS: Spontaneous bacterial peritonitis. Mayo Clin Proc 70:365–370, 1995; Sort P, et al: Effect of intravenous albumin on renal impairment and mortality in patients with cirrhosis and spontaneous bacterial peritonitis. N Engl J Med 341:403–409, 1999.

Catheter-related Infections

I. Central venous catheters coated with silver sulfadiazine and chlorhexidine have been shown to have a significant decrease in catheter colonization and catheter-related infections.

II. The catheter insertion tract (between the skin or tissue and catheter) is the major route of entry of microorganisms. Thus, site preparation before insertion and aseptic maintenance of the catheter are important measures in preventing infections.

III. Arterial pressure monitoring systems are generally at greater risk than central venous catheters for infections because of transducer colonization due to stagnant blood and multiple blood sampling.

IV. Routine replacement of central venous catheters every 3–4 days may prevent infections but complication rates increase. The decision to exchange catheters over a guidewire (possibly associated with an increased risk of bloodstream infection) vs. a new stick (with the potential increased risk of mechanical complications) must be weighed. A study comparing (1) replacement every 3 days at a new site, (2) replacement every 3 days by exchange over a guidewire, (3) replacement only when clinically indicated at a new site, or (4) replacement only when clinically indicated over a guidewire found that routine replacement every 3 days is not warranted. Thus, catheters should be changed only when clinically indicated. The decision whether to change over a wire (greater risk of bloodstream infection) or to use a new site (more mechanical complications) must be weighed for each patient.

V. A positive catheter tip culture is ≥ 15 colonies; colonization is defined as < 15 colonies on a semiquantitative culture. Catheter-related septicemia requires recovery of the same organism from the peripheral blood.

VI. The leading causes of infections from IV devices are coagulase-negative staphylococci (*S. epidermidis*), *S. aureus*, and enterococci. The coagulase-negative staphylococci produce a capsular polysaccharide that allows adhesion to the catheter surfaces. Another organism that may colonize hospitalized patients and thus may cause line-infections is *Corynebacterium jeikeium*. Vancomycin is used to treat these organisms, but isolated cases of resistant organisms have been reported.

VII. Lipid administration is associated with an increased risk not only of staphylococcal infection but also of fungemia with *Candida albicans* and with unusual organisms such as *Malassezia furfur*.

VIII. The appearance of uncommon pathogens causing catheter-related sepsis, such as *Enterobacter*, *Citrobacter*, or *Serratia* spp., should raise suspicion of contaminated infusate.

IX. In catheter-related sepsis due to routine central venous catheters, the catheters should be removed and intravenous antibiotics given for 7–10 days. Vancomycin is the empiric drug of choice.

X. In catheter-related sepsis due to a Hickman or Broviac catheter, antibiotics should be given sequentially through each of the ports.

Key References: Cobb DK et al: A controlled trial of scheduled replacement of central venous and pulmonary-artery catheters. N Engl J Med 327:1062–1068, 1992; Farr BM: Prevention and management of vascular catheter infections. Contemp Intern Med 6:29–42, 1994.

Septic Shock

I. Septic shock is a subset of the systemic inflammatory response syndrome (SIRS) and is usually (but not always) due to a bacterial, fungal, viral, rickettsial, or parasitic infection. The response consists of fever or hypothermia, tachycardia, tachypnea, and dysfunction of at least 1 organ (e.g., altered mental status, hypoxemia, increased lactate, or oliguria) due to inadequate tissue perfusion. Aspirin overdose also may cause a syndrome consistent with sepsis syndrome.

II. **Mechanisms of shock**
1. Excessive fluid loss (cholera, toxic shock syndrome)
2. Myocardial cell invasion and pump failure (meningococcemia, viral myocarditis, diphtheria)
3. Endocarditis
4. Decreased venous return to the heart (Gram-negative sepsis)

III. **Clinical manifestations**
1. **Skin:** cellulitis, erythema multiforme, petechial and purpuric lesions of disseminated intravascular coagulation (DIC), endocarditis-associated (Janeway lesions, Osler nodes), ecthyma gangrenosum (*Pseudomonas* sepsis: reddish macules → bull's eye erythematous halo surrounding a central vesicle or ulcer).
2. **Cardiovascular:** although high cardiac output and low systemic vascular resistance are the classic findings with septic shock, patients also may present with a concomitant depressed left and right ventricular ejection fraction (EF) and dilated ventricles. In fact, in some patients the EF is so depressed that cardiac output is decreased, requiring inotropic support.
3. **Pulmonary:** hyperventilation (respiratory alkalosis) is an early sign of sepsis. The development of adult respiratory distress syndrome (ARDS) signifies a high mortality rate (~ 50%). Respiratory muscle failure may result in ventilatory failure.
4. **Hematologic:** marked leukocytosis or neutropenia (the latter is seen with intracellular pathogens, viral infections, and overwhelming bacteremia), thrombocytopenia, DIC (microvascular thromboses due to fibrin deposition), and presence of Döhle bodies, toxic granulation, and vacuolization of neutrophils are clues to possible bacteremia.
5. **Renal insufficiency** is mostly due to acute tubular necrosis but may be glomerular in origin (e.g., endocarditis).
6. **Gastrointestinal bleeding and liver dysfunction** (cholestatic jaundice) may occur. Hyperbilirubinemia more commonly associated with *Bacteroides* spp. infections. A rapid rise in transaminases to very high levels typically indicates shock liver. Hypoglycemia may occur.

IV. **Therapy**
1. **Broad-spectrum antibiotics** covering the most likely pathogens based on setting of infection and host factors (e.g., encapsulated organisms such as *Streptococcus pneumoniae, Hemophilus influenzae*, and *Neisseria meningitidis* in asplenic individuals). Search for occult sites of infection if the

source is not apparent, e.g., urinary tract (perinephric abscess), biliary tract, pelvis, and retroperitoneum.

2. **Oxygen and ventilatory support** (see Managing Adult Respiratory Distress Syndrome in Pulmonology Section).
3. **Intravenous fluids.** There is no clear advantage with either colloids or crystalloids. For crystalloids, normal saline or lactated Ringer's solution should be used. A typical fluid challenge is 1–1.5 L over 15–20 min. Patients may not be able to tolerate IV fluids well because of myocardial depression, which may be seen in some cases of septic shock.
4. **Vasopressors**, such as dopamine (5–20 μg/kg/min) or norepinephrine (0.5–30 μg/min), and **inotropes**, such as dobutamine (5–20 μg/kg/min), may be required. (See Common Intravenous Cardiac Drug Dosages in Cardiology Section.)
5. Certainly in patients with shock and hypotension, a **pulmonary artery catheter** may help not only in managing fluids based on intracardiac filling pressures but also in diagnosing myocardial depression. It is recommended that pulmonary arterial wedge pressure be maintained at ~ 12–15 mmHg to maintain filling pressure and maximize cardiac output. However, the pulmonary artery catheter has not been shown to improve mortality.
6. There is **no** role for corticosteroids in managing septic shock.

Key References: Hines DW, Bone RC: Septic shock. In Gorbach SL, Bartlett JG, Blacklow NR (eds): Infectious Diseases. Philadelphia, W.B. Saunders, 1992, pp 544–548; Parker MM, McCarthy KE, Ognibene FP, Parrillo JE: Right ventricular dysfunction and dilatation, similar to left ventricular changes, characterize the cardiac depression of septic shock in humans. Chest 97:126–131, 1990.

Serologic and Immunologic Diagnosis of Infectious Pneumonias

Organism	Serologic and immunologic tests	Comments
Mycoplasma pneumoniae	Complement fixation (IgG)	≥ 4-fold rise in titer
	Enzyme immune assay (IgG and IgM)	More specific than CF
	Cold-agglutinin (IgM autoantibodies)	Although not specific, titers ≥ 1:32 are suggestive
Legionella pneumophila	Serum IFA	4-fold rise in titer may take up to 6–9 wk
	Sputum DFA	Fluorescein-labeled antibody; experience required for interpretation
	Urinary antigen (RIA or ELISA)	Sensitivity ~ 90%, specificity ~ 100% Detects only serogroup 1, but it accounts for ~90% of cases
Chlamydia pneumoniae (TWAR)	Microimmunofluorescence test (IgM)	Presumptive diagnosis if initial titer is ≥ 1:32
	Complement fixation (IgG)	Presumptive if IgG ≥ 1:512 In both cases, significant seroconversion may take ≥ 4 wk
Influenza	Hemagglutinin-inhibition titers	Obtain 10–14 days apart
Adenovirus	Serum antibody titers by CF, CF, neutralization, ELISA, and RIA	

(Table continued on next page.)

Organism	Serologic and immunologic tests	Comments
Histoplasma capsulatum	Immunodiffusion or CF antibody titers	Even in endemic areas, background rates of seropositivity are < 1% by ID and ~ 5% by CF. Both tests are positive in ~ 90% with active symptomatic histoplasmosis, although seroconversion may take 4–6 wk
Coccidioides immitis	Immunodiffusion (IgM to tube precipitin) Latex particle agglutination reaction (IgM but less specific than ID)	In both ID and LPA, they are seldom detected > 6 mo after infection, have no prognostic value, and are not useful in CSF. Both are good screening tests for acute infection.
	Complement fixation (IgG against coccidioidin antigen	Positive several weeks after infection; titers > 1:16 often indicate chronic pulmonary *coccidioides* pneumonia or dissemination; detection of CFA in CSF is diagnostic for meningitis

CF = complement fixation, IFA = indirect fluorescent antibody, DFA = direct fluorescent antibody, RIA = radioimmunoassay, ELISA = enzyme-linked immunosorbent assay, ID = immunodiffusion, LPA = latex particle agglutination, CSF = cerebrospinal fluid, CFA = complement-fixing antibody.

Necrotizing Fasciitis

I. **Definition**: necrotizing fasciitis (NF) is also known as necrotizing soft-tissue infections because it is characterized by rapidly progressing inflammation and necrosis of the skin, subcutaneous fat and fascia, and sometimes muscle. NF is also known as Fournier's gangrene when it involves the male genital organs. Underlying risk factors for NF: diabetes mellitus, peripheral vascular disease, intravenous drug use, obesity, and malnutrition.

II. **Bacteriology**: based on culture results, NF may be divided into type I (mixed anaerobic and facultative bacteria including Enterobacteriaceae and non-group A streptococci) and type II (group A streptococcus alone or with staphyococci).
   1. Streptococci are the most common causative organism.
   2. *Escherichia coli* and *Proteus* spp. are prevalent in the postsurgical setting.
   3. Anaerobes: *Bacteroides* spp and *Peptostreptococcus* spp.
   4. Other less common etiologic agents of NF: *Vibrio vulnificus*, group B streptococci, *Aeromonas hydrophila*. Consider group C and G β-hemolytic streptococci after podiatric surgery.

III. **Case definition of group A streptococcal NF**
   1. **Definite**
      a. **Necrosis of soft tissues with involvement of the fascia** *plus*
      b. **Serious systemic disease** including at least one of the following:
         - Death
         - Shock (systolic pressure < 90 mmHg)
         - Disseminated intravascular coagulopathy
         - Failure of organ system (respiratory, liver, renal) *plus*
      c. Isolation of group A streptococcus from normally sterile body site.
   2. **Suspected**
      a. a + b above + serologic diagnosis of group A streptococcus (ASLO or DNAse B)
      b. a + b above + histologic confirmation of gram-positive cocci in a necrotic soft tissue infection.

IV. **Clinical manifestations**
1. NF can affect any body part but is more common in the **extremities**. It is mainly acquired by open wounds, abrasion, and intravenous drug use. NF may also complicate episiotomy and cesarean section and after dental and pharyngeal infection. It may also be idiopathic without obvious portal of entry.
2. Marked **systemic toxicity** with fever, tachycardia, tachypnea, and hypotension.
3. Affected area: red, hot, shiny, swollen, and painful out of proportion to local findings → blue-grey ill-defined patches on overlying skin → cutaneous bullae and necrosis → anesthesia of area due to thrombosis of blood vessels and destruction of superficial nerves. Fascial necrosis is accompanied by widespread undermining of the skin.

V. **Differential diagnoses**
1. Erysipelas: sharply demarcated borders with lymphangitis and lymphadenopathy.
2. Cellulitis: typically does not have marked toxicity out of proportion to local findings.

VI. **Laboratory (nonspecific)**
1. Immatute leukocyte forms in peripheral blood
2. Anemia may be secondary to bone marrow depression or severe hemolysis.
3. Mild hypocalcemia may be secondary to binding of calcium to fatty acids formed from degradation of subcutaneous fat by bacterial lipases.
4. Hyponatremia and hypoproteinemia.

VII. **Diagnosis**
1. Lack of resistance to a probe along a fascial plane.
2. Frozen section biopsy: necrosis, dense neutrophil infiltration to deep dermis and fascial plane, and vascular thrombosis.

VIII. **Treatment and prognosis**
1. **Fluid and electrolyte resuscitation**
2. **Surgical debridement** of necrotic skin and nonviable fascia. Re-exploration is recommended in 24 hr as needed.
3. **Empiric antibiotics** should cover streptococci, anaerobes, enteric gram-negative bacilli, and staphylococcus: (1) ampicillin, aminoglycoside, and metronidazole; (2) clindamycin and aminoglycoside, or (3) β-lactam-β-lactamase (e.g., ampicillin-sulbactam). Tetracycline should be used for *V. vulnificus*.
4. Consider hyperbaric oxygen therapy.
5. **Mortality ranges from 9–74%**. Mortality is increased with diabetes, delay in diagnosis, advanced age, and certain sites of involvement (e.g., mortality is greater with perianal vs. urogenital involvement and with abdominal vs. extremity involvement).

Key Reference: Chapwick EK, Abter EI: Necrotizing soft-tissue infections. Infect Dis Clin North Am 10:835–855, 1996.

Hantavirus Pulmonary Syndrome

I. Hantavirus pulmonary syndrome (HPS) is a clinical disorder caused by the hantavirus. In the U.S., there are at least three distinct hantaviruses: (1) Sin Nombre virus (Southwestern U.S.), (2) Black Creek Canal virus (Florida), and (3) Bayou virus (Louisiana, Texas).

II. **Epidemiology**
1. Transmitted horizontally by rodents through their saliva, urine, and feces. Acquisition is via inhalation or direct contact.
2. Increased moisture in the winter increases the food supply for rodents in the summer, leading to increased prevalence of hantavirus.

III. **Clinical manifestations**
1. **Prodromal phase** lasting 3–6 days: fevers, myalgias, nausea, vomiting, and abdominal pain.
2. **Cardiopulmonary phase** lasting 24–48 hr: fever, cough, dyspnea, and hypotension.
3. **Convalescent phase:** with improvement in oxygenation and blood pressure.

IV. **Laboratory features**
1. Abnormalities typically occur in the cardiopulmonary phase and include the classic hematological tetrad of neutrophilia, hemoconcentration due to capillary leak syndrome, thrombocytopenia, and circulating immunoblasts. Other laboratory abnormalities include increased prothrombin time, lactate dehydrogenase, liver transaminases, and lactic acidosis.
2. Bronchoalveolar lavage is remarkable for the absence of inflammatory cells but may show large amounts of proteinaceous fluid.
3. Hemodynamic monitoring may reveal decrease cardiac output, increased systemic vascular resistance, and normal pulmonary capillary wedge pressure, suggesting intravascular volume depletion (due to capillary leak).

V. **Radiographic and pathologic findings**
1. Chest radiograph may show interstitial edema, Kerley B lines, alveolar infiltrate, and pleural effusions.
2. Edematous lung is due to interstitial and intraalveolar edema, interstitial lymphocytic infiltrates, minimal hyaline membrane formation, and serous pleural effusions.

VI. **Diagnosis**
1. Mu capture IgM
2. IgG ELISA
3. Hantavirus antigen testing by immunohistochemistry
4. RT-PCR to detect viral DNA

VII. **Treatment**
1. **Careful fluid resuscitation** to support blood pressure; a pulmonary artery catheter may be necessary to prevent volume overload.
2. **Ribavirin**, 33 mg/kg IV load, followed by 16 mg/kg IV every 6 hr for 4 days, then 8 mg/kg IV every 8 hr for 3 days. Monitor for ribavirin-induced anemia.
3. **Extracorporeal membrane oxygenation** (ECMO) – anecdotal reports suggest that this form of aggressive treatment may be helpful in selected cases.

Key References: Crowley M, et al: Successful treatment of adults with severe Hantavirus pulmonary syndrome with extracoporeal membrane oxygenation. Crit Care Med 26:409–414, 1998; Doyle T, et al: Viral hemorrhagic fevers and hantavirus infections in the Americas. Infect Dis Clin North Am 12:95–107, 1998.

Pseudomembranous Colitis

I. Pseudomembranous colitis is associated not only with antibiotic use but also with antivirals and anticytotoxics. Diarrhea may not be prominent or may occur weeks after the antibiotics are discontinued. Fulminant cases may cause toxic megacolon and mixed flora sepsis.

II. **Diagnosis** is made by *Clostridium difficile* culture and toxin in the stool. However, a positive assay for *C. difficile* is not specific for pseudomembranous colitis because 3% of healthy adults and 10–20% of hospitalized patients are colonized with this organism. Fecal leukocyte is positive in only 50% of cases. Although pseudomembranes may be grossly found on sigmoidoscopy, a normal-appearing mucosa does **not** rule out the diagnosis because microscopic examination may reveal mucosal inflammation and pseudomembranous degeneration.

III. **Treatment**

1. **Metronidazole**, 250 mg PO or IV (if PO is impossible) 4 times/day, *or*
2. **Vancomycin**, 125 mg PO 4 times daily for 7–14 days
3. **Cholestyramine**, 4 gm PO 3 times daily may be added in refractory cases. Antiperistaltic agents and barium enemas are contraindicated. Relapses may occur from reactivation of latent spores.

Reference: Bartlett JG: *Clostridium difficile*: Clinical considerations. Rev Infect Dis 12:S243–S251, 1990.

Culture-negative Infective Endocarditis

I. **Estimates of the prevalence** of sterile blood cultures among patients with infective endocarditis varies from ~ 2.5% to 31%. Causes of culture-negative endocarditis include:

1. Previous antibiotic therapy
2. Right-sided endocarditis
3. Fastidious and slow-growing organisms

II. **Organisms to consider in culture-negative endocarditis** (the first five form the acronym **HACEK**)

1. *Haemophilus parainfluenzae, H. aphrophilus, and H. paraphrophilus*
2. *Actinobacillus actinomycetemcomitans*
3. *Cardiobacterium homonis*
4. *Eikenella corrodens*
5. *Kingella kingae*
6. *Bartonella* species
7. *Chlamydia* species
8. *Coxiella burnetii*
9. Whipple disease bacterium (*Tropheyma whippelli*)

III. **Clinical manifestations**

1. All HACEK organisms produce a similar clinical syndrome that is often insidious in onset. Findings include fever, splenomegaly, embolic phenomenon, and a new or changing murmur.
2. Preexisting structural valvular disease is common.
3. Recent prior dental procedure is not uncommon.
4. In a report of 4 patients with endocarditis due to Whipple's bacterium, none had overt gastrointestinal disease. Clinically, the most common valvular abnormality was aortic regurgitation. All four patients had arthralgia that resolved with antibiotic treatment.

IV. **Diagnosis**

1. **Serologic examination** for suspected organisms should be undertaken for presumed diagnosis of culture-negative endocarditis because fastidious organisms are often intracellular pathogens.

2. **Special stains** on tissue specimens (e.g., cardiac valves)
   a. Whipple bacterium: periodic acid-Schiff (PAS)
   b. *Bartonella* species: Warthin-Starry stain
   c. *C. burnetii*: Gimenez stain
3. **Whipple's bacterium**: although polymerase chain reaction (PCR) technology has been developed for this bacterium, it is susceptible to contamination. Therefore, the diagnosis of Whipple disease based on a positive PCR is not absolute in the absence of histologic lesions confirmed by PAS staining.

V. **Causes of noninfective endocarditis**
1. **Associated with neoplasms**: atrial myxoma, marantic endocarditis (adenocarcinoma), neoplastic disease (lymphoma, rhabomyosarcoma), carcinoid.
2. **Associated with autoimmune disease**: rheumatic heart disease, Libman-Sacks endocarditis of systemic lupus erythematosus, antiphospholipid antibody syndrome, polyarteritis nodosa, and Behçet's disease.
3. **Postvalvular operation**: thrombus, sutures.
4. **Miscellaneous**: eosinophilic heart disease, ruptured mitral chordae, myxomatous degeneration.

Key References: Berbari EF, Cockerill FR, Steckelberg JM: Infective endocarditis due to unusual or fastidious microorganisms. Mayo Clin Proc 72: 532–542, 1997; Gubler JGH, et al: Whipple endocarditis without overt gastrointestinal disease: Report of four cases. Ann Intern Med 131:112–116, 1999.

Epiglottitis

I. **Epiglottitis** is an unusual cause of acute upper airway obstruction that can result in acute cardiopulmonary arrest. Although epiglottitis is characterized by inflammation and edema of the epiglottis, other supraglottic structures, including the aryepiglottic folds, arytenoids, pharynx, and uvula, may be involved.

II. **Clinical manifestations**
1. **Sore throat** and **odynophagia** are the most prominent symptom.
2. Other signs and symptoms include fever, dysphagia, drooling, muffled voice, respiratory difficulty, and stridor, with or without neck cellulitis.
3. **Course may be fulminant** in both children and adults.
4. **Sitting erect and presence of stridor** are predictive of airway compromise.
5. **Local complications** include spread of the infection into the retropharyngeal area and epiglottic abscess formation. **Systemic complications** include bacteremia, pneumonia, meningitis, arthritis, and cellulitis.

III. **Diagnosis**
1. **Indirect laryngoscopy** with a mirror or **direct laryngoscopy** with a laryngoscope: edema/erythema of the uvula, tongue base, vallecula, epiglottis, and aryepiglottic folds. One important caveat to remember is that pharyngitis may coexist with epiglottitis; therefore, if a diagnosis of pharyngitis is made, epiglottitis may still be present in the clinically suspicious patient.
2. **Lateral neck films** may show enlargement of the epiglottis and edema of other supraglottic soft tissue, but their usefulness is limited by insufficient sensitivity and specificity.
3. **Blood cultures** are positive in only 20–35% of cases (*Haemophilus influenzae* > *Streptococcus pneumoniae* > *H. parainfluenzae*).

IV. **Treatment**
1. Adult patients without evidence of airway compromise may be watched closely in the ICU without prophylactic intubation. However, airway obstruction may

occur abruptly; thus, plans must be made for rapid and successful intubation of the trachea. A tracheotomy may be required.

2. A **broad-spectrum antibiotic,** such as a third-generation cephalosporin, may be given empirically because *H. influenzae* is the most common pathogen, even in adults.
3. Corticosteroids have not been shown to be helpful and are generally not recommended.

Key Reference: Chan ED, Hodges TN, Parsons PE: Sudden respiratory insufficiency in a previously healthy 47-year-old man. Chest 112:1419–1422, 1997.

Intravenous Dosages of Common Antimicrobials

Note: Dosages are given in total dose per day; if given more than once per day, divide the total dose by the frequency to determine the dose of each administration. Dosages may need to be adjusted for patients with renal or hepatic failure.

Drug	Daily dosage
Acyclovir	15–30 mg/kg/day IV over 1 hr every 8 hr
Amikacin	15 mg/kg/day IV daily or every 8–12 hr
Ampicillin sodium	2–12 gm/day IV every 4–6 hr
Ampicillin + sulbactam (Unasyn)	4–8 gm ampicillin/day IV every 6 hr
Aztreonam	1.5–6 gm/day IV every 6–8 hr
Cefazolin (Ancef)	2–6 gm/day IV every 8 hr
Cefotaxime (Claforan)	2–12 gm/day IV every 6–8 hr
Cefotetan (Cefotan)	2–4 gm/day IV every 12 hr
Cefoxitin (Mefoxin)	2–12 gm/day IV every 4–6 hr
Ceftazidime (Fortaz)	3–6 gm/day IV every 8–12 hr
Ceftriaxone (Rocephin)	1–2 gm/day up to 4 gm/day IV every 12–24 hr
Cefuroxime (Zinacef)	2.25–4.5 gm/day IV every 6–8 hr
Ciprofloxacin	400–800 mg/day IV every 12 hr
Clindamycin phosphate	1.8–2.7 gm/day IV every 6–8 hr
Erythromycin	1–4 gm/day IV every 6 hr
Fluconazole	100–400 mg/day IV or orally every 24 hr
Foscarnet	40–60 mg/kg IV every 8 hr (induction) 90–120 mg/kg IV daily (maintenance)
Ganciclovir	5 mg/kg IV twice daily (induction) or daily (maintenance)
Gentamicin	3–5 mg/kg/day IV daily or every 8 hr
Imipenem-cilastatin (Primaxin)	1–4 gm/day IV every 6 hr
Meropenem	500 mg–2 gm IV every 8 hr
Metronidazole (Flagyl)	0.75–2 gm/day IV every 6–12 hr
Nafcillin	2–12 gm/day IV every 4–6 hr
Penicillin G	2–20 million U/day IV every 4–6 hr
Pentamidine	4 mg/kg/day IV daily (treatment) 300 mg/mo (prophylaxis)
Piperacillin	6–24 gm/day IV every 4–6 hr

(Table continued on next page.)

Drug	Daily dosage
Piperacillin + tazobactam (Zosyn)	12:1.5 gm/day IV in 4 doses = 3:0.375 gm every 6 hr
Teicoplanin (Targocid)	6 mg/kg IV at 0 and 12 hr, then 6–12 mg/kg/day (use lower end of dosage range for less serious infections)
Doxycycline (Vibramycin)	200 mg/day IV every 12–24 hr
Ticarcillin (Ticar)	4–24 gms/day IV every 4-6 hr
Ticarcillin + clavulanic acid (Timentin)	12–24 gm ticarcillin/day IV every 4–6 hr
Tobramycin	3–5 mg/kg/day IV daily or every 8 hr
Trimethoprim-sulfamethoxazole (Bactrim, Septra)	2–20 mg/kg/day of trimethoprim IV every 6–8 hr
Vancomycin	1–2 gm/day IV every 12 hr

Key Reference: Bartlett JG: Pocket Book of Infectious Disease Therapy. Baltimore, Williams & Wilkins, 1996.

Hemodynamic Monitoring

Pulmonary Artery Catheter

I. The utility of the pulmonary artery (PA) catheter continues to be debated. As with any invasive procedure, its use should be considered carefully and individualized for each patient, taking into account the need for diagnosing or managing a particular disorder plus the risks involved in placement. A recent study indicated that critically ill patients in whom the PA catheter was used had a higher mortality rate than patients in whom no catheter was placed. This article prompted a letter by the American College of Chest Physicians and the American Thoracic Society, stating, among other things, that prospective, randomized, controlled trials of the use of the PA catheter are needed.

References: Chernow B: Pulmonary artery flotation catheters. A statement by the American College of Chest Physicians and the American Thoracic Society. Chest 111: 261–262, 1997; Conner AF, Speroff T, Dawson NV, et al: The effectiveness of right heart catheterization in the initial care of critically ill patients. JAMA 276:889–897, 1996; Taylor R (ed): Controversies in pulmonary artery catheterizations. New Horizons 5:1–296, 1996.

II. **Abbreviations**

RA, LA: right atrium, left atrium
RV, LV: right ventricle, left ventricle
PA: pulmonary artery
PAD: pulmonary artery diastolic pressure
PAWP: pulmonary artery wedge pressure
LVEDV, LVEDP: left ventricular end-diastolic volume and pressure
dV/dP: change in volume over change in pressure = compliance
P_A: alveolar pressure
Pv: pulmonary venous pressure
P_a: mean pulmonary artery pressure
Pc: capillary hydrostatic pressure
P_{pl}: pleural pressure
Patm: atmospheric pressure
EKG: electrocardiogram
PEEP: positive end-expiratory pressure
CI: cardiac index
CO: cardiac output
SVI: stroke volume index
LVSWI: left ventricular stroke work index
RVSWI: right ventricular stroke work index
MAP: mean arterial systemic blood pressure
SVR: systemic vascular resistance
SVRI: systemic vascular resistance index
CVP: central venous pressure
PVRI: pulmonary vascular resistance index
PAP: peak airway pressure
$\dot{D}O_2$: oxygen delivery
$\dot{V}O_2$: oxygen utilization
O_2ER: oxygen extraction ratio
SaO_2: arterial oxygen saturation
$S\bar{v}O_2$: mixed venous oxygen saturation

III. **Pressure waveforms.** The peak systolic pressure of the PA coincides with the T wave on the EKG, and the waveform displays the characteristic dicrotic notch of the PA pressure tracing.

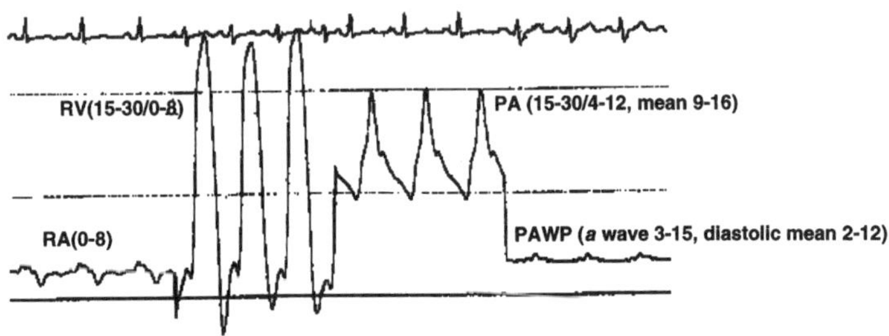

Adapted from Sprung CL: The Pulmonary Artery Catheter, 2nd ed. Closter, NJ, Critical Care Research Associates, 1993.

IV. **General pearls**

1. Because ventricular fibrillation and ventricular tachycardia may occur with insertion, a defibrillator should be present.
2. Right internal jugular or left subclavian veins are preferred sites of insertion.
3. The right atrium is reached at about 10–15 cm.
4. If < 1.3 ml of air in the balloon is required to wedge the pulmonary artery, pull back the catheter slightly.
5. Obtain a daily chest radiograph for PA catheter position.
6. LVEDV α transmural ventricular pressure (intracavitary pressure – juxtacardiac pressure) and α compliance (dV/dP) of the myocardium.
7. In rapidly breathing patients with a sudden or unexplained increase in PAWP, consider auto-PEEP as the cause.
8. Signs that the balloon is in a non-zone 3 region include marked respiratory variation in pressure tracings or an increase in PAWP by ≥ 50% of the PEEP applied.

V. **The normal atrial pressure tracing.** The peak of the *a* wave follows the peak of the p wave on the EKG, and the peak of the *v* wave follows the peak of the T wave.

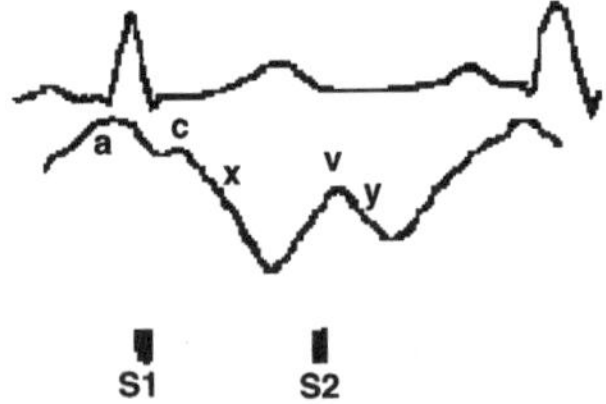

1. The ***a* wave** = atrial contraction (i.e., follows the p wave of the EKG and is presystolic). A large *a* wave indicates that the atrium is contracting against increased resistance (e.g., tricuspid stenosis, pulmonary hypertension, pulmonic stenosis, or atrioventricular (AV) dissociation seen with ventricular tachycardia (VT) or complete atrioventricular block (AVB). The *a* wave is absent in atrial fibrillation.
2. The ***c* wave** coincides with the beginning of ventricular systole and is produced by the bulging of the tricuspid valve into the atrium.
3. The **x descent** is due to a combination of atrial relaxation and downward displacement of the tricuspid valve (TV) during ventricular systole. Cardiac tamponade and constrictive pericarditis are associated with an increase in the slope of the x descent. In TV regurgitation, the x descent is often reversed (i.e., upsloping) due to the regurgitant jet.

4. The ***v* wave** occurs during late systole with filling of the atria (see below for causes of large *v* waves).
5. The **y descent** = rapid ventricular filling with opening of the AV valves. A rapid, deep y descent in early diastole occurs with severe TV regurgitation and constrictive pericarditis. It is absent or diminutive in cardiac tamponade and is often absent in right ventricular infarction.

VI. **Assumptions and problems with pressure measurements**

1. The PAWP is an estimate of the LVEDV, which in turn is a measure of preload:

   PAD ↔ **PAWP** ↔ Pc ↔ Pv ↔ P_{LA} ↔ **LVEDP** ↔ LVEDV ↔ preload

2. **Distinction between PAWP and Pc.** The pulmonary veins account for at least 40% of the total resistance in the pulmonary circulation. Therefore, the pressure drop across the pulmonary veins ($Pc - P_{LA}$) = 0.4(Pa – PAWP). In healthy subjects, Pc ≈ PAWP because Pa is low (e.g., Pc = 10 + 0.4(15–10) = 12). In adult respiratory distress syndrome (ARDS), where Pa may be doubled and pulmonary venous resistance is increased by 50%, Pc > PAWP (e.g., Pc = 10 + 0.6(30–10) = 22). Such a discrepancy probably accounts for the common observation of hydrostatic edema in the face of normal PAWP and presumably intact endothelium. Predisposing disorders in some fashion obliterate the pulmonary vascular channels: pulmonary veno-occlusive disease, emphysema, and recurrent pulmonary emboli.
3. **Although PAWP ≈ LVEDP in most settings, exceptions occur:**
   a. **Conditions that cause P_{LA} ≠ LVEDP:**
      - Decreased LV compliance (ischemia, pericardial disease): LA contraction → large increase in LVEDP with less effect on $P_{LA,diastolic}$ → PAWP underestimates LVEDP; (the clinical significance is that LV preload may be augmented without as much risk of pulmonary edema).
      - Severe aortic insufficiency → PAWP underestimates LVEDP.
      - In mitral stenosis or regurgitation, PAWP or P_{LA} overestimates LVEDP.
      - Respiratory failure: PAWP > LVEDP secondary to hypoxic pulmonary vasoconstriction.

   b. **Conditions that result in Pv (and thus PAWP) overestimating P_{LA} (and thus LVEDP)** include those with an obstruction between the occluded balloon and the left atrium (e.g., left atrial myxoma, thoracic tumors, or mediastinal fibrosis).
   c. **Conditions that cause PAWP ≠ Pv** result in zone 1 (P_A > Pa > Pv, e.g., PEEP) or zone 2 (Pa > P_A > Pv, e.g., hypovolemia) in the lungs. In both zones 1 and 2, P_A is > Pv during balloon occlusion, collapsing alveolar vessels and giving a falsely elevated PAWP. Thus PAWP is a valid measure of Pv only when Pa > Pv > P_A (zone 3). There are (at least) three surrogate markers that the catheter tip is **not in zone 3:**
      - Tip is located above the left atrium.
      - The PAWP wave tracing is unusually smooth.
      - PAD < PAWP

   d. **PAD ↔ PAWP** relationship: in tachycardia (especially > 120) and pulmonary hypertension, PAD overestimates PAWP.
4. **Effect of respiration and positive pressure ventilation (PPV) on PA catheter measurements**
   a. Because $P_{pl} \approx P_{atm}$ at end-expiration (except with PEEP), **vascular readings should be taken at end-expiration.**
   b. In patients with increased respiratory rate (RR), the estimation of vascular pressures is difficult. This problem may be ameliorated by obtaining simultaneous respiratory and pressure tracings (or switching the wedge digital

reading from "mean" to "diastolic" during mechanical ventilation since the lowest measured PAWPs during PPV are found near end-expiration).

c. In PEEP, when the P_{pl} remains positive at end-expiration, transmural pressure is < measured intraluminal pressure. Thus, PAWP overestimates LVEDP. Usually PEEP causes a net decrease in LV transmural pressure, despite an increase in PAWP because the P_{pl} will increase more than intravascular pressure due to decreased venous return with PEEP. However, in patients with stiff lungs, PEEP up to 30 cmH_2O may not affect PA catheter pressure measurements.

d. In patients without stiff lungs, PEEP > 10 may overestimate the true PAWP. This may be corrected by using either of the following formulas:

$PAWP_{calc} = PAWP_{measured} - (PEEP)(C_{lung})/(C_{lung} + C_{chest\ wall})$ where C_{lung} and $C_{chest\ wall}$ are the lung and chest wall compliances. Normally, these values are equivalent, so $PAWP_{calc} = PAWP_{measured} - \frac{1}{2}$ PEEP. **With stiff lungs**, as in ARDS (low C_{lung}), this ratio drops (approaches zero), and **$PAWP_{calc} \sim PAWP_{measured}$. With a stiff chest wall**, as in a burn with circumferential eschar formation (low $C_{chest\ wall}$), this ratio approaches 1 and **$PAWP_{calc} \sim PAWP_{measured} - PEEP$**.

VII. **Interpreting pressures**

1. Measure pressure during end-expiration when $P_{pl} = P_{atm}$.
2. A PAWP change (from the baseline) ≥ 4 mmHg is considered significant.
3. PAWP should never exceed the PAD. When PAD is < PAWP, either the balloon is overinflated or excessive P_A has occurred (no longer in zone 3).
4. PAD may be falsely increased if the heart rate (HR) is > 120 beats/min because of insufficient time for pressure to return to baseline.
5. In the presence of a large *v* wave, the PAWP tracing does not appear atrial and the mean PAWP ~ mean Pa ("ventriculization"). This may lead to excessive feeding of the catheter in an attempt to "wedge," which in turn may lead to pulmonary infarction or pulmonary artery rupture. Differentiating a PAWP tracing with a large *v* wave from a true PA tracing with a *v* wave is based on two criteria: **morphology** of the wave form and **timing** of the wave with respect to the EKG:

a. The PA tracing with a large *v* wave is bifid (see figure below), with the *v* wave usually appearing earlier than the dicrotic notch. As the catheter wedges, the bifid contour changes into a monomorphic *v* wave.

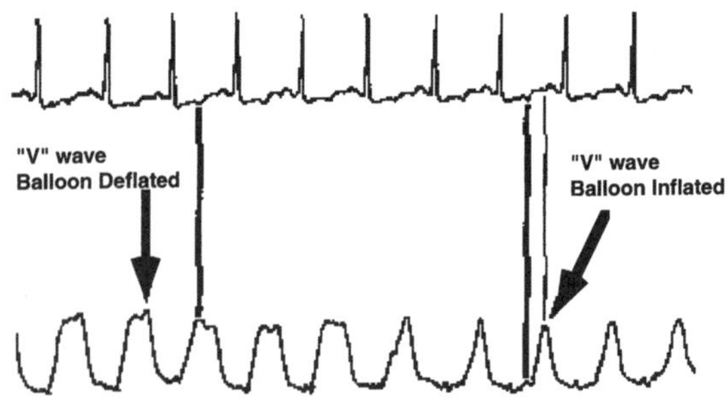

b. The PA systole is synchronous with the T wave on the EKG, whereas the *v* wave is seen later in the cardiac cycle after the T wave.
Adapted from Sprung CL: The Pulmonary Artery Catheter, 2nd ed. Closter, NJ, Critical Care Research Associates, 1993.

c. **Differential diagnosis of a large *v* wave** on a PAWP tracing (one pearl to remember is that severe mitral regurgitation may occur with trivial *v* waves, and large *v* waves may occur without significant mitral regurgitation):

- Mitral regurgitation
- Noncompliant or overdistended LA: remember that the normal *v* wave is due to passive filling of the left atrium from the pulmonary veins during late ventricular systole.
- Increased pulmonary blood flow resulting in increased LA filling (e.g., ventricular septal defect).

6. **Other examples of pressure tracings** in various cardiac disorders
   a. **Tricuspid or mitral stenosis** is associated with a large *a* wave due to increase in atrial pressure during atrial systole against a stenotic atrioventricular valve.

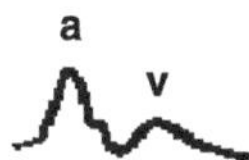

   b. **Constrictive pericarditis** is associated with increased RA pressure, increased PAWP, "dip and plateau" (square root sign) in RV and LV pressures (because virtually all filling of the ventricles occurs early in diastole), and M- or W-shaped atrial pressure tracing with steep y (and occasionally also x) descent. The prominent y descent is due to rapid atrial emptying. In contrast, a steep x descent and absent or attenuated y descent (because cardiac compression limits RV filling) in the atrial pressure tracing, pulsus paradoxus, and absent square root sign in the ventricular pressure tracing are consistent with cardiac tamponade.

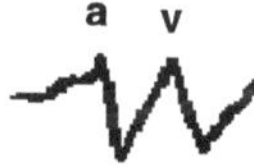

   c. **Tricuspid regurgitation** is associated with a large RA *v* wave and a steep y descent. Typically, there is a broad *cv* wave. Mean RA pressure is elevated and may increase with inspiration (Kussmaul's sign); thus, both the positive *cv* wave and the negative y descent are augmented with inspiration. In patients with RV infarction, the RA pressure is also elevated, and there may be steep x and y descents as well as Kussmaul's sign.

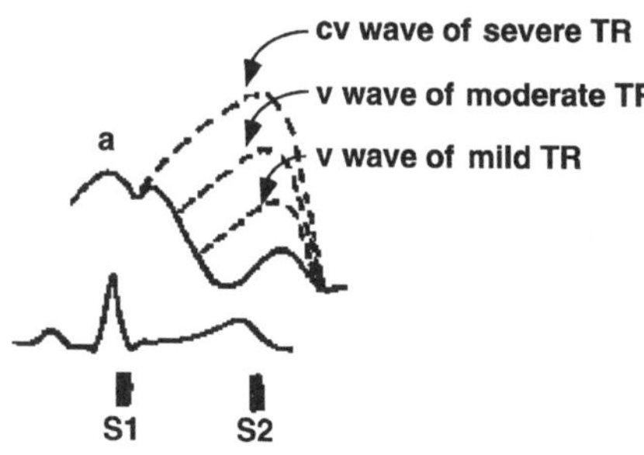

   d. **Complete AV block.** Note the cannon *a* waves associated with atrioventricular dissociation.

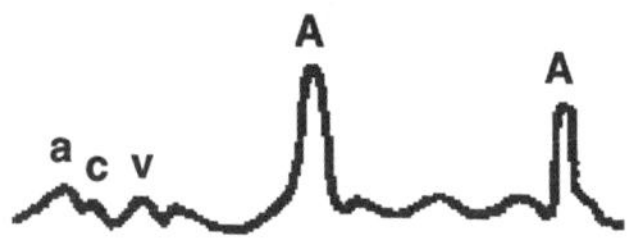

e. **Atrial fibrillation.** Note the absence of α waves.

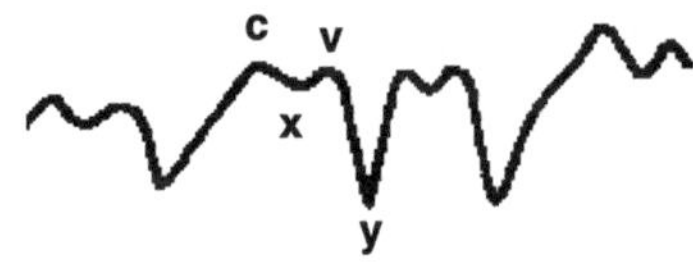

VIII. **Derived parameters**

Formula	Normal range
CI = CO/body surface area	2.6–4.2 L/min/m^2
SVI = (CI/HR) × 1000 ml/L	35–40 ml/contraction/m^2
LVSWI = (MAP – PAWP) × SVI × 0.0136	44–56 gm-m/m^2
RVSWI = (mean Pa – CVP) × SVI × 0.0136	7–10 gm-m/m^2
SVR = 80 × (MAP – CVP)/CO	1200 dynes/cm^2
SVRI = 80 × (MAP – CVP)/CI	1200–2500 dynes-sec/cm^2/m^2
PVRI = 80 × (mean PAP – PAWP)/CI	80–240 dynes-sec/cm^2/m^2
$\dot{D}O_2 = CI \times CaO_2 = 1.36(CI)(Hb)(SaO_2)(10)$	500–600 ml/min-m^2
$\dot{V}O_2 = CI(CaO_2 - CvO_2) = 1.36(CI)(Hb)(SaO_2 - SvO_2)(10)$	110–160 ml/min-m^2
$O_2ER = \dot{V}O_2/\dot{D}O_2$	22–32%
AV O_2 difference = $1.36(Hb)(SaO_2 - S\bar{v}O_2)$	3–5.5 volume %

IX. **Ventricular dysfunction profile**

Parameter	Right ventricle	Left ventricle
Preload	CVP	PAWP
Stroke output*	SVI	SVI
Afterload	PVRI	SVRI

* SV is used instead of CO to eliminate influence of HR. In patients with cardiac dysfunction, the goal is to increase CO but to decrease stroke work.

X. **Hypotension profile**

The relationship MAP = CI × SVRI helps to distinguish between cardiogenic, septic, and hypovolemic shock (see Use of the PA Catheter to Diagnose Shock Etiology).

XI. **Peripheral O_2 balance profile**

	$\dot{D}O_2$	$\dot{V}O_2$	O_2ER
Hemorrhagic shock	low	low	high
Septic shock	high	low-normal	low
Cardiogenic shock	low	low	high

XII. **Causes of low $S\bar{v}O_2$:** $S\bar{v}O_2 = SaO_2 - [\dot{V}O_2/(13.6 \times CI \times Hb)]$
1. Hypoxemia
2. Increased metabolic rate
3. Anemia
4. Low CO

XIII. **Causes of high $S\bar{v}O_2$**
1. High-output states (sepsis, hyperthyroidism, or liver failure) increase $\dot{D}O_2$
2. Decreased extraction of O_2 by tissues (sepsis) decreases $\dot{V}O_2$
3. Left-to-right intracardiac shunt
4. Severe mitral regurgitation (? by left-to-right shunt)
5. Cyanide poisoning
6. Nitroprusside toxicity
7. Hypothermia
8. Wedged pulmonary artery catheter (artifactual increase in $S\bar{v}O_2$)

XIV. **Complications of insertion and placement**

1. **Arrhythmias** (risks for ventricular tachycardia are hypoxia, acidosis, and myocardial ischemia)
2. **Right bundle-branch block** or complete heart block in patients with preexisting left bundle-branch block
3. **Pulmonary infarction, pulmonary artery pseudoaneurysms and rupture** (major risks are pulmonary hypertension and overwedging with an inflated balloon). **Pulmonary artery rupture** may occur when the pulmonary artery (PA) catheter has been left constantly in the wedge position (inflated or deflated) or when the balloon is inflated in a small distal PA (i.e., requiring < 1.5 cc of air to wedge). The wedge position is identified by (1) bifid waveform of *a* and *v* waves; (2) pulmonary artery wedge pressure < mean PA pressure; and (3) *v* wave of wedge tracing after the Tw on EKG or the peak PA tracing occurring before or coincident with the Tw on the EKG.
4. **Catheter knotting, endocardial damage** and endocarditis of tricuspid or pulmonic valve, and **tricuspid regurgitation**
5. **Complications at insertion site** (pneumothorax, air embolism, thrombosis, arterial puncture).

Key References: Leatherman JW, Marini J: Pulmonary artery catheter: Pressure monitoring. In Sprung CL: The Pulmonary Artery Catheter, 2nd ed. Closter, NJ, Critical Care Research Associates, 1993, pp 119–156; Marino PL: The ICU Book. Philadelphia, Lea & Febiger, 1991; Wiedemann HP, Matthay MA, Matthay RA: Cardiovascular-pulmonary monitoring in the intensive care unit (Pts. 1 and 2). Chest 85:537–549, 656–668, 1984.

Use of the PA Catheter to Diagnose Shock Etiology

Diagnosis	PAWP	CO	SVR	Comments
Cardiogenic shock				
Myocardial dysfunction	↑	↓	↑	Major MI, cardiomyopathy, myocarditis
Acute VSD	±↑	↓LVCO (RVCO > LVCO)	↑	Oxygen step-up at RV
RV infarct	±↓	↓	↑	↑ Right sided pressures with low/normal PAWP
Acute MR	↑	↓ Forward CO	↑	*v* wave on PAWP
Pericardial tamponade	↑	↓	↑	Equalization of mean P_{RA}, RVEDP, PAD, and PAWP
Massive PE	±↓	↓	↑	Prolonged or overwedging of catheter may further decrease pulmonary blood flow
Oligemic shock	↓	↓	↑	Often obvious and usually does not require PA catheter to diagnose or to manage unless there is concomitant (severe) cardiopulmonary disorder

(Table continued on next page.)

Diagnosis	PAWP	CO	SVR	Comments
Septic shock	±↓	↑ (rarely ↓)	↓	Myocardial depressant factor (?tumor necrosis factor) may cause low CO
Anaphylaxis	±↓	±↑	↓	Epinephrine is mainstay of treatment

VSD = ventricular septal defect, MR = mitral regurgitation, PE = pulmonary embolism, MI = myocardial infarction, CMP = cardiomyopathy, RVEDP = right ventricular end-diastolic pressure, PAD = pulmonary artery diastolic pressure, TNF = tumor necrosis factor.

Key Reference: Parrillo JE: Shock. In Isselbacher KJ, Braunwald E, Wilson JD, et al (eds): Harrison's Principles of Internal Medicine, 13th ed. New York, McGraw-Hill, 1994, pp 187–192 (source of table).

Methods for Calculating Venous-to-Arterial Shunts

I. **Derivation of the shunt equation:** requires use of the PA catheter. The amount of oxygen in the total arterial blood (Q_T) = amount of oxygen in blood that has traversed pulmonary capillaries (Qc) + amount of oxygen in shunted blood (Qs):
   1. $(CaO_2) \times Q_T = (CcO_2) \times Qc + (CvO_2) \times Qs$
      where $Qc = Q_T - Q_S$
   2. $Qs = Q_T\,(CcO_2 - CaO_2) / (CvO_2 - CcO_2)$
      where CaO_2 = arterial oxygen content, CcO_2 = capillary oxygen content, and CvO_2 = mixed venous arterial content.

II. **Estimation of shunt after breathing 100% oxygen:** for every 2% shunt, PaO_2 is expected to decrease by 35 mmHg. At sea level, the expected PaO_2 on 100% oxygen is 673 mmHg ($= 760 - P_A(H_2O) - P_ACO_2$) ~ $760 - 47 - 40 = 673$. In Denver, the expected PaO_2 on 100% oxygen is $618 - 47 - 40 = 531$.

III. **A calculated and simplified approach:** no need for PA catheter or mixed venous sample.

   Reference: Vora S, Wildrick K: Determination of intrapulmonary shunt: A simplified approach. Presented at ACCP Meeting, October 30–November 3, 1994, in New Orleans.

   % shunt = {700 – [a:A ratio × (713 – $PaCO_2$/0.8)]} / 20

   where a:A ratio = PaO_2/P_AO_2

   For example, given a $PaCO_2$ of 40 mmHg and a PaO_2 of 180 mmHg on 80% oxygen:
   1. $P_AO_2 = 0.8(760 - 47 - 40/0.8) = 530.4$
   2. a:A ratio = 180 / 530.4 = 0.339
   3. % shunt = {700 – [0.339 × (713 – 40/0.8)]} / 20 = 23.76%

Electrolyte Disorders

Hyponatremia

I. **Differential diagnoses**

1. Most cases of hyponatremia are due to decreased osmolality. It is less commonly associated with normal or increased osmolality.
2. Osmolality = 2Na + BUN/2.8 + glucose (mg/dl)/18, where Na = sodium (mEq/L), and BUN = blood urea nitrogen (mg/dl). Normal: 282–292 mOsm/kg. Alternatively, SI formula: Osmolality (mmol/kg) = 2Na (mmol/L) + urea (mmol/L) + glucose (mmol/L).
3. **Hyposmolar hyponatremia**
   a. **Increased extracellular fluid (ECF) volume and edema** (excessive total body sodium + larger excess of total body water): congestive heart failure (CHF), cirrhosis, nephrosis/renal failure
      - Diagnosis: $U_{Na} \leq 20$ mmol/L for cirrhosis and CHF; $U_{Na} > 20$ mmol/L with acute renal failure, where U_{Na} = urinary sodium concentration.
      - Treatment: correction of underlying disorder, diuretics, water restriction

   b. **Normal ECF volume and no edema** (excessive total body water): syndrome of inappropriate antidiuretic hormone (SIADH; see below), psychogenic polydipsia, hypothyroidism
      - Diagnosis: $U_{Na} > 20$ mmol/L
      - Treatment: water restriction, demeclocycline, correction of underlying disorder

   c. **Decreased ECF volume** (deficit of total body water + larger deficit of total body sodium): salt/water losses replaced with hypotonic fluids
      - Diagnosis: may be renal ($U_{Na} > 20$ mmol/L) or extrarenal ($U_{Na} < 10$ mmol/L) in origin
      - Treatment: isotonic fluids
4. **Normosmolar hyponatremia** (pseudohyponatremia): hyperlipidemia, hyperproteinemia
5. **Hyperosmolar hyponatremia:** mannitol, hyperglycemia (for every increase of 100 mg/dl (5.5 mmol/L) of glucose → decrease of 1.5 mmol/L of Na)
6. **Determining the volume of water excess**
   Current volume (L) = 0.6 (current weight, kg)
   Total body solute (mOsm) = measured osmolality (mOsm/L) × current volume
   Normal volume = total body solute/desired osmolality
   Excessive water = current volume – normal volume
7. **Criteria for diagnosis of SIADH:** ADH secretion is independent of osmotic or hemodynamic stimuli.
   a. Hyposmolar hyponatremia
   b. Normovolemic
   c. Less than maximally dilute urine (urine osmolality > 300 mOsm/L [or mmol/kg]): in contrast, in the **absence** of ADH, urine osmolality may fall to 50 mOsm/kg. Assuming 1000 mOsm of solute excretion, a maximally dilute urine allows excretion of 20 L/day of urine.
   d. $U_{Na} > 20$ mmol/L
   e. Normal renal, adrenal, and thyroid function
   f. No diuretics

g. Causes: major categories include carcinomas, pulmonary disorders, and CNS disorders, drugs

II. **Emergencies and treatment pearls**

1. The principal danger of **rapid-onset hyponatremia** (drop of ≥ 0.5 mEq/L/hr) is **brain edema**. The two lines of defense against brain swelling are (1) loss of interstitial fluid and Na into the cerebral spinal fluid and (2) loss of intracellular solute (potassium, organic osmolytes).
2. Dangers of **rapid correction** of hyponatremia (especially in chronic hyponatremia)
   a. **Brain shrinkage**
   b. **Osmotic demyelination syndrome** with histopathology of central pontine myelinolysis occurs after initial improvement in hyponatremic symptoms. Symptoms range from behavioral changes, seizures, movement disorders, or akinetic mutism to pseudobulbar palsy, quadriparesis, and unresponsiveness.
3. **Approach to acute hyponatremia**
   a. **Psychogenic polydipsia.** Most patients recover uneventfully with interruption of the polydipsia by medical intervention or neurologic event.
   b. **Parenteral water intoxication.** Women are at greater risk because of lower total body water content (women are smaller and have more fat). Risk is higher in the postoperative period due to administration of hypotonic fluids and release of ADH with anesthesia/surgery. Treatment: diuretics may be required. Carefully replace sodium chloride, potassium, and magnesium losses and limit the increase in serum sodium by no more than 0.5-1.0 mEq/L/hr.
   c. **Postprostatectomy syndrome** is due to absorption of electrolyte-free irrigating solutions. Isotonic hyponatremia occurs because the solutes in the irrigant are confined to the extracellular space. Treatment: diuretics. (See Postprostatectomy Syndrome in Nephrology Section.)
4. **Approach to chronic hyponatremia**
   a. Hyponatremia due to **volume depletion** is treated with isotonic saline.
   b. Hyponatremia due to **thiazides** is susceptible to rapid correction because correction of hypokalemia also raises [Na]. Serum [Na] = (total body Na + total body K)/total body water.
   c. In **SIADH**, isotonic saline may result in a more concentrated urine, worsening the hyponatremia. Loop diuretics impair the ability to concentrate the urine, but fluid restriction is the mainstay of therapy.
   d. In **edematous states**, loop diuretics are the mainstay of therapy.
5. **Hypertonic saline (guidelines): use extreme care.**
   a. **Rapid infusion: 3% saline at 1–1.5 ml/kg/hr for 2–3 hr.**
      Indications: seizure/coma (except when urine is dilute and urine output > 300/hr: in such patients (psychogenic polydipsia and acute water intoxication from IV fluids), hyponatremia will self-correct.
   b. **Slow infusion:** 3% saline at 15 ml/hr.
      Indications: slow response to water restriction and with acute symptoms (e.g., in SIADH, combine with furosemide) and inability to take oral salt.
   c. **Cautions:** avoid correction by more than 12 mEq/L/day; also use furosemide for patients at risk for congestive heart failure.

Key References: Berl T: Treating hyponatremia: What is all the controversy about? Ann Intern Med 113:417–419, 1990; Cluitmans FHM, Meinders AE: Management of severe hyponatremia: Rapid or slow correction? Am J Med 88:161–166, 1990; Dunagan WC, Ridner ML: Manual of Medical Therapeutics, 26th ed. Boston, Little, Brown, 1989.

Hypernatremia

I. In general, patients who are hypernatremic are also hyperosmolar.
   1. Normal serum osmolality = 282–292 mOsm/kg (mmol/kg)
   2. Osmolality = 2(Na) + BUN/2.8 + glucose/18
   3. Na > 160 mEq/L: irritability, anorexia, ataxia, cramping
   4. Na > 180 mEq/L: confusion, stupor, seizure

II. **General classification**
   1. **Hypernatremia with increased volume:** due to hypertonic saline or sodium bicarbonate ($NaHCO_3$). Treatment: diuretics and replacement with water.
   2. **Hypernatremia with normal volume:** nephrogenic or neurogenic diabetes insipidus, sweat or lung loss of fluid that is relatively solute-free replaced with inadequate amounts of water. Treatment: water.
   3. **Hypernatremia with decreased volume:** diarrhea.

III. **Water depletion (L) ≈ 0.6 × (current body weight in kg) × [(P_{Na}/140) – 1],** where P_{Na} = plasma sodium in mEq/L
   1. Replace ½ of the deficit over the first 24 hr and remainder over the next 1–2 days.
   2. If Na > 175 mEq/L, monitor osmolality and Na hourly until 155 mEq/L, allowing a decline of at most 2 mOsm/hr or Na drop of ≤ 2 mEq/hr.

IV. **Diabetes insipidus (DI):** lack of production or response to antidiuretic hormone (ADH). ADH normally allows the collecting tubules to be permeable to water.
   1. **Criteria:** polyuria > 4 L/day (polydipsia if alert), high Na, high plasma osmolality, low urine osmolality (< 300 mOsm/kg [mmol/kg]).
   2. **Neurogenic DI:** idiopathic, CNS infection, CNS injury (e.g., surgery, postanoxic, postpartum necrosis), CNS neoplasia, CNS vascular disease, systemic disease (sarcoidosis, histiocytosis X, and Wegener's granulomatosis).
   3. **Nephrogenic DI:** drugs (amphotericin B, colchicine, demeclocycline, chlorpropamide, lithium, methoxyflurane, propoxyphene, prostaglandin, vinblastine), primary renal (Fanconi syndrome, chronic interstitial disease, polycystic kidney disease, chronic obstructive uropathy, nephrocalcinosis), systemic disease (amyloidosis, hypercalcemia, hypokalemia, multiple myeloma, sarcoidosis, sickle cell disease, Sjögren's syndrome).
   4. **DI may be masked in patients with adrenal insufficiency** because cortisol is necessary to excrete maximally dilute urine. Corticosteroid administration may unmask the DI.

V. **Differential diagnosis of polyuria with low urine osmolality**
   1. Neurogenic DI
   2. Nephrogenic DI
   3. Psychogenic polydipsia

Key Reference: Marsden PA, Halperin ML: Pathophysiological approach to patients presenting with hypernatremia. Am J Neph 5:229–235, 1985.

Hypokalemia

I. Normal serum potassium [K] = 3.3–4.9 mEq/L.

II. In general, the lower the K, the greater the total body deficiency of K:
   [K] of 3.0–3.5 mEq/L → 150–300 mEq K deficit
   [K] of 2.5–3.0 mEq/L → 300–500 mEq K deficit
   For each additional decrease in [K] of 1 mEq/L, there is a 200–400 mEq additional deficit.

III. **Causes of hypokalemia**

1. **Hypokalemia with metabolic alkalosis:** vomiting, nasogastric suctioning, hyperaldosteronism, Bartter's syndrome, Cushing's syndrome, thiazide and loop diuretics, fludrocortisone, 11β-hydroxysteroid dehydrogenase deficiency (may be hereditary or due to licorice ingestion)
2. **Hypokalemia without potassium depletion** (due to shifts of K into cells): β_2-adrenergic agonists (epinephrine, pseudoephedrine, albuterol), theophylline, tocolytics (ritodrine, nylidrin), caffeine, verapamil overdose, chloroquine intoxication, familial hypokalemic periodic paralysis, hyperthyroidism-associated (especially in Asians), insulin, glucose, and barium ingestion (blocks K exit from cells). Both insulin and β_2-adrenergic catecholamines increase cellular K uptake by stimulating cell-membrane Na/K-ATPase.
3. **Hypokalemia without acid–base disturbance:** osmotic diuresis, penicillin or carbenicillin (causes obligate K loss due to excretion of anions), magnesium deficiency, low dietary intake (due to obligatory urinary loss of K especially when intake is < 1 gm (25 mmol) / day), theophylline; aminoglycosides, cisplatin, foscarnet, and amphotericin B all cause renal K wasting by inducing magnesium depletion. Renal K wasting can be seen with acute myelogenous, monomyeloblastic, or lymphoblastic leukemia.
4. **Hypokalemia with metabolic acidosis:** diarrhea and laxative abuse, types I and II renal tubular acidosis (toluene abuse is a cause of hypokalemia by this mechanism), diabetic ketoacidosis, and acetazolamide.

IV. **Clinical manifestations:** proximal muscle weakness, fatigue, cramps, rhabdomyolysis (K < 2.5 mmol/L), hyporeflexia, ascending paralysis that may impair respiratory function (K < 2.0 mmol/L), ileus, constipation, orthostatic hypotension, hypertension, arrhythmias (especially with digoxin), T-wave flattening, U wave, ST-segment depression.

V. **Treatment**

1. For non–life-threatening hypokalemia, oral replacement therapy with KCl is the best and safest in a patient who is able to take medications enterically. The liquid preparation is less well tolerated. Among the two oral preparations, a wax matrix formulation and a microencapsulated formulation, the risk of gastrointestinal ulceration may be lessen with the latter preparation. In general $KHCO_3$ is only recommended when K depletion occurs in the setting of metabolic acidosis. Consider a K-sparing diuretic such as amiloride, triamterene, or spironolactone in a patient with continuing loss.
2. **Intravenous therapy**
   a. For most situations that require IV therapy, KCl may be given at a rate up to **10 mmol/hr in concentrations up to 30 mmol/L.**
   b. **For dire emergencies** (e.g., [K] < 2 mmol/L with severe EKG or neuromuscular complications), KCl may be given through **two** peripheral lines at a rate up to **15–20 mmol/hr in concentrations up to 60 mmol/L** in each iv (**total: 30–40 mmol/hr**) with continuous EKG monitoring and frequent check of [K]. For acute treatment of severe hypokalemia, use glucose-free solutions. Glucose may decrease serum [K] further by driving K into the intracellular compartment from the actions of glucose and insulin.

Key References: Gabow PA, Peterson LN: Disorders of potassium metabolism. In Schrier RW (ed): Renal and Electrolyte Disorders. Boston, Little, Brown, 1986, pp 207–249; Gennari FJ: Hypokalemia. N Engl J Med 339:451–458, 1998.

Hyperkalemia

I. Hyperkalemia may be spurious (pseudohyperkalemia), due to increased redistribution from the intracellular space to the extracellular space, or due to a true increase in total body potassium (K).

II. **Pseudohyperkalemia:** hemolysis, prolonged tourniquet application, marked leukocytosis (> 10^5/µl) or thrombocytosis (> 10^6/µl)

III. **Redistributative hyperkalemia:** systemic acidosis, insulin deficiency

IV. **True hyperkalemia:** renal failure (acute > chronic: serum K usually does not rise until creatinine clearance < 10 ml/min, provided urine output is adequate), potassium-sparing diuretics (spironolactone, triamterene, amiloride), heparin, angiotensin-converting enzyme inhibitor, digitalis intoxication, β-blockers, potassium penicillin, NSAIDs, rhabdomyolysis, primary K secretory defect of renal tubules (renal transplantation, systemic lupus erythematosus, sickle cell anemia, urinary tract obstruction).

V. **Clinical symptoms:** weakness, flaccid quadriplegia, paresthesias, areflexia, paralysis, hypotension, cardiac arrest

VI. **EKG findings:** tall peaked T waves, loss of P waves, increased PR interval, increased QRS (to sine wave), depressed ST, increased QT, ventricular fibrillation

VII. **Treatment.** Calcium lowers the resting potential of cardiac muscles, rendering them less arrhythmogenic. Insulin and $NaHCO_3$ cause K to enter the cells; both act within minutes.

1. Calcium gluconate 10%, 5–10 ml IV over 5 min, repeat in 5 min if no improvement. Relative contraindication: digitalis-induced hyperkalemia.
2. D50, 1 ampule, + 5–10 U regular insulin IV; repeat every 15 min as needed.
3. $NaHCO_3$, 1 ampule (50 mmol) over 5 minutes; repeat in 10 minutes if no EKG improvement. In patients with end-stage renal disease, administration of $NaHCO_3$ has only a slight effect on the transcellular distribution of K.
4. β2-adrenergic receptor agonist such as 2.5 mg nebulized albuterol (0.5 ml of 0.5% solution + 2.5 ml sterile saline) also drives K intracellularly.
5. Kayexalate, 15–30 gm in 20 ml sorbitol, + 100 ml H_2O every 3–4 hr orally or 50 gm + 200 ml H_2O as retention enema (held for 1–2 hr).
6. Hemodialysis, which can remove 25–30 mmol/hr of K, is indicated when hyperkalemia is complicated by volume overload, severe uremia, or acidosis.

Key Reference: Gabow PA, Peterson LN: Disorders of potassium metabolism. In Schrier RW (ed): Renal and Electrolyte Disorders. Boston, Little, Brown, 1986, pp 207–249.

Hypercalcemia

I. **Causes**

1. Parathyroid disorders (adenoma, multiple endocrine neoplasia [MEN], familial hypercalciuria, lithium)
2. Malignancy (solid tumor with metastases or humoral mediation, hematologic)
3. Vitamin D-associated (intoxication, granulomatous disorders)
4. High bone turnover (hyperthyroidism, immobilization, thiazides, excessive vitamin A)
5. Associated with renal failure (aluminum intoxication, tertiary hyperparathyroidism, milk-alkali)

II. **Treatment**

1. **0.9 N or 0.45 N saline:** 250–500 ml/hr, assuming normal renal and cardiac function

2. **Furosemide:** 20–40 mg IV every 2 hr once volume repleted
3. **Glucocorticoids:** Hydrocortisone, 250–500 mg IV every 8 hr → 10–30 mg/day orally. **Pearl:** useful for hypercalcemia associated with myeloma, lymphoma, or increased vitamin D.
4. **Phosphate:** Phospho-soda (600 mg phosphorus/5 ml), 1 tsp orally 3 or 4 times/day or Neutra-Phos (250 mg phosphorus/capsule), 2–3 capsules orally 3 or 4 times/day as needed. **Pearl:** limit use to patients with low phosphate levels (e.g., primary hyperparathyroidism).
5. In general, one of the following more specific calcium-lowering medications is required for longer lasting control of hypercalcemia:
   a. **Etidronate disodium**, 7.5 mg/kg/day IV over 4 hr for 3–7 days (oral therapy to maintain normocalcemia: 20 mg/kg/day for 30 days). Warnings: diarrhea, nephrotoxicity, decrease dose with renal insufficiency.
   b. **Pamidronate**, 15–45 mg/day slow IV for 3 days or 90 mg IV over 24 hr
   c. **Calcitonin**, 4–8 IU/kg every 12 hr SQ or IM (use IM if volume > 2 ml; 200 IU/ml). Warnings: skin testing before use: 10 IU + 1 ml 0.9 N NaCl → 0.1 ml intracutaneously. If positive reaction (erythema or wheal) in 15 min, do not use. Pearl: most rapid onset of action, but effects wear off quickly. Salmon calcitonin is measured in IU, human calcitonin in mg; calcitonin also has potent analgesic properties.
   d. **Plicamycin (mithramycin)**, 25 μg/kg IV for 1 dose over 4–6 hr, then 10 μg/kg IV BIW as needed. Contraindications: thrombocytopenia, overt hepatic or renal dysfunction, decreased clotting factors Pearl: treatment should not be repeated until hypercalcemia recurs because toxicity is proportional to frequency and dose.

Key Reference: Bilezikian JP: Management of acute hypercalcemia. N Engl J Med 326:1196–1203, 1992.

Hypocalcemia

I. **Definition:** total [Ca] < 8.5 mg/dl (2.12 mmol/L) (with normal albumin) or ionized calcium (Ca_i) < 0.96 mmol/L (normal [Ca_i]: 0.96–1.4 mmol/L or 4.1–5.1 mg/dl). Correction factor: albumin decrease of 1 gm/dl → decrease of 0.8 mg Ca/dl. However, this correction factor is *inferior* to Ca_i determination. Measure Ca_i anaerobically and do **not** correct pH to 7.4.

II. **Causes:** hypoalbuminemia (pseudohypocalcemia), hypomagnesemia, hypermagnesemia (Mg may mimic Ca and suppress parathyroid hormone [PTH]), acute respiratory alkalosis (decreased Ca_i due to increased binding to protein), vitamin D deficiency, liver and renal disease (decreased hydroxylation of vitamin D), PTH deficiency, hyperphosphatemia (e.g., Na phosphate enema overdose), osteoblastic metastases, blood transfusion*, albumin (binds Ca), $NaHCO_3$ (decreases Ca_i by binding to albumin), radiocontrast media (chelation), toxic shock syndrome, fat embolism, plasma exchange (due to loss of albumin and chelation by anticoagulant citrate dextrose solution [ACDS] used to anticoagulate the blood during the exchange), and sepsis (due to increased binding of Ca to albumin by free fatty acids [FFA]†, PTH insufficiency, or vitamin D deficiency).

* When citrate clearance is impaired (liver/renal disease) and transfusion is rapid, the increased citrate may cause hypocalcemia by chelation.

† Free fatty acids may be increased in the stress response by epinephrine, heparin, glucagon, growth hormone, corticotropin, IV lipids, norepinephrine, isoproterenol, or alcohol ingestion. Normal FFA ≈ 250 μmol/L, overnight fast ≈ 400–600 μmol/L, severe stress ≈ 3000 μmol/L.

III. **Manifestations**

1. **Cardiovascular:** hypotension, heart failure, arrhythmias (bradycardia, ventricular fibrillation, electrical mechanical dissociation), insensitivity to drugs that act through calcium-related mechanisms (digoxin, norepinephrine, dopamine), increased QT interval, T wave inversion
2. **Respiratory:** laryngospasm, bronchospasm, apnea
3. **Neurologic:** tetany (Chvostek's and Trousseau's signs), spasms (including laryngeal), seizures, hyperreflexia, cramps
4. **Psychiatric:** anxiety, dementia, depression, psychosis, irritability

IV. **Treatment of acute symptomatic hypocalcemia** (100–200 mg of elemental calcium): calcium administration may precipitate digitalis toxicity.

1. 10% Ca gluconate (93 mg Ca/10-ml ampule): 1–2 amps IV over 10–15 min

   or

2. 10% $CaCl_2$ (272 mg Ca/10-ml ampule): 1 amp over 10–15 min

V. **Treatment of severe hypocalcemia requiring continuous IV infusion of Ca (1–2 mg/kg/hr):** for a 70-kg person at 1 mg/kg/hr: 5 amps 10% Ca gluconate (≈ 500 mg) in 500 ml D_5W at 70 ml/hr

VI. **Treatment of subacute/chronic hypocalcemia**

1. Oral preparations (generally require 2–4 gm of elemental Ca/day)
   $CaCO_3$ (Os-Cal 250–500 mg Ca/tablet)
   Ca lactate (1–2 gm 3 times/day)
2. Vitamin D preparations: ergocalciferol, 50,000 U/day or calcitriol, 0.25–1.0 µg/day

Key Reference: Zaloga GP, Chernow B: Hypocalcemia in critical illness. JAMA 256:1924–1929, 1986.

Magnesium

I. **Normal levels:** 1.4–2.2 mEq/L or mmol/L

II. **Hypomagnesemia**

1. **Causes:** malabsorption syndromes, starvation, alcoholism, severe diarrhea, nasogastric suction, parathyroid surgery, hypophosphatemia, diuresis (diuretics, osmotic, postobstructive or post-ATN) primary hyperaldosteronism (increased Mg excretion due to volume expansion), Bartter's syndrome, renal tubular acidosis, diabetic ketoacidosis, hyperthyroidism, digitalis toxicity, aminoglycoside (causes renal Mg wasting), cisplatin, and cyclosporine.
2. **Hypomagnesemia may cause hypokalemia** (from increased renal loss by mechanism not well-established) and **hypocalcemia** (parathyroid hormone [PTH] secretion depends on calcium-sensitive, magnesium-dependent adenylate cyclase system and PTH action requires magnesium).
3. **Manifestations**
   a. **Cardiovascular:** coronary vasospasm (by potentiating the actions of vasoconstrictors), premature ventricular contractions, prolonged PR and QT intervals, T wave flattening, atrial fibrillation, torsades de pointes, and congestive heart failure.
   b. **Respiratory:** failure due to respiratory muscle weakness.
   c. **Neurologic:** parathesias, spasms, seizures, tetany, confusion, obtundation, positive Chvostek's sign, hyperreflexia, and coma.
   d. **Metabolic:** refractory hypokalemia, hypocalcemia.
   e. **Digitalis toxicity is markedly potentiated by hypomagnesemia.**

4. **Treatment**
   a. Hypomagnesemic tetany: with normal renal function, 6 gm of $MgSO_4$ in 1 L D5W over 6 hr
   b. Oral magnesium oxide, 250–500 mg 4 times/day

III. **Hypermagnesemia** (rare in patients with normal renal function)
   1. **Causes:** renal failure (acute or chronic), administration of high Mg doses for toxemia, and Mg-containing antacids or enemas in patients with renal insufficiency.
   2. **Signs and symptoms:** areflexia (at levels ~ 5 mmol/L), nausea, vomiting, hypotension, confusion, lethargy, muscular weakness, respiratory depression (occurs at level ~ 7.5 mmol/L), increased QT interval, peaked T waves, atrioventricular block, intraventricular conduction defect, and asystolic arrest.
   3. Hypermagnesemia may suppress PTH → hypocalcemia (as seen and reported in preeclamptic women). Thus increased Mg may suppress PTH secretion, whereas decreased magnesium may either stimulate (mimicking hypocalcemia) or suppress (see above) PTH secretion.
   4. **Treatment:** cardiovascular toxicity and respiratory depression of hypermagnesemia may be antagonized by 1 gm IV calcium gluconate until hemodialysis or peritoneal dialysis is instituted.

Key Reference: Reinhart RA: Magnesium metabolism: A review with special reference to the relationship between intracellular content and serum levels. Arch Intern Med 148:2415–2420, 1988.

Phosphorus

I. **Normal values:** 2.5–4.5 mg/dl or 0.81–1.45 mmol/L

II. **Hypophosphatemia**
   1. **Causes:**
      a. **Increased urinary excretion:** hyperparathyroidism, renal tubular defects, diuretic phase of acute tubular necrosis, postobstructive diuresis, diuretics, renal transplant, extracellular fluid volume expansion, corticosteroids, xanthine derivatives, aldosteronism.
      b. **Decreased gastrointestinal absorption:** malabsorption, malnutrition-starvation, administration of phosphate binders.
      c. **Abnormal vitamin D metabolism** resulting in vitamin D deficiency.
      d. **Shifts to the intracellular space:** treatment of diabetic ketoacidosis, respiratory alkalosis, metabolic alkalosis, alcohol withdrawal, recovery phase of starvation, initiation of hyperalimentation, administration of glucose, insulin, epinephrine, glucagon, or corticosteroids.
   2. **Manifestations:** muscular weakness (diaphragmatic dysfunction), rhabdomyolysis, hemolysis, platelet dysfunction, tissue hypoxemia due to shift of O_2-dissociation curve to the left (due to decreased 2,3-diphosphoglycerate), myocardial depression, and neurologic abnormalities (paresthesias, Guillain-Barré-like syndrome, seizures, and coma).
   3. **Treatment of mild hypophosphatemia** (1–2.5 mg/dl) or 0.32–0.81 mmol/L
      a. **Neutra-Phos** (250 mg phosphorus and 7 mmol each of Na and K capsule, 2 capsules orally 2 or 3 times/day.
      b. **Phospho-Soda** (129 mg phosphorus, 4.8 mmol Na/ml): 5 ml orally 2 or 3 times/day.

4. **Treatment of severe hypophosphatemia** (< 1 mg/dl) or < 0.32 mmol/L
   a. **Na_3PO4 or K_3PO4** (4 mEq Na or K and 93 mg phosphorus/ml):
      2.5–5 mg elemental phosphorus/kg IV over 6–8 hr as initial dose, then as needed (~ 200 mg or ~ 2 ml diluted in saline for 70-kg patient).
   b. Complications of IV phosphate therapy: hyperphosphatemia, precipitation of calcium phosphate (if Ca × P > 60), and symptomatic hypocalcemia.

III. **Hyperphosphatemia**

1. **Causes:** renal insufficiency, hypoparathyroidism, pseudohypoparathyroidism, acromegaly, tumor lysis, rhabdomyolysis, phosphate enemas, Paget's disease of the bone, and treatment with diphosphonates (e.g., for Paget's disease).
2. **Manifestations:** related to secondary hypocalcemia (see Hypocalcemia section).
3. **Treatment**
   a. **Dietary restriction** to 0.7–1.0 gm/day (impractical because PO_4 is ubiquitous).
   b. **Phosphate binders:** Amphojel (aluminum hydroxide) or Basaljel (aluminum carbonate gel), 5–10 ml or 1–2 tabs orally 3 times/day before meals.
   c. **$CaCO_3$, alone or in combination with aluminum agents** also may be used in patients with renal failure to avoid aluminum toxicity (keep Ca-phosphate product < 70 to minimize soft tissue calcification).

Key Reference: Halevy J, Bulvik S: Severe hypophosphatemia in hospitalized patients. Arch Intern Med 148:153–155, 1986.

Toxicology

Approach to the Poisoned Patient

I. **Phone number of nearest poison control center:** ____________________ .

II. **Initial therapy for patients with altered mental status**
   1. **Oxygen**—assess airway and ventilation
   2. **Thiamine**, 50–100 mg IM or IV
   3. **Glucose**, 25–50 gm IV, to rule out hypoglycemia (unless blood glucose is immediately available and is elevated, as in hyperosmolar nonketotic coma)
   4. **Naloxone**, 2 mg IV

III. **Drugs in which levels are needed on an emergent basis**
   1. Salicylate
   2. Methanol
   3. Ethylene glycol
   4. Iron
   5. Theophylline
   6. Lithium
   7. Carbon monoxide

IV. **History and physical exam**
   1. The history may be unreliable in the poisoned patient. However, symptom complexes, called **toxic syndromes**, with abnormalities in sensorium, motor signs, ocular findings, or odor of breath may lead to a toxin-pattern recognition that is extremely useful in initial treatment (see also Common Toxic Syndromes).
   2. **Behavior and hallucinations**
      a. Lilliputian hallucinations: atropine
      b. Peripheral vision hallucinations: cocaine
      c. Complex hallucinations with paranoid psychosis: phencyclidine (PCP)
      d. Illusions, hallucinations and pseudohallucinations (knowing when one is hallucinating): LSD
      e. Synesthesia (e.g., hearing colors): LSD, marijuana, morning glory seeds, magic mushrooms
      f. Well-formed auditory hallucinations: usually indicative of schizophrenia
   3. **Motor signs**, such as tremors, hyperreflexia, and nature of seizures, may be helpful diagnostic findings. For example, generalized seizures in an alert patient may indicate strychnine poisoning. Some toxin-induced seizures have a specific unconventional therapy: isoniazid seizure, pyridoxine; theophylline seizure, rarely responds to one drug and phenytoin is contraindicated.
   4. **Vital signs**
      a. Sympathomimetics and anticholinergics cause an increase in all vital sign values.
      b. Organophosphates, opiates, barbiturates, β-blockers, benzodiazepines, alcohol, and clonidine may result in hypothermia, respiratory depression, and bradycardia.
   5. **Ocular findings**
      a. **Pupillary signs: mydriasis** (dilatation) with sympathomimetics and anticholinergics (with cocaine, pupils respond to light; with anticholinergics, no response to light); **myosis** (constriction) with organophosphate insecticides, narcotics, bromide, acetone, clonidine, and nicotine. PCP may cause either.
      b. **Nystagmus:** horizontal nystagmus with alcohols, lithium, carbamazepine, solvents, meprobamate, quinine, and primidone. Combined vertical, horizontal, and rotatory nystagmus suggests PCP, phenytoin, and sedative hypnotics. Ping-pong gaze (periodic disturbances) suggests monoamine oxidase inhibitors.

6. **Odors** emanating from the patient may give clues about the intoxication. For example, garlic suggests arsenicals, phosphorus compounds, or organophosphate pesticides; rotten egg odor suggests hydrogen sulfide or disulfiram.

V. **Common radiopaque ingestions** (a negative finding does not exclude such ingestion) can be remembered with the mnemonic **CHIPE**:

C—Chloral hydrate, **c**ocaine condoms, **c**alcium
H—Heavy metals (arsenic and lead)
I—Iron, **i**odides
P—Phenothiazines, **p**sychotropics (tricyclic antidepressants), **p**otassium
E—Enteric-coated tablets, slow-release capsules

VI. **Clinical laboratory evaluation** includes assessment of three gaps:

1. **Anion gap:** $[Na^+ - Cl^- - HCO_3] > 12$ mEq/L is most commonly due to ketoacidosis, uremia, salicylates, methanol, ethylene glycol, alcohol, lactic acidosis.
2. **Osmolar gap:** measured – calculated osmolality ($2 \times Na^+$ + urea/2.8 + blood glucose/18) > 10 mOsm/kg is mostly seen in intoxications with one of the exogenous alcohols and glycols.
3. **Oxygen saturation gap:** > 5% difference between pulse oximetry and oxygen saturation in arterial blood is seen with carbon monoxide, cyanide, hydrogen sulfide, and methemoglobin.

VII. **Decontamination**

1. **Terminate exposure:** stop ingestion of agent, stop dermal exposure by removing clothing and irrigating affected area with copious amounts of tap water. Irrigate ocular exposures with tap water.
2. **Gastrointestinal tract decontamination:** absorbants such as charcoal, gastric lavage, cathartics, and/or whole bowel irrigation. Inducing emesis with ipecac is generally **not** recommended for adults as charcoal is clearly superior.
   a. **Activated charcoal** is effective in preventing absorption of many poisons from the GI tract. Small-molecular-weight drugs or chemicals (e.g., iron or lithium) are not absorbed by the charcoal.
      i. **Dose:** children, 30–50 gm orally; **adults**, 50–100 gm orally (1 gm/kg) with 60 ml sorbitol. If ingestion involves a large amount of toxin or is life-threatening or if sustained-release products have been ingested or drugs that undergo enterohepatic recirculation (e.g., digoxin, phenobarbital, carbamazepine, theophylline), repeated doses of charcoal may be necessary every 2–4 hr in patients with no evidence of GI obstruction.
      ii. **Pearls for activated charcoal:**
         - Contraindicated in caustic ingestion.
         - May bind N-acetylcysteine but not clinically significant.
         - Ineffective in alcohol (e.g., methanol), simple ions (e.g., iron, lithium, cyanide), or strong acid or base ingestions.
         - Pulse doses every 2–4 hr effective for drugs with significant enterohepatic recirculation, but must ensure that GI tract is functional and charcoal being eliminated; otherwise, drug may be reabsorbed.
   b. **Gastric lavage** should be used within 60 min of most ingestions (with agents causing delayed gastric emptying or in overdoses associated with considerable morbidity and mortality, such as TCAs, cyanide, and calcium channel blockers, gastric lavage should be tried even after 60 min). Use Ewald tubes (24–26 Fr for children; 36–40 Fr for adults) with lavages of 2–3 cc/kg aliquots. Typically, lavage is limited to serious ingestions of agents not bound to charcoal, such as intentional lithium or iron ingestions or symptomatic patients with potentially life-threatening ingestions. You should have a low threshold for intubating patients with mental status changes prior to lavage.

c. **Cathartics** may aid in elimination of the toxin bound to charcoal: sorbitol, 1–1.5 g/kg, or magnesium citrate, 4 ml/kg.

d. **Whole bowel irrigation.** When activated charcoal will not bind the toxin, undertake whole bowel irrigation to eliminate the toxin. Administer isosmotic GoLytely solution at a rate of ~2 L/hr until the rectal effluent is roughly the same color as the administered solution (at least 10 L of fluid is usually required). This technique should not be used in patients who have an ileus or are at risk for GI perforation, bleed, or obstruction.

VIII. **Antidotes:** See Antidote section.

IX. **Other modes of enhanced elimination**

1. **Cholestyramine resin**, 4 gm every 8 hr, may enhance elimination of digoxin, phenobarbital, warfarin, lorazepam, methotrexate, or lindane.
2. **Forced diuresis.** The use of saline diuresis with or without ion trapping has theoretical benefits. A urine flow rate of 3 ml/kg/hr should be achieved using isotonic fluid administration and diuretics. One may achieve urinary alkalinization with 50–100 mEq of $NaHCO_3$ per liter of half normal saline. Titrate to urine pH ≥ 7.5. Monitor potassium with alkalinization.
3. **Extracorporeal techniques**

   a. **Hemodialysis** is especially good for correcting electrolyte disturbances and metabolic acidosis. It is also ideal for substances that are of low molecular weight (< 500 daltons) or water-soluble or have a small volume of distribution (< 1 L/kg), low lipid solubility, and low protein binding. Common drugs or toxins that are effectively removed by hemodialysis include **methanol, ethylene glycol, salicylate, theophylline, lithium, phenobarbitol,** and **ethanol.**

   b. **Charcoal hemoperfusion** increases elimination of drugs that are adsorbed (e.g., theophylline, phenytoin).

X. **Toxic gas inhalation** (see Inhalational Injury by Irritant Gases)

XI. **Criteria for admission of poisoned patient to ICU**

1. Need for hemofiltration, hemodialysis, or extracorporeal membrane oxygenation
2. Respiratory depression ($PaCO_2 > 45$ mmHg)
3. Possible, impending, or required intubation
4. Seizures
5. Cardiac: arrhythmia, hypotension (systemic blood pressure < 80 mmHg), or heart block (second or third degree)
6. Decreased consciousness, unresponsiveness to verbal stimuli
7. Increasing metabolic acidosis
8. TCA or phenothiazine overdose with anticholinergic signs, neurologic abnormality, QRS duration > 0.12 sec, or QT > 0.5 sec (prolonged QTc)
9. Administration of pralidoxime in organophosphate toxicity
10. Pulmonary edema secondary to drugs or toxic inhalants
11. Drug-induced hypothermia or hyperthermia, including neuroleptic malignant syndrome
12. Digoxin overdose with hyperkalemia or need for digoxin-immune antibody Fab fragments
13. Body packers and stuffers
14. Emergency surgical intervention
15. Antivenom administration
16. Need for continuous infusion of naloxone

Key References: Eilers MA, Garrison TE: General management principles. In Rosen P, Barkin RM (eds): Emergency Medicine, 3rd ed. St. Louis, Mosby, 1992; Krenzelok, EP, Leikin JB: Approach to the poisoned patient. Dis Month 42(9):509–608, 1996; Leikin JB, Pauloucek FP: Poisoning and Toxicology Compendium with Symptom Index. Hudson, OH, Lexi-Comp Inc, 1998.

Common Toxic Syndromes

I. **Anticholinergic syndromes**
   1. **Common signs:** delirium with mumbling speech, hallucinations, tachycardia, dry/flushed skin, dilated pupils, visual blurring, myoclonus, slightly increased temperature, urinary retention, decreased bowel sounds (ileus), hypertension. Seizures, choreoathetosis, toxic psychosis coma, respiratory failure, dysrhythmias, and cardiovascular collapse may occur in severe cases.
   2. **Common causes:** antihistamines, antiparkinson medication (benztropine [Cogentin], atropine, scopolamine), amantadine, antipsychotics (butyrophenones [Haldol], phenothiazines), tricyclic antidepressants, antispasmodics, mydriatics, skeletal muscle relaxants, and many plants (notably jimson weed and *Amanita muscaria*).
   3. **Treatment:** sedation with benzodiazepines and supportive care.

II. **Sympathomimetic syndromes**
   1. **Common signs:** excess of speech and motor activity, delusions, paranoia, tachycardia (or bradycardia if the drug is a pure alpha-adrenergic agonist), hypertension, hyperpyrexia, diaphoresis, piloerection, mydriasis, and hyperreflexia. Seizures, hypotension, and dysrhythmias may occur in severe cases.
   2. **Common causes:** cocaine, amphetamine, methamphetamine, phenylpropanolamine, ephedrine, pseudoephedrine, LSD, phencyclidine (PCP), methylphenidate, nicotine. Similar findings with theophylline and caffeine overdoses due to release of endogenous catecholamines.
   3. **Treatment:** benzodiazepines.

III. **Opiate, sedative, or ethanol intoxication**
   1. **Common signs:** stupor, coma, respiratory depression, miosis, hypotension, bradycardia, hypothermia, pulmonary edema, decreased bowel sounds, hyporeflexia, and needle marks. Seizures may occur after overdoses of some narcotics, notably propoxyphene.
   2. **Common causes:** narcotics (opiates, dextromethorphan, pentazocine, propoxyphene, methaqualone, meprobamate), barbiturates, benzodiazepines, ethchlorvynol, glutethimide, methyprylon, ethanol, clonidine, and guanabenz.
   3. **Treatment:** supportive, especially of the airway; naloxone (opiates); flumazenil (benzodiazepines); urinary alkalinization (barbiturates).

IV. **Cholinergic syndromes**
   1. **Common signs:** confusion, CNS depression, weakness, salivation, lacrimation, urinary and fecal incontinence, GI cramping, emesis, diaphoresis, muscle fasciculations, pulmonary edema, miosis, bradycardia or tachycardia, and seizures.
   2. **Common causes:** organophosphate and carbamate insecticides, pilocarpine, physostigmine, edrophonium, and some mushrooms.
   3. **Treatment:** atropine.

V. **Extrapyramidal syndromes**
   1. **Common signs:** choreoathetosis, hyperreflexia, trismus, opisthotonos, rigidity, and tremor.
   2. **Common causes:** haloperidol, phenothiazines.
   3. **Treatment:** diphenhydramine, benztropine.

VI. **Solvent syndrome**
   1. **Common signs:** lethargy, confusion, dizziness, headache, restlessness, incoordination, derealization, depersonalization.
   2. **Common causes:** acetone, chlorinated hydrocarbons, hydrocarbons, naphthalene, trichloroethane, toluene.
   3. **Treatment:** avoid catecholamines.

Key References: Krenzelok EP, Leikin JB: Approach to the poisoned patient. Dis Month 42:509–608, 1996; Kulig K: Initial management of ingestions of toxic substances. N Engl J Med 326:1677–1681, 1992.

Antidotes Commonly Used in Overdoses

Toxin	Antidote	Dose and Comments
Opiates	Naloxone	Start at 2 mg IV. More may be needed (if no response in 5–15 min, give 10 mg IVP); withdrawal possible in addicts. May also be given IM, SQ, or endotracheally.
Methanol or ethylene glycol	Fomepizole	Load: 15 mg/kg iv over 30 min, then 10 mg/kg q 12 hrs for 4 doses, then 15 mg/kg q 12 hrs until EG levels are below 20 mg/dL (< 3.32 mmol/L).
	Ethanol	Load: 10 ml/kg of 10% solution in D5W IV over 30 min to 1 hr; maintenance: 1.5 ml/kg/hr of 10% solution. Oral load: 600–700 mg/kg; oral maintenance: 125–150 mg/kg/hr (may mix as 20% drink). Maintain blood alcohol level of 100–200 mg/dl (21.7–43.4 mmol/L). Double maintenance dose with dialysis. Continue until [MeOH] < 20–25 mg/dl (6.2–7.8 mmol/L).
Anticholinergics	Physostigmine	1–2 mg IV over 5 min every 30–60 min. Use only with severe delirium, cardiac dysrhythmia refractory to lidocaine, and with extreme caution (may cause seizures); maximal dose: 4 mg/30 min. Contraindicated in asthmatic patients.
	Benzodiazepine	Lorazepam 2 mg iv q 5 min up to 30 mg or more to control anticholinergic delirium is **safer and easier to use than physostigmine** with the caveat that endotracheal intubation may be necessary.
Organic phosphate or carbamate insecticides (essentially cholinergic poisoning)	Atropine	Test dose: 2 mg IV (IM, SQ) Repeat every 5–30 min as needed till drying of pulmonary secretions occurs (may require ~ 200 mg in first hr and 50 mg/hr infusion for days). Atropine effective at muscarinic and not nicotinic sites.
	Pralidoxime (2-PAM)	1 gm IV (or PO) over 15–30 min every 8–12 hr for 3 doses as needed. Handle patients with gloves (skin absorption).
Isoniazid, hydrazine	Pyridoxine	Give gram-per-gram equivalent doses to what was ingested. Start with 5 gm over 30–60 min if amount ingested is unknown.
Beta blockers, hypoglycemic agents	Glucagon	5–10 mg IV over 2 min. Titrate to normalization of vital signs: 2–10 mg/hr as needed as IV infusion. For hypoglycemia, 0.5–1 mg SQ/IM/IV; may repeat in 15 min (requires liver glycogen stores).
Tricyclic antidepressant (TCA)	Bicarbonate	1–2 mmol/kg IV for substantial cardiac conduction delay or ventricular dysrhythmias; titrate to response/pH.
Digitalis	Digoxin-specific antibody fragments	No. vials = (mg digoxin ingested)(0.8)/0.6. Unknown amount: give 10–20 vials IV with life-threatening arrhythmia.

(Table continued on next page.)

Toxin	Antidote	Dose and Comments
Digitalis *(cont.)*	(Digibind)	No. vials = [Dig (ng/ml)](5.6)(wt_{kg})/600 if digoxin level is known.
Benzodiazepines	Flumazenil	0.2 mg over 30 sec, then 0.3 mg as needed, then 0.5 mg every 1 min as needed for a total dose of 3 mg. Should not be given with concomitant TCA overdose or history of seizures.
Iron	Deferoxamine	Indications: > 30 mg/kg elemental Fe, serum Fe > 300 mg, or serum Fe > TIBC. Therapeutic dose: 1 gm IM or IV, then 500 mg every 4 hr for 2 doses. Then 500 mg every 4–12 hr as needed (no more than 6 gm in 24 hr).
Acetaminophen	N-Acetylcysteine	Load: 140 mg/kg PO *or* 150 mg/kg IV over 15 min. Maintenance: 70 mg/kg every 4 hr for 17 doses PO; *or* 150 mg/kg IV over 30-60 min, followed by 50 mg/kg in 500 ml D_5W over 4 hr, then 100 mg/kg in 1 liter D_5W over 16 hr.
Calcium channel blockers, fluorides, hydrofluoric acid	Calcium	1 gm $CaCl_2$ over 5 min Repeat for life-threatening situations but monitor [Ca] after third dose.

TIBC = total iron-binding capacity; MeOH = methanol.

Key References: Dunagan WC, Ridner ML: Manual of Medical Therapeutics, 26th ed. Boston, Little, Brown, 1989, pp 490–501; Krenzelok EP, Leikin JB: Approach to the poisoned patient. Dis Month 42:509–608, 1996; Kulig K: Initial management of ingestions of toxic substances. N Engl J Med 326:1677, 1992 (source of table).

Treatment of Hypotension Associated with Drug Poisoning

I. **Calcium channel antagonists.** The dihydropyridines (e.g., nifedipine, amlodipine, isradipine) exert their effects mainly on vascular tone and may cause reflex tachycardia. In contrast, diltiazem and verapamil overdoses often result in sinoatrial and atrioventricular slowing and negative inotropy.
   1. **Gastric lavage, charcoal 1 gm/kg.**
   2. With sustained-release forms, perform **whole bowel irrigation** with GoLytely, 2 L/hr.
   3. **Hypotension associated with the dihydropyridines: fluid resuscitation** because the primary problem is vasodilation.
   4. **Hypotension associated with diltiazem or verapamil** often is accompanied by poor cardiac contractility; therefore, patients may not tolerate fluid resuscitation. Thus calcium (**$CaCl_2$, 1 gm over 5–10 min IV**, repeated once or twice, to a total dose of 5 gm) is the therapeutic agent of choice. If calcium is unsuccessful, give **glucagon, up to 5 mg IV slowly over 30 sec.** Glucagon enhances inotropy via non–β-adrenergic mechanism. Thus, glucagon is useful for myocardial depression associated with verapamil or diltiazem overdoses, but use is limited with dihydropyridine toxicity. If no response to fluid, calcium, or glucagon, administer **norepinephrine**.

II. **Tricyclic antidepressants.** TCAs may produce hypotension by two different mechanisms: (1) sodium channel blockade → cardiotoxicity and (2) α-adrenergic blockade → vasodilation → hypotension.

Treatment of hypotension

1. **Sodium bicarbonate** for hypotension or cardiac conduction toxicity
2. **Fluid resuscitation**
3. **Norepinephrine** (0.5–30 μg/min) or **phenylephrine** (10 mg/100 ml at 100 ml/hr). Titrate to blood pressure (dopamine may not work because presynaptic stores of catecholamines may be depleted).

III. **Theophylline.** At high toxic doses, β-adrenergic effects predominate over α-adrenergic effects, producing tachycardia (β_1) and hypotension (β_2). The phosphodiesterase inhibition results in increased cAMP → increased β-adrenergic tone.

Treatment of hypotension (see also Theophylline Toxicity)

1. **Fluid resuscitation**
2. Cautious use of calcium channel blockers to treat supraventricular tachycardia because blood pressure may drop.
3. **Alpha-pressors** (e.g., norepinephrine or phenylephrine).
4. **Beta blockers** (use propranolol, which has β_2-blocking effects).
5. **Charcoal hemoperfusion**

Key Reference: Nelson L: What to do when drug poisoning causes hypotension. J Crit Illness 11:88–92, 1996.

Carbon Monoxide Poisoning

I. Carbon monoxide (CO) is an odorless, colorless, tasteless, and nonirritating gas; therefore, insidious exposure is not uncommon.

II. The **principal toxicity** associated with CO poisoning is its **strong binding to hemoglobin** (COHb), competing with oxygen and causing widespread tissue hypoxemia. In addition CO **displaces the oxyhemoglobin dissociation curve to the left** (impeding oxygen unloading in tissues) and **binds to cytochrome A**, thereby inhibiting oxidative metabolism and cellular respiration.

III. The **half-life of COHb** is 1/α to the FiO_2: 5 hr on room air, 90 min with 100% O_2 at 1 atm, and 20 min with 100% at 2 atm.

IV. **Clinical diagnosis.** The "cherry red lips" of CO poisoning may not be present in all patients; they may mask cyanosis in some patients. The two major organ systems affected by CO poisoning are **neurologic** (manifested in varying ways but may include irritability, disturbed judgment, confusion, seizures, and strokes; patients may appear intoxicated) and **cardiac** (arrhythmias and ischemia). Other signs and symptoms include headache, shortness of breath, and visual disturbances (decrease in acuity, retinal venous engorgement, retinal hemorrhages).

V. **Laboratory diagnosis.** Do not delay empiric treatment with 100% O_2 based on clinical suspicion.

1. **[COHb] is directly measured on a co-oximeter.** In general COHb < 10% is asymptomatic (cigarette smokers may have levels of ~ 5–10%). Confusion occurs at levels of 30–50%, and the incidence of rapid fatality is high at 70–80%. Patients with underlying cardiopulmonary disease are often affected at lower levels. Because PaO_2 is a reflection of dissolved O_2, the PaO_2 often is normal, although the O_2 content [CaO_2] in blood is very low.
2. **Metabolic acidosis** due to tissue hypoxemia (may also signal concomitant cyanide poisoning in the case of smoke inhalation).

VI. **Treatment**

1. **100% O_2 is the best form of treatment for CO poisoning.** It should be given until COHb is < 20% and patient has no symptoms related to hypoxemia.

Supplemental oxygen is beneficial for two reasons: (1) the increase in PaO_2 (dissolved oxygen) increases the rate of elimination of COHb and (2) although the amount of dissolved O_2 in plasma is low when breathing room air, it may increase to ~ 2 vol % on 100% O_2, which is enough O_2 to supply one-third of the O_2 demand of the body.

2. **Hyperbaric oxygen therapy** (consider strongly in all patients with a history of loss of consciousness). 100% O_2 at 2–2.5 atm for 1 hr; even with 100% COHb, adequate tissue oxygenation may be achieved because of the markedly elevated amount of dissolved oxygen (as reflected by the increase in PaO_2).

Key Reference: Crocker PJ: Carbon monoxide poisoning, the clinical entity and its treatment: A review. Milit Med 149:257–259, 1984.

Illicit Drugs and Controlled Substances of Abuse

I. **Cocaine**

1. Many pharmacologic effects of cocaine are due to intense vasoconstriction, which results from increased levels of catecholamines because of blocked reuptake at secretory adrenergic synapses, inhibition of monoamine oxidase, and direct anticholinergic effects.
2. **Cardiac effects**
   Myocardial ischemia (coronary vasospasm, coronary thrombosis)
   Myocarditis
   Rupture of ascending aorta, aortic dissection
   Atrial and ventricular tachyarrhythmia
   Hypertension
   Transient myocardial depression
3. **Neurologic effects**
   Dysphoric agitation, delirium
   Seizures
   Stroke
   Cerebral vasculitis, subarachnoid hemorrhage
4. **Pulmonary effects**
   Barotrauma
   Pulmonary edema with diffuse alveolar hemorrhage (crack lung)
   Nasal septal necrosis
5. **Other**
   Rhabdomyolysis
   Hyperthermia
   Intestinal ischemia
6. **Treatment** is mainly supportive. Benzodiazepines have been found to be especially useful in controlling the stimulatory effects of cocaine. Relatively high doses may be required, e.g., lorazepam 2 mg in q 5 min up to 30 mg with the caveat that endotracheal intubation may be required. Antipsychotics such as haloperidol may be used but may lower the seizure threshold. For hypertensive crisis and myocardial infarction, pure beta blockers are contraindicated due to unopposed alpha-stimulation.

Key References: Mark H, Cregler LL: Medical complications of cocaine abuse. N Engl J Med 315: 1495–1500, 1986; Murray RJ, Albin RJ, Mergner W, Criner GJ: Diffuse alveolar hemorrhage temporally related to cocaine smoking. Chest 93:427–429, 1988.

II. **Narcotic (Opiate) Overdose**

1. May occur with both prescription and illicit opiates.
2. **Clinical presentation:** somnolence, respiratory depression, cyanosis, possibly pulmonary edema, hypothermia, pinpoint pupils.
3. **Treatment**
   a. Airway management; gastric lavage and charcoal with oral overdose.
   b. Naloxone, 2 mg IV, for somnolent or comatose patient with respiratory depression. More may be needed (if no response in 5–15 min, give 10 mg IVP); repeated doses every 20–60 min may be needed, although withdrawal is possible in addicts. Naloxone drip may be used if a response is seen and patient starts to drift back into respiratory depression. One important caveat is that if the airway/oxygenation is controlled, then reversing the effects of the opiates may be more problematic in regard to agitation and its adverse sequelae.

III. **Benzodiazepine overdose**

1. Death from benzodiazepine overdose is rare. When it occurs, it is often accompanied by a mixed overdose. Therefore, toxicology screening is essential to rule out ingestion of other common drugs such as aspirin or acetaminophen.
2. **Clinical presentation:** somnolence, (mild) respiratory depression, and hypothermia.
3. **Treatment**
   a. Airway management
   b. Gastric lavage, charcoal
   c. Give naloxone to rule out (concomitant) narcotic overdose. If no response to naloxone, then give flumazenil 0.2 mg IV over 30 sec, then 0.3–0.5 mg IV every 1 min as needed for a total dose of 3 mg. Flumazenil should only be used with caution and avoided in benzodiazepine addicts or if tricyclic antidepressant is co-ingested because of the risk of precipitating a seizure.

IV. **Sedative-hypnotic overdose**

1. May be divided into **barbiturates** and **nonbarbiturates** (e.g., chloral hydrate or methaqualone).
2. **Clinical presentation:** lethargy, hypotonia, vertigo, ataxia, nystagmus, somnolence, coma, respiratory suppression, hypothermia, and hypotension. Deep tendon reflexes and pupillary responses are usually normal.
3. **Toxic barbiturate levels**

Drug	Toxic level	Drug	Toxic level
Amobarbital	> 40 μmol/L	Pentobarbital	> 40 μmol/L
Barbital	> 170 μmol/L	Phenobarbital	> 170 μmol/L
Butabarbital	> 45 μmol/L	Secobarbital	> 6 μmol/L
Butalbital	> 45 μmol/L		

4. **Treatment**
   a. Airway management, gastric lavage, multiple-dose activated charcoal. Barbiturates are long acting; therefore, mechanical ventilation is more common.
   b. Fluids ± diuretics, forced alkaline diuretics for phenobarbital and barbital.
   c. Hemodialysis or hemoperfusion
   d. Physical tolerance of barbiturates occurs with long-term use. Acute withdrawal of tolerant individuals may lead to significant symptoms: delirium, hallucination, hyperpyrexia, seizures, and death. Consider phenobarbital loading in patients with seizures, hyperthermia, or major delirium.

V. **Stimulant-induced pulmonary toxicity**

1. **Barotrauma (pneumomediastinum, pneumothorax, pneumopericardium, or subcutaneous emphysema)** is caused by an increased alveolar-interstitial pressure gradient from cocaine inhalation with mouth-to-mouth positive pressure

and Valsalva maneuver. Hamman's sign may be heard. Most cases resolve spontaneously and can be managed expectantly.

2. **Pulmonary edema** (cardiogenic and noncardiogenic) may be the result of either cocaine or amphetamines.
3. **Crack lung** is characterized by fever, diffuse alveolar infiltrates, pulmonary and systemic eosinophilia, and alveolar damage with hyaline membrane formation 1–48 hr after heavy cocaine smoking.
4. **Asthmalike symptoms** may be seen after smoking crack but are difficult to sort out from concomitant tobacco or marijuana smoking.
5. **Diffuse alveolar hemorrhage**—more likely with crack

Key References: Albertson TE et al: Stimulant-induced pulmonary toxicity. Chest 108:1140–1149, 1995; Seaman ME: Barotrauma related to inhalational drug use. J Emerg Med 8:141–149, 1990.

Alcohol Withdrawal

I. The severity of alcohol withdrawal is variable and depends on the duration and intensity of alcohol exposure. Mild reactions consist of insomnia, irritability, and tremor. Severe withdrawal reactions include delirium tremens. Stress responses often accompany withdrawal, resulting from excessive catecholamine release, and consist of tachycardia, perspiration, and increased blood pressure. Alcohol withdrawal is a common and often overlooked problem in the ICU, especially in post-trauma or postoperative patients.

II. **Indications for hospitalization**
   1. Presence of other medical or surgical conditions requiring treatment
   2. Hallucinations, tachycardia > 110 bpm, dysrhythmias, severe tremor, extreme agitation, or history of severe withdrawal symptoms
   3. Fever > 38°C
   4. Ataxia, nystagmus, confusion, and ophthalmoplegia (Wernicke's encephalopathy)
   5. Confusion or delirium
   6. Seizures: generalized seizures occurring for the first time in the withdrawal state, focal seizures, status epilepticus, seizure in patient withdrawing from a combination of alcohol and other drugs
   7. Recent history of head injury with loss of consciousness
   8. Physical dependence on other drugs

III. **Assess for other medical conditions that occur in alcoholics:** infection, trauma, pancreatitis, dehydration, electrolyte abnormalities, hypoglycemia, hyperthermia, aspiration, and dysrhythmias.

IV. **Management of severe alcohol withdrawal.** Delirium tremens may have mortality rate as high as 15–20%. There is autonomic activity with fever, tachycardia, tremors, diaphoresis, seizures, hallucinations, and agitation. It usually occurs 3–4 days after last drink, although it may occur as late as 1 week later.
   1. Hydrate and correct electrolytes such as potassium, magnesium (magnesium sulfate, 2 gm IV 4 times/day for 3 days), and phosphate as needed.
   2. Place patient in a quiet room, reassure him or her, and dim the lights.
   3. Cardiac monitor if dysrhythmias are present.
   4. Thiamine, 100 mg/day IV for 3 days
   5. The goal of **sedation therapy** is to achieve a level of sedation equivalent to a score of 2–4 on the Ramsey Sedation Scale (see below).
      a. **Lorazepam:** start with **1–2 mg PO or IV every 1 hr as needed**, adjusting dosing interval to severity of the symptoms. If patient requires an increasing

dose (> 24 mg/day) or frequency of every hour for 2–3 hr because of increasing agitation, consider using a continuous lorazepam drip. Because lorazepam may cause significant respiratory depression, patients must be monitored carefully. However, lorazepam has some advantages in patients with liver disease because it conjugates with glucoronic acid to form an inactive metabolite. This conjugation is not influenced by alcoholic cirrhosis.

or

Diazepam, 5 mg IV every 5–10 min until symptoms are controlled; then 5–10 mg every 2–6 hr as needed.

b. **Haloperidol.** Consider adding haloperidol at 2.5–5 mg PO or IV (IV route is not FDA-approved) 2 times/day. This butyrophenone has antihallucinatory activity in alcohol withdrawal. It also lowers the seizure threshold and should be used with caution until risk of seizures has diminished (i.e., 3 days after cessation of drinking).

c. **Beta blocker or central alpha agonist (clonidine).** May be used in conjunction with lorazepam or haloperidol if the patient has no contraindication.

6. Modified Ramsey Sedation Scale
   - 1 = Anxious and agitated/restless
   - 2 = Cooperative, oriented, and tranquil
   - 3 = Responds to commands only
   - 4 = Brisk response to a light glabellar tap or loud auditory stimulus
   - 5 = Sluggish response to 4
   - 6 = No response to 4

V. **Management of alcohol withdrawal seizures.** Seizures during alcohol withdrawal are generally grand mal type, nonfocal, one or two in number, between 12 and 60 hr after cessation of drinking. Patients with no seizure history need a seizure work-up. Treatment with benzodiazepines alone usually controls seizures. In patients with seizure history, prophylactic treatment with phenytoin is indicated, 10 mg/kg load at a rate not exceeding 50 mg/min, then 300 mg/day PO for 5 days.

Key Reference: Devenyi P, Reeves JL: Addiction Research Foundation Clinical Institute Physicians Manual, 4th ed. 1986.

Medical Complications of Alcoholism

I. **Neurologic complications**

1. **Wernicke-Korsakoff syndrome.** Characterized by Wernicke's triad (confusion, ataxia, ophthalmoplegia) and Korsakoff psychosis (severe recent memory impairment with confabulation). Thiamine deficiency plays a prominent role.
2. **Peripheral neuropathy.** Associated with thiamine and other nutritional deficiencies. It is symmetrical, distal sensorimotor neuropathy of legs > arms. Loss of ankle jerks is an early sign.
3. **Cerebral atrophy.** The clinical organic brain syndrome associated with brain atrophy ranges from minimal cognitive and intellectual impairment to severe dementia.
4. **Cerebellar degeneration.** Involves mainly the vermis. Thus, the main clinical picture is ataxic gait with relative preservation of tone and coordination.
5. **Pseudoparkinsonism.** Tremor, rigidity, and bradykinesia may be present but resolve with abstinence.
6. **Subdural hematoma.** More likely in alcoholics after trivial head injury (secondary to stretching of subdural veins by cortical atrophy). Maintain high index of suspicion because the symptoms may be subtle (headache, intellectual deterioration, unexplained drowsiness, or bizarre neurologic picture) and fluctuating. Signs of raised intracranial pressure are rare.

II. **Gastrointestinal complications**

1. **Alcoholic liver disease.** Includes three distinct but often overlapping diseases: (1) **fatty liver**, which is mostly reversible with abstinence; (2) **alcoholic hepatitis**, which ranges from asymptomatic to florid acute illness with fever, jaundice, abdominal pain, and death; and (c) **cirrhosis**. Indicators of **poor prognosis** include persistent jaundice, decreased albumin, prolonged prothrombin time, and anemia.
2. **Alcoholic gastritis and esophagitis**
3. **Alcoholic pancreatitis.** Pancreatic pain is often worse when the patient is recumbent and relieved when sitting up. Pancreatitis may be complicated by shock and acute tubular necrosis. Diagnosis is clinical with the following features: increased serum amylase and lipase, with or without pancreatic calcification on abdominal film, elevated left hemidiaphragm, pleural effusion, ascites (increased amylase), and hypocalcemia. Treat pain with meperidine, 100 mg IV every 3–4 hr as needed; replace fluid and electrolytes; avoid oral ingestion; and use nasogastric suction.

III. **Hematologic complications**

1. **Anemias.** Often multifactorial, including iron and folate deficiencies. Ethanol may cause macrocytosis.
2. **Toxic thrombocytopenia.** Reversible with abstinence.
3. **Leukocytosis.** May be due to alcoholic hepatitis, infection, or alcohol itself.

IV. **Endocrine and metabolic complications**

1. **Alcoholic hypoglycemia and ketosis.** The characteristics of alcoholic ketoacidosis include female predominance, history of alcohol consumption plus starvation with or without vomiting, anion gap acidosis (mainly due to β-hydroxybutyrate), normoglycemia, or mild hypoglycemia. The combination of starvation (depletes glycogen stores) plus alcohol (inhibits gluconeogenesis) results in hypoglycemia. Hypoglycemia decreases insulin secretion, which results in increased mobilization of free fatty acids (glucagon effect). The free fatty acids are incompletely metabolized to ketoacids in the liver. Treatment is with IV fluids containing glucose, repletion of electrolytes and magnesium; treat intercurrent illness, and feed the patient.
2. **Pseudo-Cushing syndrome.** Transient Cushingnoid features in alcoholics are due to stimulation of the pituitary-adrenal axis by ethanol.
3. **Hyperuricemia**
4. **Hypogonadism**

V. **Cardiorespiratory complications**

1. **Alcoholic cardiomyopathy.** Congestive heart failure and atrial tachyarrhythmias.
2. **Hypertension.** Often present in withdrawal period.
3. **Obstructive sleep apnea.** Aggravated by alcohol.

VI. **Infections**

1. **Pneumonias.** *Streptococcus pneumoniae* is most common, but *Klebsiella* sp. (upper lobe) and anaerobic infections are more common in this group. Consider pneumovax for all alcoholics.
2. **Spontaneous bacterial peritonitis** (see section in Infectious Diseases).

Digitalis Toxicity

I. Digoxin (the most common formulation) is excreted two-thirds by the kidney and one-third by the liver.

II. For any given level, risk of toxicity is increased by hypokalemia, hypomagnesemia, hypothyroidism, hypercalcemia, increased age, renal insufficiency, hypoxemia, ischemia, and amyloid.

III. Drugs that increase digoxin concentration: quinidine, amiodarone, verapamil, propafenone, and spironolactone. Some patients may be digitalis-toxic with normal levels.

IV. **Manifestations:**
   1. **Gastrointestinal:** anorexia, nausea, vomiting, diarrhea
   2. **Central nervous system:** fatigue, headache, agitation, delirium, lethargy, seizures
   3. **Visual:** Scotoma, color perception changes, halos
   4. **Hyperkalemia** (Note that hypokalemia may increase digitalis-induced arrhythmia, but overdose of digitalis may cause hyperkalemia.)

V. **Arrhythmias.** Many of the arrhythmias associated with digoxin toxicity may be predicted by its ability to increase the refractory period in the atrioventricular (AV) node (causing conduction blocks) and automaticity in the Purkinje fibers (causing ventricular tachyarrhythmias). Other arrhythmias include atrial premature contractions, paroxysmal atrial tachycardia with block, junctional tachycardia, premature ventricular contractions, ventricular tachycardia, sinoatrial block, AV block (type 1, second degree), and atrial fibrillation with regular ventricular response.

VI. **Treatment for life-threatening arrhythmias** (heart block, ventricular tachycardia, bradyarrhythmias) or hyperkalemia
   1. **Digoxin-specific antibody** is the treatment of choice. Clinical improvement begins within 30–60 min of administration. Each vial is reconstituted in 4 ml sterile water. Give dose over 30 min.
      a. **Acute ingestion:** No. vials = (mg of digoxin ingested) (0.8) / 0.6
      b. **Chronic ingestion:** No. vials = (Digoxin level in ng/ml) (wt in kg) / 100
      c. **Unknown acute ingestion:** 20 vials (12 mg)
      d. Digoxin toxicity may recur after 24 hr of treatment and require repeat dosing. Also, repeat dose if toxicity has not been reversed after several hours.
      e. Monitor potassium; hypokalemia usually develops during therapy.
   2. **Lidocaine**, 75 mg IV over 1 min, then 50 mg IV every 5 min for 3 doses as needed (if ventricular arrhythmia persists) to a total dose of 225 mg. Also begin IV infusion at 1–4 mg/min (start at 2 mg/min). Reduce loading and maintenance doses by 50% in patients with congestive heart failure, hepatic dysfunction, and age > 70 yr.
   3. **Phenytoin**, 100 mg every 5 min at rate not exceeding 50 mg/min, as needed, until atrial or ventricular tachyarrhythmia is abolished or a total of 1 gm is given.
   4. **Avoid** sympathomimetics (e.g., bretylium or isoproterenol) because they may worsen ventricular arrhythmias by increasing norepinephrine levels.

Key Reference: Freed M, Grines C: Essentials of Cardiovascular Medicine. Birmingham, MI, Physicians' Press, 1994, pp 73–74.

Calcium Channel Blocker Toxicity

I. **Calcium blocker formulations**

Drug	Unique features
Nifedipine (Procardia, Adalat)	Potent vasodilator and thus may cause substantial hypotension; may but less likely to cause ↑ [digoxin] than diltiazem
Diltiazem (Cardizem)	May increase digoxin, β-blocker, and cyclosporine concentrations; diltiazem levels may be increased by H_2 blockers
Verapamil (Verelan, Calan)	More likely to cause myocardial depression and conduction blocks than nifedipine or diltiazem. May also increase digoxin levels.
Amlodipine (Norvasc)	Similar to nifedipine

II. **Clinical features** include profound hypotension, conduction abnormalities (mainly seen with verapamil and diltiazem), bradyarrhythmias, decreased level of consciousness, lactic acidosis, hyperglycemia, and hypokalemia. Most cardiac effects occur within 6 hr of ingestion, unless a sustained-release preparation has been ingested, in which case toxicity may not be evident for 12 hr or more. Many of the effects are due to blockade of L-type calcium channels in myocardial cells, smooth-muscle cells, and beta cells.

III. **Treatment**

1. **Establish airway, gastric lavage, activated charcoal.**
2. **Consider prophylactic pacemaker.**
3. **$CaCl_2$**, 1 ampule (272 mg Ca/10 ml ampule) over 10–15 min (contraindicated in patients with hypertrophic cardiomyopathy).
4. **Atropine**, 0.5 mg IV every 5 min until desired rate is achieved.
5. **Sympathomimetics** such as dopamine, dobutamine, or norepinephrine.
6. **Glucagon** (increases cardiac output by increasing cAMP), 5–10 mg IV bolus followed by continuous infusion at 0.07 mg/kg/hr.
7. **Hyperinsulinemia-euglycemia therapy** improves inotropy and peripheral vascular resistance and reverses acidosis, possibly by improving carbohydrate uptake by myocytes and smooth-muscle cells. Dose for regular insulin is 0.5 units/kg/hr IV ± glucose infusion to maintain euglycemia.
8. **4-aminopyridine**, neuromuscular blockade reverser not yet available in U.S.

Key References: Doyon S, et al: The use of glucagon in a case of calcium channel blocker overdose. Ann Emerg Med 22:1229–1233, 1993; Yuan TH, et al: Insulin-glucose as adjunctive therapy for severe calcium channel antagonist poisoning. J Toxicol Clin Toxicol 37:463–474, 1999.

Acetaminophen Hepatotoxicity

I. A single dose of 10–15 gm (e.g., twenty 500-mg tablets) can produce liver injury; classically, fulminant hepatic failure (FHF) is associated with ≥ 25 gm ingestion.

II. Ingestion even of therapeutic doses (as low as 2.5 gm/day) of acetaminophen (AAP) with **acute or chronic alcohol** (or possibly phenobarbital) ingestion increases the risk of hepatotoxicity.

III. **Distinguishing AAP hepatotoxicity in chronic alcoholics from hepatotoxicity in suicide ingestion**

	Alcoholic/AAP toxicity	AAP toxicity (suicide)	Alcoholic hepatitis
AST	↑↑↑	Normal, then ↑↑↑	Usually < 300
ALT	↑↑	Normal, then ↑↑↑	Normal to slight ↑
AST/ALT	> 2	< 2	> 2
Prothrombin time	↑↑↑	Normal, then ↑↑↑	↑ (usually < 20)
AAP level	Normal to ↑	↑↑	None

AST = aspartate aminotransferase, ALT = alanine aminotransferase.

IV. **Mechanism of hepatotoxicity**

1. AAP is normally detoxified by conjugation to glutathione.
2. With overdose, the glutathione stores are depleted.
3. The excess AAP is then metabolized by P-450 mixed function oxidase system (MFOS) to N-acetylimidoquinone (toxic).
4. Alcohol and fasting deplete glutathione levels, and alcohol increases MFOS activity.

V. **Clinical course**
1. First few hours after overdose: nausea, vomiting, with or without obtundation, right upper quadrant pain, or diarrhea.
2. Symptoms disappear 24 hr after ingestion and patient appears well.
3. 24–72 hr after ingestion: onset of liver failure with or without acute tubular necrosis or cardiotoxicity with increased prothrombin time, bilirubin, and transaminases.
4. **Poor prognostic signs:** coagulopathy, acidosis, increased creatinine, hypophosphatemia (due to renal loss), encephalopathy.
5. Elevated bilirubin levels actually correlate with increased survival; i.e., those with highest bilirubin levels survive early complications (cerebral edema, hypotension) of fulminant hepatic failure (FHF).

VI. **Treatment**
1. Caveats to treatment
   a. Give 50 gm of activated charcoal to adult patients if < 1 hr since overdose.
   b. If AAP levels are not available, give NAC if > 150 mg/kg (≈ 10 gm) ingested.
   c. If > 24 hr after overdose, give a course of NAC if > 150 mg/kg ingested, patient is symptomatic, or has abnormal liver function tests.
2. **N-acetylcysteine (NAC, Mucomyst):** most effective when given ≤ 12–20 hr after ingestion
   a. 140 mg/kg PO, then 70 mg/kg PO every 4 hr for 17 doses *or*
   b. 150 mg/kg in 200 ml D5W over 15 min, then 50 mg/kg in 500 ml D5W over 4 hr, then 100 mg/kg in 1 liter D5W over 16 hr (increased risk of anaphylaxis with IV therapy).
   c. NAC also has positive inotropic and potent vasodilator properties. The increased $\dot{D}O_2$ (due to increased cardiac index) and $\dot{V}O_2$ (resulting in an increased O_2 extraction ratio [O_2ER]) in response to NAC may account for some of its beneficial effect on survival in patients with FHF due to AAP.

VII. The nomogram serves as a guide to therapy but should not be used to exclude therapy with NAC. The typical nomogram treatment line is also known as the 150 line (it joins 150 mg/L at 4 hr with 4 mg/L at 24 hr. It has been suggested that in alcoholics, a 100 line cut-off be used (joining 100 mg/L at 4 hr and 15 mg/L at 15 hr).

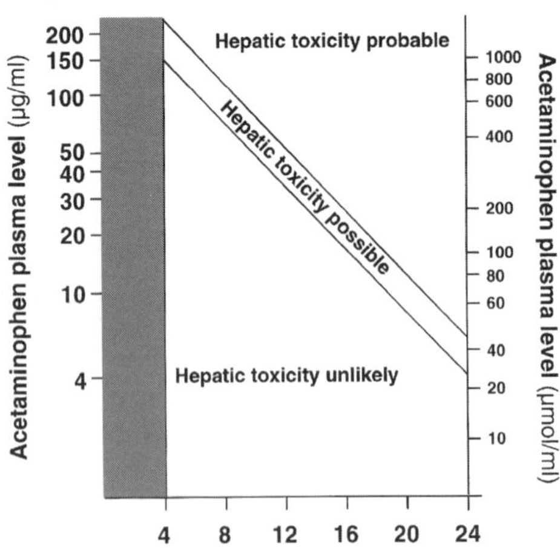

Adapted from Rumack BH, Matthew H: Acetaminophen poisoning and toxicity. Pediatrics 55:871, 1975.

Key References: Kumar S, Rex DK: Failure of physicians to recognize acetaminophen hepatotoxicity in chronic alcoholics. Arch Intern Med 151:1189–1191, 1991; Smilkstein

MJ, Knapp GL, Kulig KW, Rumack BH: Efficacy of oral N-acetylcysteine in the treatment of acetaminophen overdose. N Engl J Med 319:1557–1562, 1988; Vale JA, Proudfoot AT: Paracetamol (acetaminophen) poisoning. Lancet 346: 547–552, 1995.

Salicylate Overdose

I. Classically, intoxication is divided into **acute** (younger patients as a suicide gesture, mortality rate ≈ 1–2%) and **chronic** (older patients, mortality rate ≈ 25% due to low index of suspicion and delay in treatment).

II. Therapeutic levels: 15–30 mg/dl (1.1–2.2 mmol/L)
Toxic levels: > 30 mg/dl (> 2.2 mmol/L)

III. **Primary pathophysiologic effects of salicylates**
1. Direct stimulation of medullary respiratory center
2. Uncoupling of oxidative phosphorylation
3. Inhibition of Kreb cycle enzymes
4. Interference with hemostatic mechanisms
5. Stimulation of gluconeogenesis, glycolysis, and lipid metabolism

IV. **Clinical signs and symptoms: tinnitus, vertigo, hearing loss, nausea, vomiting, disorientation, lethargy, seizures, coma, hyperglycemia** (interference with carbohydrate metabolism) followed by **hypoglycemia** (due to depletion), **fever** (heat production from inefficient/uncoupling of oxidative phosphorylation), **respiratory alkalosis** (medullary respiratory center stimulation), **metabolic acidosis** (lactic acid and ketoacid production from inhibition of Kreb cycle enzymes with activation of glycolysis and lipid metabolism), **noncardiogenic pulmonary edema** (? due to capillary leak syndrome), **hepatocellular necrosis**, and **cerebral edema**. May also see **paradoxical aciduria** (i.e., aciduria due to ketoacids, lactic acid, amino acids, and other organic acids despite alkalemia from predominant respiratory alkalosis). Progressive dehydration → **prerenal azotemia** and **acute tubular necrosis**. **Hematologic problems** include increased prothrombin time, decreased platelet adhesiveness, thrombocytopenia, and increased capillary fragility.

V. **Treatment**
1. **Gastric lavage**
2. **Activated charcoal**, 50–100 gm diluted in water
3. **Hydration, correction of electrolytes.** Hypokalemia must be treated aggressively to succeed in urinary alkalinization (hypokalemia prevents preferential tubular excretion of H^+).
4. **Alkalinization of urine.** Consider if [salicylate] > 35 mg/dl (> 2.53 mmol/L); corrects metabolic acidosis, promotes excretion, and decreases passage of salicylate into tissues by forming ion forms. Maintain UpH ~ 8–8.5 by adding sodium bicarbonate, 50–100 mEq to 1 liter of 0.45% saline at 250–500 ml/hr.
5. **Mechanical ventilation as needed.** May be required for cerebral edema or airway protection.
6. **Hemodialysis.** Specific indications: levels > 100 mg/dl (> 7.24 mmol/L) in acute ingestion and > 70 mg/dl (> 5 mmol/L) in chronic toxicity, rising levels, and CNS or pulmonary abnormalities.

VI. **The Done nomogram for acute salicylate overdose** is most useful for acute salicylate intoxication. It is not accurate for chronic salicylate intoxication or acute intoxication with enteric preparations.

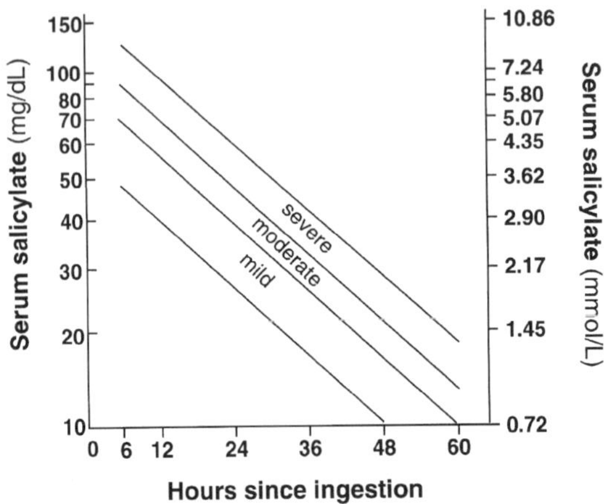

Adapted from Done AK: Salicylate intoxication: Significance of salicylate in blood in cases of acute ingestion. Pediatrics 26:800–807, 1960.

Key Reference: Proudfoot AT: Toxicity of salicylates. Am J Med 75:99–103, 1983.

Tricyclic Antidepressant Overdoses

I. **General issues**
   1. Peak serum concentration of tricyclic antidepressants (TCAs) may be delayed because of delayed gastric emptying due to anticholinergic effects of the drug.
   2. Hypoalbuminemia and acidemia increase free-drug concentration.
   3. TCAs have potent anticholinergic (antimuscarinic) and antihistaminic effects.
   4. **Diagnosis is clinical.** No correlation between TCA concentration and symptoms of serious poisoning. Patients may display an **anticholinergic syndrome** (see Common Toxic Syndromes).

II. **Cardiac toxicity** (major cause of mortality): **sinus tachycardia**; terminal Rw in lead AVR and Sw in leads I and AVL on EKG; prolonged QTc interval and **widened QRS** (≥ 0.10 sec; some studies suggest increased QRS or QTc > 0.5 sec correlates with seizures and ventricular arrhythmias); **ventricular ectopy**; idioventricular rhythm (poor sign), first-degree atrioventricular block, bundle-branch block, complete heart block, supraventricular tachycardia, **hypotension** (due to myocardial depression from inhibition of fast sodium channels, vasodilatation from α-blockade, and depletion of norepinephrine (NE) from continued inhibition of NE reuptake), **bradycardia** (late).

III. **Central nervous system:** anticholinergic excitation (confusion, hallucination, ataxia), seizures (common, brief, usually in the first 6–8 hr after presentation), stupor, coma. Initial level of consciousness is good predictor of serious toxicity.

IV. **Respiratory toxicity:** depression, adult respiratory distress syndrome (risk increases with hypotension).

V. **Treatment**
   1. **Gastric evacuation.** Lavage with a 36–40 Fr orogastric tube.
   2. **Endotracheal intubation.** May be necessary before lavage.
   3. **Activated charcoal**, 1 gm/kg with 60 ml sorbitol, oral or per NG, then 0.5–1 gm/kg every 4–8 hr if bowel is functional.

4. **$NaHCO_3$.** Sodium, rather than pH, may be the crucial factor in reversing the cardiotoxicity by counteracting the inhibition of fast sodium channels. 1–2 mEq/kg IV bolus, then 150 mEq in 850 ml D_5W to maintain pH of 7.45–7.50. Clear indications include **marked acidosis, refractory hypotension, prolonged cardiac conduction (QRS ≥ 0.16), ventricular arrhythmia, and cardiac arrest.**
5. **Lidocaine** for ventricular arrhythmia. Procainamide, disopyramide, and quinidine are **contraindicated**.
6. **For refractory hypotension:** norepinephrine (NE) and phenylephrine have theoretical advantages over dopamine. TCAs are known to deplete NE stores, which are released by dopamine.
7. **Caveats for cardiac arrests:** (1) Use HCO_3 early; (2) do not use type 1A or 1C antiarrhythmic agents; and (3) prolonged resuscitation (at least 1 hr) should be attempted, because good outcome may still result.
8. **Symptomatic bradycardia.** Isoproterenol or pacemaker; do not use atropine, which may increase anticholinergic effects.

Key References: Krenzelok EP, Leikin JB: Approach to the poisoned patient. Dis Month 42:509–608, 1996; Pimentel L, Trommer L: Cyclic antidepressant overdoses: A review. Emerg Clin North Am 12:533, 1994.

Monoamine Oxidase Inhibitor Overdose

I. Monoamine oxidase inhibitors (MAOIs) are antidepressants that irreversibly bind the MAO enzyme, thus preventing degradation of catecholamines and resulting in an increased level of serotonin, norepinephrine, epinephrine, and dopamine in the central nervous system.

II. Many **food and drug interactions** with MAOIs are likely to produce a hypertensive or a hyperthermic crisis. Implicated foods typically contain high tyramine, such as cheese and red wines. Other foods include fava beans, liver, and tofu. Implicated drugs include **meperidine (Demerol)**, tricyclic antidepressants, dextromethorphan, L-tryptophan, amphetamines, and disulfiram.

III. **Clinical manifestations** of MAOI overdose vary during the course of presentation:

1. **Phase 1:** asymptomatic or latent period; typically lasts 6–12 hr after ingestion.
2. **Phase 2: neuromuscular excitation** with irritability, hyperreflexia, restlessness, facial grimacing, trismus, myoclonus, and muscle fasciculations; **sympathetic hyperactivity** with moderate increase in blood pressure and hyperpyrexia, with initial warm dry skin progressing to profuse diaphoresis and flushing.
3. **Phase 3: CNS depression** with confusion, hallucination progressing to coma, muscle rigidity, decerebrate posturing, opisthotonos, and seizures; **cardiovascular collapse** with hypotension and cold, clammy skin.
4. **Phase 4: secondary complications**, including acute renal failure, rhabdomyolysis, coagulopathy, hemolysis, pulmonary edema, and cardiac arrest due to ventricular tachyarrhythmias.

IV. **Treatment** is generally supportive and symptomatic because there is no specific antidote. Dialysis and hemoperfusion are of no proven benefit. Patients should be monitored for at least 24 hr after ingestion for delayed toxicities.

1. **Gastric emptying, lavage, activated charcoal.**
2. **Muscular rigidity:** sedation with benzodiazepines; neuromuscular-blocking agents may be required if the neuromuscular excitability is severe enough to cause respiratory and metabolic acidosis and rhabdomyolysis.

3. **Hyperthermia:** acetaminophen; external cooling; dantrolene, 2.5 mg/kg IV every 6 hr.
4. **Hypertension:** nitroprusside or phentolamine IV.
5. **Hypotension:** norepinephrine; avoid dopamine if possible because it may cause the release of excess norepinephrine stores, resulting in severe hypertension.

Key Reference: Linden CH, et al: Monoamine oxidase inhibitor overdose. Ann Emerg Med 13:1137–1444, 1984.

Arsenic Poisoning

I. **Pearl:** consider in anyone with severe gastrointestinal symptoms and/or shock.

II. **Source: insecticides**, herbicides, fungicides, rodenticides, wood preservatives, compounds in dye/ceramic/glass manufacturing. Although seafoods contain arsenic, it is in an organic and **nontoxic** variant.

III. **Metabolism:** absorbed through the skin, lungs, and GI tract. 90–95% is excreted through the urine: may be detected for 7–21 days after an overdose.

IV. **Mechanism of toxicity**

1. Arsenic binds to dihydrolipoic acid, a cofactor of pyruvate dehydrogenase, inhibiting the first step in gluconeogenesis and the Kreb cycle.
2. Arsenic also competes with phosphate binding to ADP.
3. Arsenic binds to tissue protein -SH groups, causing denaturation (especially kidneys → ATN)

V. **Clinical toxicity** (lethal dose for adult: 130–300 mg)

1. **GI tract** (symptoms due to vasculitis): dysphagia, garlic breath odor, metallic taste in mouth, nausea, vomiting, profuse/watery diarrhea, colicky abdominal pain.
2. **Cardiorespiratory:** respiratory failure due to respiratory muscle weakness, ARDS, hypotension (due to capillary leak and dehydration), arrhythmia (usually ventricular).
3. **Central nervous system:** delirium, coma, seizures, Guillain-Barré-like syndrome.
4. **Peripheral neuropathy**
5. **Kidneys:** acute tubular necrosis
6. **Heme:** hemolytic anemia, pancytopenia
7. **Chronic toxicity:** hyperpigmentation, hyperkeratosis, Mees lines, polyneuritis, bronchitis, tracheitis, laryngitis.

VI. **Laboratory:** although arsenic is radioopaque and may be detected in nails/hair, **the only reliable test is a 24-hr urinary collection for arsenic.** Arsenic is detectable in blood only during the first 2–4 hr after ingestion. **Normal U_{As} is < 20 μg/day (< 267 mmol/day);** be suspicious with levels > 100 μg/day. Unfortunately in patients who have eaten seafood within the past 1–2 days, U_{As} may be as high as 50–2000 μg/day (or 668–26,700 mmol/day): fractionation of arsenic into the inorganic (toxic) and organic (nontoxic) forms can be performed by a cation-exchange cartridge and absorption spectrophotometry.

VII. **Treatment**

1. Acute ingestion: ipecac (alert) or gastric lavage (obtunded).
2. Correct dehydration and electrolyte disorder.
3. Urinary alkalinization (pH ≈ 7.5) to prevent tubular deposition of RBC products.
4. **Dimercaprol**, 3–5 mg/kg IM every 6 hr for 24 hr, then every 12–24 hr for 10 days *or*
5. Penicillamine, 25 mg/kg 4 times/day (up to 1 gm/day) for 5 days *or*
6. Hemodialysis (particularly useful with renal failure).

Key Reference: Moyer TP: Testing for arsenic. Mayo Clin Proc 68:1210–1211, 1993.

Cyanide Poisoning

I. **Pearl:** consider cyanide (CN) poisoning in anyone with unexplained cardiovascular collapse and coma.
II. **Sources: rodenticide**, chemicals used in photography, metallurgy, electroplating, metal and jewelry polishing, and ore refining; **fruit seeds:** apple, plum, apricot (**Laetrile**); **smoke inhalation**, because cyanide is a common byproduct during combustion of many synthetic materials (elevated [lactate] may be a clue to cyanide toxicity).
III. **Inhibits cytochrome oxidase** and oxidative phosphorylation, resulting in lactic acidosis.
IV. Cyanide is rapidly absorbed from the stomach, lungs, mucosal surfaces, and skin.
V. **Clinical signs:** headache, faintness, vertigo, anxiety, burning sensation in mouth and throat, dyspnea, tachycardia, hypertension, nausea, vomiting, diaphoresis, bitter almond breath, erosion of gastric mucosa. **Late effects:** coma, convulsions, opisthotonos, trismus, paralysis, respiratory depression, pulmonary edema, arrhythmia, bradycardia, and hypotension.
VI. **Associated laboratory findings: lactic acidosis and high $S\bar{v}O_2$** (low AVO_2 difference).
VII. **Diagnosis:** correlation between blood CN levels and symptoms is imperfect: 20–40 μmol/L (flushing, tachycardia), 40–100 μmol/L (obtundation), and 100–200 μmol/L (coma, respiratory depression)
VIII. **Treatment (Lilly cyanide antidote kit):** nitrite is used to induce methemoglobinemia (which has a high affinity for CN); thiosulfate removes CN from metHb to form thiocyanate (renally excreted).
   1. **Gastrointestinal decontamination and oxygen** (competes with CN)
   2. **Amyl nitrite** (inhale 30 sec of each minute while preparing sodium nitrite)
   3. **Sodium nitrite (3%)**, 10 ml (300 mg) over 4 min while monitoring blood pressure to produce ≈ 25% metHb. **Sodium nitrite is a potent vasodilator and thus may cause severe hypotension**; if severe hypotension already exists, use thiosulfate alone, although it is less effective.
   4. **Sodium thiosulfate (25%)**, 50 ml (12.5 gm) over 10–12 min
   5. Hydroxocobalamin (B_{12}) has been used (combines with CN to yield cyanocobalamin, which is excreted in urine).

Key References: Baud FJ, Barriot P, Toffis V, et al: Elevated blood cyanide concentrations in victims of smoke inhalation. N Engl J Med 325:1761–1769, 1991; Hall AH, Rumack BH: Clinical toxicity of cyanide. Ann Emerg Med 15:1067–1074, 1986.

Iron Poisoning

I. Iron is a much more common toxin in children than in adults; however, because it is readily available, suicide attempts with iron medications are not uncommon in adults. Toxicity stems from effects on gastrointestinal mucosa; delayed effects on Krebs cycle enzymes, which cause lactic acidosis; and generation of free radicals causing cellular damage. Free iron is toxic to vasculature and mitochondria and causes release of vasoactive substances such as histamine.
II. **Toxic dose:** 60 mg/kg of elemental iron. Total body stores 4–5 gm (60% in Hb, 25% of stores in liver as ferritin and hemosiderin). Absorption converts ferrous to ferric form.

III. **Five clinical stages of iron poisoning:**
   1. **½–6 hr after ingestion:** GI symptoms due to corrosive effect of iron: nausea, vomiting, pain, bleeding, lethargy, hypotension (due to vasodilatation), metabolic acidosis, leukocytosis, or hyperglycemia.
   2. **6–24 hr:** latent period with symptom quiescence.
   3. **6–48 hr:** metabolic and systemic derangement develops with cardiovascular collapse, coma, seizures, coagulopathy, and congestive heart failure.
   4. **2–7 days:** hepatotoxicity, coagulopathy, metabolic acidosis, renal failure.
   5. **1–8 wk:** primary delayed GI tract complications with fibrosis, obstruction.

IV. **Diagnosis: toxic serum iron levels** that require chelation: > 350 µg/dl (> 62.7 µmol/L) in patients with symptoms, > 500 µg/dl (> 89.6 µmol/L) in patients without symptoms.

V. **Treatment.** Hemodialysis is **not** helpful, and activated charcoal does **not** bind iron.
   1. **Gastric lavage** with $NaHCO_3$, which converts iron into less absorbable ferric form.
   2. **Abdominal flat plate** and, if iron visible, whole bowel irrigation with GoLytely at 2 L/hr.
   3. **Hydration** because of third space losses in abdomen; dopamine or norepinephrine if no response to fluid.
   4. **Monitor serum iron levels** and clearing of *vin rosé* color in urine.
   5. Sodium bicarbonate for severe acidosis.
   6. **Deferoxamine mesylate** (specific iron chelator) for any serum iron level > 500 µg/dl (> 89.6 µmol/L). After iron is bound, it is excreted in kidney, giving urine a wine-rose coloration. **Therapeutic dose**, 1 gm IM or IV at a rate not to exceed 10–15 mg/kg/hr, then 500 mg every 4 hr for 2 doses, then 500 mg every 4–12 hr as needed (no more than 6 gm in 24 hr).

Key Reference: Krenzelok EP, Leikin JB: Approach to the poisoned patient. Dis Month 42(9): 509–608, 1996.

Lithium Carbonate Overdose

I. Lithium carbonate (Li^+) can substitute for other monovalent cations, such as Na^+. It is rapidly absorbed through the GI tract but forms gastric concretions in large overdoses. It is not protein-bound, but volume of distribution is vast. The halflife is 29 hr, and it is eliminated through the kidney. Approximately 80% of Li^+ is reabsorbed in the proximal tubule; thus, dehydration causes increased Na^+ and Li^+ reabsorption.

II. **Clinical symptoms (therapeutic levels: 0.6–1.2 mmol/L; levels > 1.5 mmol/L are generally considered toxic).**
   1. **Mild** acute intoxication (serum levels < 2.5 mmol/L): tremor, ataxia, nystagmus, choreoathetosis, photophobia, or lethargy.
   2. **Moderate** acute intoxication (serum levels ≤ 3.5 mmol/L): agitation, fascicular twitching, confusion, nausea, vomiting, anorexia, and diarrhea.
   3. **Severe** acute intoxication (serum level > 3.5 mmol/L): hypotension, hypovolemia from a diabetes insipidus, cardiac dysrhythmias, seizures, coma, adult respiratory distress syndrome, acute renal failure. In chronic Li^+ poisoning there is no correlation between drug levels and clinical presentation.

III. **Laboratory tests:** Serum Li^+ level is important to direct management. A low anion gap with increased bicarbonate may be a clue to severe Li^+ toxicity. Increased serum [Na^+] with increased urine output is seen with nephrogenic diabetes insipidus.

IV. **Treatment.** Charcoal does **not** bind Li^+.
   1. **Gastric lavage** (concretions with sustained-release forms)
   2. **Fluid hydration** with normal saline is the mainstay of therapy.
   3. **Kayexalate** (sodium polystyrene sulfonate) binds lithium.
   4. **Whole bowel irrigation** with polyethylene glycol (2 L/hr for 5 hr) is useful to eliminate sustained-release preparations.
   5. **Hemodialysis** for Li^+ levels > 3.5 mmol/L in acute ingestion and > 2.5 mmol/L for chronic ingestion with symptoms of decreased consciousness, seizures, cardiovascular symptoms, or renal failure. There is a rebound effect after hemodialysis due to the redistribution of Li^+ from tissues into plasma. Protracted and repeated hemodialysis may be necessary to reach a goal Li^+ level of 1 mmol/L 8 hours after dialysis. It may be more effective to use bicarbonate (35 mmol/L) dialysis bath than acetate.
   6. **Monitor serum Li^+** levels for evidence of a decrease.

Key References: Krenzelok EP, Leikin JB: Approach to the poisoned patient. Dis Month 42:509–608, 1996; Simard M, Gumbiner B, Lee A, et al: Lithium carbonate intoxication: A case report and review of the literature. Arch Intern Med 149:36–46, 1989.

Serum Osmolality

I. Principal use in the ICU is to screen for the presence of foreign low-molecular-weight substances in the blood.

II. **Osmolality** is a measure of the total number of particles in the solution. For nonpolar solutes, 1 mol = 1 Osm. For salts that dissociate into 2 ions (NaCl), 1 mol = 2 Osm.

III. **Calculated osmolality = 2 × sodium + (glucose/18) + blood urea nitrogen/2.8 + [ethanol]/4.5** (normal 286 ± 4 mOsm/kg water).

IV. If (measured – calculated) osmolality > 10 mOsm/kg water (osmolar gap), one of the following diagnoses should be considered:
   1. **Decreased serum water content** (hyperlipidemia, hyperproteinemia) → pseudohyponatremia. **Calculated osmolality is low, but measured osmolality is normal.**
   2. **Additional low–molecular-weight substances in serum. Calculated osmolality is normal, but measured osmolality is high.**
      a. With elevated anion gap: suspect methanol, ethylene glycol, propylene glycol, or ethanol (EtOH), but increased osmolar gap may be associated with alcoholic lactic acidosis, diabetic (DKA) or alcoholic (AKA) ketoacidosis, chronic renal failure (no dialysis), shock (with lactic acidosis). **Note: DKA, AKA, and lactic acidosis may have an elevated osmolar gap.**
      b. With normal anion gap: ethanol, acetone, isopropanol, ethyl ether, trichloroethane, methanol or ethylene glycol with ethanol (EtOH prevents methanol and ethylene glycol metabolism), infusion of mannitol, bladder irrigation with glycine solution.

V. Acetoacetic acid, β-hydroxybutyric acid, and lactic acid are the principal acids involved in DKA, AKA, and lactic acidosis. Because these acids have a low pKa, they are dissociated at physiologic pH. Serum HCO_3 decreases, the total concentration of anions and cations remains constant, and there is no effect on serum osmolality.

VI. **Algorithm** for patient with (1) **anion gap metabolic acidosis**, (2) **osmolal gap**, and (3) **suspected toxic alcohol ingestion:**
   1. Begin EtOH at 10 ml/kg of 10% solution in D_5W, then 1.5 ml/kg/hr of 10% solution to maintain [EtOH] ~ 100 mg/dl.

2. Obtain toxicology screen. If positive, continue EtOH drip and consider hemodialysis; if negative, discontinue EtOH drip.
3. If toxicology screen is unavailable, consider EtOH drip/hemodialysis if the osmolal gap > 25 mmol/kg (specificity is ~ 88% using this higher threshold). Increase (~ 2×) EtOH infusion rate during dialysis.

Key References: Gennari FJ: Serum Osmolality. N Engl J Med 310:102–105, 1984; Schelling JR, Howard RL, Winter SD, Linas SL: Increased osmolal gap in AKA and DKA. Ann Intern Med 113:580–582, 1990.

Ethanol Poisoning

I. The level of ethanol does not always correlate with clinical severity. Compared with ethanol-tolerant individuals, significantly lower levels of ethanol may produce the same deleterious effect in ethanol-naive individuals.

II. **Correlation of blood levels and symptoms**

Blood ethanol levels	Manifestation
100–200 mg/dl (21.7–43.4 mmol/L)	Signs of intoxication: slurred speech, incoordination, ataxia, impaired
250–400 mg/dl (54.3–86.8 mmol/L)	Coma, respiratory depression
> 450 mg/dl (> 97.7 mmol/L)	Death; significantly lower levels have been associated with death in children; and in persons who are tolerant to ethanol, the LD 50 may be > 600 mg/dl (130.3 mmol/L).

III. Estimation of **blood EtOH level = osmolar gap χ 4.3.**

IV. **Treatment. Supportive therapy**, including protecting the airway, is the principal treatment. Charcoal is **not** useful. **Electrolyte replacement** (e.g., potassium, magnesium, phosphate) may be required. **Hypoglycemia** may be severe. **Hemodialysis** may be tried in severe cases.

Key Reference: Morgan DL, et al: Severe ethanol intoxication in an adolescent. Am J Emerg Med 13:416–418, 1995.

Ethylene Glycol Poisoning

I. Ethylene glycol (EG) is found in detergents, antifreeze, and polishes. The toxic metabolite, glycolic acid, is responsible for the metabolic acidosis, anion gap, and osmolar gap. Later, renal insufficiency contributes to the acidosis.

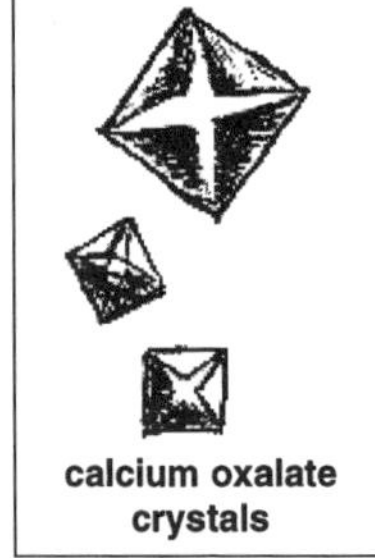
calcium oxalate crystals

II. **Clinical presentation**
1. **Stage 1 (30 min–12 hr)** is predominated by **CNS findings:** intoxication without ethanol odor, slurred speech, ataxia, hallucinations, seizures, tetany, or coma. Mild tachycardia, nausea, and vomiting may be seen.
2. **Stage 2 (12–24 hr)** is characterized by **cardiopulmonary findings** with hypertension, tachycardia, pulmonary edema, with or without myositis.
3. **Stage 3 (24–72 hr): renal findings** with flank pain, calcium oxalate dihydrate (envelope shaped) and monohydrate (needle shaped) crystalluria, with or without oliguria or anuria.

III. **Laboratory findings:** anion gap metabolic acidosis, hypocalcemia (due to calcium precipitation by oxalate and with increased QT interval), elevated osmolal gap, calcium oxalate crystalluria (see figure), proteinuria, hematuria, pyuria, cylinduria, leukocytosis (10–40 K, mainly polymorphonuclear neutrophils), elevated creatine phosphokinase, detection of sodium fluorescein (present in antifreeze) by Wood's lamp in urine, stomach content, or on the skin.

IV. **Treatment:** serum level < 10 mg/dl (< 1.61 mmol/L), supportive care; 20–50 mg/dl (3.22–8.05 mmol/L), IV EtOH; > 50 mg/dl (> 8.05 mmol/L), hemodialysis.

1. **Gastric lavage**
2. **Hemodialysis.** Indications for early dialysis include confirmed intoxications, deteriorating vital signs, refractory metabolic acidosis, crystalluria, and serum EG > 50 mg/dl).
3. **Ethanol.** Affinity for alcohol dehydrogenase (ADH) is 100 times greater than EG. Loading dose, 10 ml/kg of 10% solution in D_5W IV over 30 min–1 hr, then maintenance dose 1.5 ml/kg/hr of 10% solution (to keep level ~ 100 mg/dl (21.7 mmol/L) until [EG] = 0).
4. **Fomepizole (Antizol)**, an alcohol dehydrogenase inhibitor: 15 mg/kg iv infusion over 30 min, followed by 10 mg/kg every 12 hrs for 4 doses, then 15 mg/kg every 12 hrs until EG levels are < 20 mg/dL (< 3.22 mmol/L).
5. **Sodium bicarbonate.** Unlike lactic acidosis, the acids formed by ethylene glycol metabolism (oxalic acid, glycolic acid, and glyoxalic acid) are not metabolized to HCO_3. Therefore, either $NaHCO_3$ needs to be given, or a use of the HCO_3 bath with hemodialysis (HD) is effective.
6. **Fluids**, with or without furosemide or mannitol, to maintain urine output ~ 400–500 ml/hr for the first 24 hr and 150–200 ml/hr for the second 24 hr to prevent calcium oxalate crystal deposition in the kidneys.
7. **Thiamine and pyridoxine** (100 mg/day of each) minimize oxalic acid production.
8. **Correct hypocalcemia.**

Key References: Brent J et al: Fomepizole for the treatment of ethylene glycol poisoning. N Engl J Med 340:832–838, 1999; Gabow PA: Ethylene glycol intoxication. Am J Kidney Dis 11:277–279, 1988.

Propylene Glycol Toxicity

I. An alcohol used as a vehicle in many medications, including IV nitroglycerin, IV etomidate, and sulfadiazine cream.

II. May cause anion gap, osmolar gap metabolic acidosis.

Key Reference: Demey HE, Daelemans RA, Verpooten DA: Propylene glycol induced side effects during intravenous nitroglycerin therapy. Intens Care Med 14:221–226, 1988.

Methanol Poisoning

I. Methanol (MeOH) is found in antifreeze, sterno, cleaners, paints.

II. **Toxicity.** Only 10 cc is necessary for blindness. MeOH is metabolized to formic acid (an optic nerve toxin). Minimal lethal dose is 1–5 gm/kg. Lethal blood level ~ 80 mg/dl (24.9 mmol/L).

$$\text{MeOH} \xrightarrow{\text{ADH}} \text{Formaldehyde} \xrightarrow{\text{ADH}} \text{Formic acid} \xrightarrow{\text{Folate}} CO_2 + H_2$$

III. **Clinical manifestations:** nausea, vomiting, abdominal pain, pancreatitis, blindness (fixed, dilated pupils, retinal edema), intoxication without ethanol odor.

IV. **Laboratory findings:** increased anion gap and osmolar gap metabolic acidosis.

V. **Treatment**

1. **Gastric lavage**
2. **Fomepizole (Antizol)**, an alcohol dehydrogenase inhibitor: 15 mg/kg IV infusion over 30 min, followed by 10 mg/kg every 12 hr for 4 doses, then 15 mg/kg every 12 hr until methanol levels are < 20 mg/dl.
3. **Ethanol.** Loading dose, 0.6 gm/kg or 10 ml/kg of 10% solution in D_5W IV over 30 min–1 hr, then maintenance dose 1.5 ml/kg/hr of 10% solution to keep EtOH level ~ 100 mg/dl (21.7 mmol/L); continue until [MeOH] < 20–25 mg/dl (< 6.24–7.8 mmol/L).
4. **Folate**, 50 mg IV every 4 hr until [MeOH] < 20 mg/dl (< 6.24 mmol/L); enhances formic acid metabolism.
5. **Sodium bicarbonate** infusion to keep pH ≥ 7.3
6. **Hemodialysis.** Indications:
   a. [MeOH] > 50 mg/dl (>15.6 mmol/L) or [formic acid] > 20 mg/dl
   b. Severe metabolic acidosis
   c. Visual impairment
   d. Renal failure

Isopropyl Alcohol Poisoning

I. Isopropanol is found in rubbing alcohol, solvents, and antifreeze.

II. **Toxicity.** Absorption is rapid, as with the other alcohols. The lethal dose is 3–4 gm/kg (~ 250 ml). Isopropyl alcohol is metabolized to acetone. Pulmonary elimination may be significant, especially in mechanically ventilated patients. The half-life is ~ 3 hr.

III. **Clinical presentation**

1. Confusion, headache, nystagmus, miotic pupils, CNS depression with respiratory arrest
2. Nausea, vomiting, abdominal pain, gastritis, pancreatitis
3. Cardiovascular depression and myocardial necrosis, arrhythmia, pulmonary edema
4. Acetone odor on breath

IV. **Laboratory findings:** increased osmolar gap, increased serum ketones and ketouria (acetoneuria). Hypoglycemia may be present. Despite the increased osmolar gap and ketones, there is usually little or no metabolic acidosis and no anion gap.

V. **Treatment**

1. Supportive care
2. Gastric lavage
3. **Hemodialysis** for refractory hypotension (poor prognostic sign), coma, lethal blood levels (> 200 mg/dl [> 33.3 mmol/L], although death has been noted with levels as low as 100–240 mg/dl [16.6–39.9 mmol/L]).

Key Reference: Rich JR, et al: Isopropyl alcohol intoxication. Arch Neurol 47:322–324, 1990.

Toluene Toxicity

I. Toluene is an aromatic hydrocarbon commonly found in paints, paint thinners, lacquers, and glues. It is one of the most heavily abused solvents by inhalation (glue and spray paint sniffing).

II. **Three symptom complexes**
   1. **Severe muscle weakness** of the extremities with sparing of the respiratory and central muscles, normal reflexes, and no sensory deficits. It may present as quadriparesis and be confused with Guillain-Barré syndrome. The weakness appears to be due to severe hypokalemia, hypophosphatemia, and nonanion gap metabolic acidosis due to a Type 1 renal tubular acidosis. Rhabdomyolysis may be due to hypokalemia, hypophosphatemia, and/or a direct toxic effect of toluene.
   2. **Gastrointestinal syndrome** consisting of abdominal pain, nausea, and vomiting. There may be associated rhabdomyolysis and electrolyte disturbances but not as severe as in the above complex.
   3. **Neuropsychiatric syndrome** includes dizziness, headaches, paresthesias, hallucinations, lethargy, cerebellar signs, seizures, or coma.

III. **Electrolyte abnormalities**
   1. **Metabolic acidosis** (normal anion gap more common than elevated anion gap and depends on how much of the hippurate has been excreted in the urine).
   2. **Urinary anion gap** (i.e., measured $U_{cations}$ [sodium, potassium] >> measured U_{anions} [chloride]); in other words, large amounts of unmeasured anion (hippurate) in urine.
   3. **Urinary osmolar gap** (i.e., measured $U_{osmolality}$ >> calculated $U_{osmolality}$, where calculated $U_{osmolality} = 2\ (Na + K) + \text{urea nitrogen}/2.8$.
   4. **Hypokalemia** due to hippurate excretion obligates sodium and potassium excretion.
   5. **Hypocalcemia** may occur with correction of fluids and electrolytes.
   6. **Hypophosphatemia**

IV. **Treatment.** There is no specific antidote for toluene toxicity. Supportive care, fluid and electrolyte replacement (potassium, calcium, phosphorus), and monitoring of respiratory and renal functions are the mainstays of therapy.

Key Reference: Streicher HZ, Gabow PA, Moss AH, et al: Syndromes of toluene sniffing in adults. Ann Intern Med 94:758–762, 1981.

Theophylline Toxicity

I. Occurs in two principal settings:
   1. Chronic intoxication due to increasing dosage or decreased clearance
   2. Acute massive ingestion as a suicide gesture or iatrogenic overdose

II. **Factors that may decrease theophylline clearance:** acute or chronic liver disease, cor pulmonale, congestive heart failure, advanced age, fever, viral infections.

III. **Drugs that may decrease theophylline clearance:** erythromycin, ciprofloxacin, cimetidine, ranitidine, oral contraceptives.

IV. **Clinical manifestations.** Many of the signs and symptoms are due to overstimulation of the β-adrenergic system by high levels of catecholamines.
   1. **Gastrointestinal symptoms** (usually the initial symptoms): nausea, vomiting, and reflux symptoms.
   2. **Central nervous system:** hyperventilation, anxiety, restlessness, tremor (may be generalized and resemble shivering), confusion, and seizures (ominous sign).
   3. **Cardiac:** tachycardia, atrial and/or ventricular tachyarrhythmia, and recalcitrant hypotension (the hypotension is hypothesized to be due to increased cyclic adenosine monophosphate from the synergistic effect of β-adrenergic hyperactivation + phosphodiesterase inhibition, which causes vascular smooth muscle relaxation).

V. **Laboratory findings**
   1. Severe **hypokalemia**
   2. Hypomagnesemia, hypophosphatemia
   3. Metabolic acidosis (probably lactate)
   4. Mild elevation of creatine phosphokinase, leukocytosis, hyperglycemia (usually well tolerated and self-limiting; if insulin is given, be certain that potassium level is not low, because insulin will further lower plasma potassium).

VI. **Treatment**
   1. Supportive therapy
   2. Gastric lavage and / or whole bowel irrigation as most theophylline preparations are sustained-release.
   3. **Activated charcoal, 30–50 gm orally or per NG every 2–3 hr with cathartic** (e.g., magnesium citrate or sorbitol), even in patients with IV overdose, because theophylline undergoes an enterohepatic circulation.
   4. **Resin hemoperfusion.** Consider in anyone with [theophylline] > 60 μg/ml (> 333 μmol/L), especially if the level is rising, because once seizure occurs, the prognosis is dismal regardless of subsequent therapy. Consider hemoperfusion if [theophylline] > 30 μg/ml (> 166.5 μmol/L) or if the patient is > 60 years old, has significant liver disease or congestive heart failure, or has ingested long-acting theophylline.
   5. **β-blockers. IV propranolol** is the most effective treatment for theophylline-induced refractory hypotension. Bronchospasm is certainly a concern in the subset of patients taking theophylline, but small IV doses appear not to have significant adverse effects, even in asthmatics. Risk-benefit ratio may warrant its use. **Dosage of propranol:** 1–3 mg IV; repeat in 2 min, then every 4–6 hr as needed. Typical oral dosage is 20–80 mg every 6 hr.

Key Reference: Biberstein MP, Ziegler MG, Ward DM: Use of β-blockade and hemoperfusion for acute theophylline poisoning. West J Med 141:485–490, 1984.

Treatment of Nerve Agent Poisoning

I. At ambient temperatures, the nerve agents likely to be used in chemical warfare or terrorist attacks **are liquids**, not gases. They are absorbed through the skin and include GA (tabun), GB (sarin), GD (soman), GF, and VX.

II. **Mechanism of action.** Nerve agents are organophosphorous compounds, similar to but much more potent than organophosphate insecticides. They **irreversibly inhibit cholinesterase**, leading to the accumulation of acetylcholine. Thus they cause toxicity by an excessive cholinergic mechanism.

III. **Clinical manifestations** include both muscarinic (increased secretions from the nose, eyes, mouth, airways, intestines) and nicotinic effects (muscle fasciculations, twitching, weakness, paralysis). Either tachycardia (nicotinic) or bradycardia (muscarinic) may be seen.
   1. **Liquid exposure:** local sweating on skin with fasciculations followed by nausea, vomiting, cramps (may be delayed). Sudden unconsciousness, convulsions, paralysis, and apnea may occur after a slight delay.
   2. **Vapor exposure:** miosis, rhinorrhea, ocular pain, conjunctivitis, dim or blurred vision, bronchoconstriction and bronchorrhea, followed by paralysis and apnea.

IV. **Treatment**
   1. Decontaminate skin with diluted household bleach (1:10) or soap and water.

2. **Atropine**, 2 mg IM for mild dyspnea, 6 mg IV or IM for severe dyspnea or multisystem signs; repeat every 5 min till secretions are minimal (miosis may persist; therefore, its resolution should not be used as a guide to therapy). Dose of Atropen Auto-Injector (with glycerin and phenol): 2 mg/0.7 ml.
3. **Pralidoxime (2-PAM)** acts primarily at nicotinic sites to normalize skeletal muscle activity. Pralidoxime reactivates (by dephosphorylation) acetylcholinesterase that had been phosphorylated by organophosphates. It should be used in conjunction with atropine. **Dose:** 1 gm IV over 20–30 min repeated at hourly interval for 1–2 additional doses. Autoinjector: 600 mg IM.
4. **Pretreatment with pyridostigmine bromide (Mestinon)**, a reversible cholinesterase inhibitor that blocks irreversible activation by the nerve agent. **Dose:** 30 mg orally every 8 hr (takes 1–2 hr to take effect; not effective alone without use of true antidotes).
5. **Anticonvulsants**, such as benzodiazepine, may be required.

Key Reference: Treatment of nerve gas poisoning. The Medical Letter 37:43–44, 1995.

Inhalational Injury by Irritant Gases

I. **Mechanisms of injury of noxious gases**

1. **Asphyxiation** may result from a fall in FiO_2 due to displacement of ambient air by the gas (e.g., CO, CO_2, NO_2, methane), altered oxygen-carrying capacity of blood (e.g., carboxyhemoglobin, sulfhemoglobin), or inhibition of cellular respiratory enzymes (e.g., cyanide).
2. **Systemic toxicity** is seen in the inhalation of fumes of oxides of various metals such as the smelting of zinc, copper, tin, nickel, and others. It causes a syndrome known as metal fume fever, characterized by thirst, metallic taste, fever, chills, myalgias, headache, weakness, and lung crackles.
3. **Immunologic effects.** Examples of sensitizers include toluene diisocyanate, methylene biphenyl isocyanate, platinum compounds, formaldehyde, and soldering flux. Sensitized patients may have bronchospasm with reexposure to low concentrations of the substance.
4. **Direct mucosal and alveolar damage.** In general, gases with the greatest solubility in water cause more eye and upper airway injury. Gases with lower solubility in water are more likely to cause greater injury in the lower respiratory tract. Thus water-soluble agents are also more likely to be noxious and thus avoided. Any gas, however, may cause lower respiratory tract injury if inhaled in high enough concentrations. Upper airway injury may manifest as upper airway obstruction and laryngotracheobronchitis. Lower respiratory tract injuries include bronchospasm, bronchiolitis, and alveolar surface injury (e.g., with phosgene, NO_2).

II. **Types of irritant gases and their characteristics**

Gas	Relative water-solubility	Uses	Distinguishing features
Chlorine (Cl_2)	High	Alkali and bleach productions; plastic industries; disinfectant for water and pools	**Phase I** (0–6 hr): coughing, wheezing, slight oropharyngeal redness **Phase II** (6 hr–8 days): upper and lower airway edema, pulmonary edema, bronchopneumonia **Phase III** (1–4 wk): gradual improvement; cough may persist

(Table continued on next page.)

Gas	Relative water-solubility	Uses	Distinguishing features
Ammonia	High	Refrigeration equipment; plastic, explosive, and fertilizer industries	Significant exposure may cause upper airway mucosal edema, bronchitis, pulmonary edema, and asphyxia.
Sulfur dioxide (SO_2)	High	Bleaching, ore smelting, paper manufacturing, refrigeration industry	SO_2 combines with water on mucosal surfaces to form sulfuric acid
Hydrogen sulfide (H_2S)	High	Natural gas making; paper pulp, sewage treatment, and tannery work	Sulfhemoglobinemia; also inhibits oxidative respiration
Nitrogen dioxide (NO_2)	Low	Arc-welding, dye and fertilizer making, farming-silage exposure	**Phase I:** cough, pulmonary edema **Phase II:** resolution **Phase III:** fever, dyspnea, hypoxemia due to bronchiolitis obliterans

III. **Treatment**

1. The major concern is **respiratory support for the airway and parenchymal compromise.** Intubation may be quite difficult due to oropharyngeal edema. Large endotracheal tubes are recommended (if possible) because of the need to aspirate copious exudates that are often present in inhalational injuries.
2. **Bronchoscopy** may help with difficult intubation, assessment of the degree of lower airway injury, and treatment of atelectasis not cleared by chest physiotherapy.
3. In exposure to oxides of nitrogen that cause methemoglobinemia, specific therapy is **methylene blue**. In addition, **corticosteroid** administration during phases I and III of NO_2 injury may prevent the development of bronchiolitis obliterans, although there are no controlled studies.
4. Although **prophylactic antibiotic is generally not recommended**, patients are susceptible to superimposed infection (due to airway injury, increased inflammatory exudate, and intubation in an ICU setting); therefore, patients should be monitored for nosocomial pneumonia and promptly treated if it develops.
5. **Inhaled bronchodilators** are useful in patients with airflow limitation.
6. Search for associated illness that may have precipitated the injury (e.g., stroke or myocardial infarction that caused accident and exposure). Also identify the cause of the exposure to prevent subsequent accidents.

Key Reference: Summer W, Haponik E: Inhalation of irritant gases. Clin Chest Med 2:273–287, 1981.

Toxins that May Be Eliminated by Multiple Dosing of Activated Charcoal

I. Human volunteer studies have demonstrated that multiple dosing of activated charcoal increases elimination of the following drugs:

Carbamazepine	Phenobarbital
Dapsone	Phenylbutazone
Digitoxin	Piroxicam
Disopyramide	Sotalol
Methotrexate	Theophylline
Nadolol	Quinine

II. Increased elimination by multiple dosing of activated charcoal is possible for the following drugs:

Acetaminophen	Phenytoin (Dilantin)
Amitriptyline	Propranolol
Cyclosporine	Salicylates
Diazepam	Valproic acid
Meprobamate	Vancomycin
Nortriptyline	

Adapted from: Krenzelok EP, Leikin JB: Approach to the poisoned patient. Dis Month 42:509–608, 1996.

Toxins or Drugs with Increased Elimination by Diuresis

I. **Toxins that may be eliminated by forced (neutral) saline diuresis:**

Barium	Iodine
Bromides	Isoniazid (?)
Chromium	Meprobamate
Cimetidine (?)	Methyliodide
Cis-platinum	Mushrooms (group 1)
Cyclophosphamide	Nickel
5-Fluorouracil (?)	Potassium chloroplatinite
Hydrazine	Thallium
Iodide	Valproic acid (?)

II. **Toxins that may be eliminated by alkaline diuresis:**

Barbital Methotrexate	
2, 4-D Chlorophenoxyacetic acid	Phenobarbital
Chlorpropamide	Primodone
Fluoride Quinolone antibiotics	
Iopanoic acid (?)	Salicylates
Isoniazid (?)	Sulfisoxazole
Mephobarbital	Uranium

Adapted from: Krenzelok EP, Leikin JB: Approach to the poisoned patient. Dis Month 42:509–608, 1996.

Drugs and Toxins that May Be Removed by Hemodialysis

Acetaminophen	Cephradine	Hydrazine (?)
Acetazolamide	Chloral hydrate	Hydrochlorothiazide
Acetone	Chloramphenicol (?)	Imipenem/cilastatin
Acetophencitidin	Chlordiazepoxide (?)	Iodides
Acetophenitidin	Chloride	Isoniazid
Acyclovir	Chlorpropamide	Isopropanol
Alkyl phosphate	Chromic acid	Kanamycin
Allopurinol	Chromium	Ketoprofen
Aluminum	Cimetidine (?)	Lead (with EDTA)

Amanita phalloides (?)
Amantadine (?)
Amikacin
Ammonia
Ammonium chloride
Amobarbital
Amoxicillin
Amphetamine
Ampicillin
Anilines
Antimony (pentavalent) (?)
Arsenic (?)
Atenolol
Azathioprine
Azlocillin
Aztreonam
Bacitracin (?)
Barbital
Boric acid
Bretylium
Bromides
Bromisoval
Butabarbital
Butalbital
Calcium
Captopril (?)
Carbamazepine
Carbenicillin
Carbromal
Carisoprodol
Cefaclor
Cefamandole
Cefazolin
Cefoperazone (?)
Cefotaxime
Cefoxitin
Ceftazidime
Cephalexin
Cephaloridine
Cephalothin
Cephapirin
Quinalbital
Quinidine
Ranitidine (?)
Rifabutin
Salicylates
Sacitoxin (?)
Secobarbital (?)
Sodium chlorate
Sodium chloride
Sodium citrate
Ciprofloxacin (?)
Colistin
Cyclobarbital
Cyclophosphamide
Cycloserine
Dapsone
Demeton-S-methyl sulfoxide
Dextropropoxyphene
Diethyl pentenamide
Dimethoxanate
Dinitro-ortho-cresol
Diquat (?)
Disopyramide
Enalapril (?)
Ergotamine
Erythromycin
Ethanol
Ethambutol
Ethchlorvynol (?)
Ethinamate
Ethosuximide (?)
Ethylene glycol
Eucalyptus oil
Famotidine (?)
Flucytosine
Fluoridem chlorate
Fluoride
5-Fluorouracil (?)
Folic acid
Formaldehyde
Foscarnet sodium
Fosfomycin
4-Methylpyrazole
Gabapentin
Gallamine triethiodide
Ganciclovir
Gentamicin
Glufosinate ammonium
Glutethimide (?)
Glycol ethers
Sotalol
Streptomycin
Strychnine
Succimer (?)
Sulfamethoxazole
Tetracycline (?)
Thallium
Theophylline
Thiocyanates
Lithium
Magnesium
Mannitol
Meprobamate
Metal-chelate compounds
Metformin (?)
Methanol
Methaqualone
Methotrexate
Methyldopa
Methylprednisolone (?)
Methyprylon
Metronidazole
Mezlocillin
Monochloroacetic acid
Nadolol (?)
Nafcillin
Neomycin
Netilmicin
Nitrates
Nitrites
Ouabain (?)
Oxalic acid
Paraldehyde
Paraquat (?)
Pargyline
Penicillin G
Pentobarbital (?)
Phenelzine (?)
Phenobarbital
Phosphate
Phosphoric acid
Piperacillin
Potassium chloride
Potassium dichromate
Practolol
Primidone
Prednisone (?)
Procainamide
Propoxyphene
Ticarcillin
Tobramycin
Tocainide
Tranylcypromine sulfate (?)
Trimethoprim
Valproic acid (?)
Vancomycin (?)
Verapamil (?)
Vidarabine

Key reference: Krenzelok EP, Leikin JB: Approach to the poisoned patient. Dis Month 42:509–608, 1996.

Drugs and Toxins that May Be Removed by Charcoal Hemoperfusion

Amanita phalloides (?)
Amobarbital
Atenolol (?)
Bromisoval
Bromoethylbutyramide
Caffeine
Carbamazepine
Carbon tetrachloride (?)
Carbromal
Chloral hydrate (trichloroethanol)
Chloramphenicol
Chlorfenvinfos (?)
Chlorpropamide
Clonidine
Colchicine (?)
Creosote (?)
Dapsone
Demeton-S-methyl sulfoxide
Digitoxin
Diltiazem (?)
Dimethoate
Disopyramide
Ethchlorvynol
Ethylene oxide
Glutethimide
Hexobarbital
Levothyroxine (?)
Lindane
Meprobamate
Methaqualone
Methotrexate
Methsuximide
Methyprylon (?)
Metoprolol (?)
Nadolol
Oxalic acid (?)
Paraquat
Parathion (?)
Phenelzine (?)
Phenobarbital
Phenytoin
Podophyllin (?)
Procainamide (?)
Quinidine (?)
Rifabutin (?)
Secobarbital
Sotalol (?)
Thallium (?)
Theophylline
Valproic acid (?)
Verapamil (?)

Adapted from: Krenzelok EP, Leikin JB: Approach to the poisoned patient. Dis Month 42:509–608, 1996.

Hematology

Transfusion Reactions

Type	Cause	Clinical	Evaluation	Therapy
Acute intravascular hemolysis	Alloantibodies, most commonly to ABO antigens C3a and C5a responsible for manifestations	Fever, chills, dyspnea, hypotension, vomiting, flushing, back pain, shock DIC, ATN	Hemoglobinuria Hemoglobinemia Low to absent haptoglobin Mild hyperbilirubinemia Positive DAT test	Stop Tx Supportive, including brisk diuresis (~ 100 ml/hr)
Acute extravascular hemolysis	Presence of IgG on RBC and/ or fixation of complement to C3 results; RBC cleared by spleen (IgG receptors) or liver (C3R)	Fever, indirect hyperbilirubinemia Patients are fairly fairly stable	Anemia, increased urine urobilinogen Positive DAT	Stop Tx Supportive care
Delayed hemolysis	Usually extravascular hemolysis due to alloantibodies against transfused RBCs; typically 1–3 weeks after transfusion	Symptoms milder than above	Mild hemoglobinemia and hemoglobinuria	Supportive care
Febrile reaction	Agglutinating antibodies in recipient's plasma reacting with transfused WBCs or platelets	Fever, chills, nausea, vomiting Often appears dramatic but often self-limiting	Diagnosis of exclusion Reconfirm ABO type Repeat cross-match Negative DAT	Stop Tx Acetaminophen Merperidine Hydrocortisone Leukocyte-depleted blood products and filters
Allergic reaction	Due to infused plasma proteins; usuallymediated by IgG even in anaphylactic reactions; IgG against IgA in IgA-deficient recipients	Mild (urticaria, confluent rash, pruritus) to anaphylaxis	Clinical diagnosis of exclusion	Stop Tx Diphenhydramine, 25–50 mg PO/IV with or without epinephrine
Micro-aggregate debris and ARDS	Dead platelets, granulocytes, fibrin strands	ARDS	Underlying illness that necessitated the transfusion probably contributes to ARDS	Microaggregate filters

(Table continued on following page.)

Type	Cause	Clinical	Evaluation	Therapy
Bacterial contamination	Usually gram-negative; *Pseudomonas*, *Yersinia*, *Enterocolitica*, *Flavobacteria* spp.	Fever/chills/ abdominal cramps, renal failure, cardiovascular collapse	Rule out hemolytic transfusion reactions	Stop Tx Antibiotics Culture untransfused blood
Noncardiogenic pulmonary edema	Donor antibodies reacting with recipient WBCs; possibly pulmonary leukostasis	Pulmonary edema with no evidence of fluid overload or heart failure	Essentially diagnosis of exclusion	Multiparous women and multiply transfused people should avoid donating blood
Hypothermia	Rapid transfusion (1 unit per 5 min)	Ventricular fibrillation	Do not warm blood under hot water or in a microwave, because "hot spots" may cause hemolysis	Most Tx do not need warming; use blood warmer if required, keep < 38°C
Electrolyte abnormalities	Citrate: may cause hypocalcemia and hypomagnesemia due to binding and hypokalemia due to HCO_3 from citrate metabolism; hyperkalemia due to stored blood		Be aware of potential electrolyte disturbances in massive transfusions and patients with renal insufficiency	Replete or treat electrolyte disorders

DIC = disseminated intravascular coagulation, ATN = acute tubular necrosis. Tx= transfusion, RBC = red blood cell, WBC = white blood cell, ARDS = adult respiratory distress syndrome, DAT = direct antiglobulin test. A positive result is due to the patient's antibody coating the donor RBCs. It is **not** an autoimmune antibody.

Key Reference: Snyder EL: Transfusion reactions. In Hoffman R, Benz EJ, Shattil SJ, et al (eds): Hematology: Basic Principles and Practice. Edinburgh, Churchill-Livingstone, 1991, pp 1644–1651 (source of table).

Transfusion of Packed Red Blood Cells

I. In addition to the potential transfusion reactions noted above and the risk of infections, transfusion of packed red blood cells (pRBCs) may not necessarily benefit patients who are critically ill and anemic.

II. In a multicenter, randomized, controlled trial of over 800 patients at 25 ICUs in Canada, patients were randomly assigned to either a liberal transfusion strategy (defined as maintaining a hemoglobin level between 10 and 12 gm/dL [100–120 gm//L]) or a restrictive strategy (hemoglobin maintained between 7–9 gm/dL (70–90 gm/L). Patients who were chronically anemic or actively bleeding were excluded. After volume resuscitation, all enrolled patients had hemoglobin ≤ 9 gm/dL (≤ 90 gm/L). Overall 30 day mortality trended to be lower in the restrictive group (p = 0.11) although in-hospital mortality was significantly lower in the restrictive group (p = 0.05). Patients in the restrictive group had lower rate of cardiac complications.

Two subgroups showed lower mortality with the restictive startegy: (i) patients < 55 years old and (ii) less severely ill patients (APACHE scores ≤ 20).

Key Reference: Hebert PC, et al: A multicenter, randomized, controlled trial of transfusion requirements in critical care. N Engl J Med 340:409–417, 1999.

Transfusion-related Acute Lung Injury

I. **Acute respiratory failure with shock** is an unusual but potentially lethal complication of hemotherapy. Transfusion-related acute lung injury (TRALI) is indistinguishable from non–transfusion-associated acute respiratory distress syndrome. TRALI has been observed with transfusion of whole blood, red cells, fresh frozen plasma, and cryoprecipitate.

II. **Pathogenesis.** The mechanism for the development of TRALI is not precisely known, but various forms of anti-HLA-A or anti-HLA-B antibodies and neutrophil-specific antibodies have been found in the donor blood products. It is hypothesized that the antibodies activate the complement cascade with aggregation of neutrophils in the pulmonary microvasculature and subsequent endothelial injury.

III. **Clinical manifestations**
1. Rapid onset of hypoxemic respiratory failure and diffuse alveolar infiltrates is typically seen 1–6 hr after transfusion.
2. Fever and hypotension.
3. Hemodynamic profile resembles sepsis: low systemic vascular resistance and a high cardiac output.

IV. **Diagnosis**
1. Exclude cardiogenic pulmonary edema, pneumonia, aspiration, anaphylaxis, and sepsis.
2. Detection of lymphocytotoxic, leukoagglutinating, or neutrophil antibodies in the donor's plasma or in the plasma-containing blood products.

V. **Treatment**
1. Supportive including respiratory support with mechanical ventilation.
2. Fluid infusion and vasopressors may be required for blood pressure support.
3. Improvement typically occurs within 24–96 hr in patients who survive; the mortality rate of TRALI is estimated at 5%.

Key Reference: Popovsky MA, et al: Transfusion-related acute lung injury: A neglected, serious complication of hemotherapy. Transfusion 32:589–592, 1992.

Fresh Frozen Plasma, Platelet, and Cryoprecipitate Transfusions

I. **Fresh-frozen plasma (FFP)** contains all of the coagulation factors as well as naturally occurring inhibitors (anticoagulants). One unit bag ~ 200–250 ml. Larger volumes of FFP (400–600 ml) are prepared by plasmapheresis from a single donor and may be preferable over 2 bags of FFP from different donors.
1. **Indications**
    a. Patients with **coagulation factor deficiency**, as documented by (1) prothrombin time (PT) > 1.5 times the midpoint of the normal range (> 18 sec) *or* (2) activated partial thromboplastin time (aPTT) > 1.5 times the top of the

normal range (> 55–60 sec) *or* (3) coagulation factor assay < 25% of activity, plus **active bleeding, planned surgery, or other invasive procedures.**

b. **Massive blood transfusion:** replacement of more than 1 blood volume (~ 5 L) with either coagulation deficiency or continued bleeding.

c. **Reversal of warfarin effect** to stop active bleeding, planned surgery, or invasive procedure when PT > 18 sec or international normalized ratio (INR) > 1.6.

d. Deficiency of antithrombin III, heparin cofactor II, protein C, or protein S.

e. **Plasma exchange for thrombotic thrombocytopenic purpura (TTP) or hemolytic uremic syndrome**; plasma from which cryoprecipitate has been removed (cryo-poor plasma) may be used in refractory TTP.

2. **Dosage**

a. If PT is 18–22 sec or aPTT is 55–70 sec, 1 unit of FFP (200 ml) may be sufficient for hemostasis. Additional FFP is based on determination of PT or aPTT after completion of transfusion. If PT is not determined within 1–2 hr after transfusion, the aPTT is a better indicator of the efficiency of therapy, because factor VII has a half-life of only 5–6 hr. In general, 4–7 units of FFP (800–1400 ml) are needed in a 70-kg person to raise coagulation factors by 10–20%.

b. If platelets are also transfused, for every 5–6 units of platelets or 1 plateletpheresis unit, the patient receives a volume equivalent of 1 bag of FFP.

II. **Platelets.** Normal count is $150 \times 10^9 - 400 \times 10^9$/L (150,000–400,000/mm^3). Platelets are obtained from whole blood donations (**1 unit = 50 ml ~ 5.5–10 × 10^{10} platelets**) or plateletpheresis donations (1 unit ~ 4×10^{11} platelets). Volume of plasma for 6 random units or 1 plateletpheresis unit is 250–350 ml.

1. **Clinical indications**

a. **Decreased platelet production** (e.g., chemotherapy, bone marrow irradiation) or both decreased production and increased destruction (e.g., acute leukemia)

- For counts ≤ **5000/mm^3**, platelets should be given regardless of apparent bleeding because the risk of spontaneous hemorrhage is high.
- For counts between **5000–30,000/mm^3**, platelets may be given prophylactically or on the basis of significant bleeding risks.
- For counts **> 50,000/mm^3**, bleeding due to platelet deficiency is exceedingly unlikely.
- The trigger for prophylactic transfusion of **leukemics** is 10,000–20,000/mm^3, although the lower number appears safe.
- For **major surgery or life-threatening bleeding**, the platelet count should be increased to 50,000/mm^3.

b. **Enhanced platelet destruction.** Limited usefulness when destruction (by antibodies or consumption) is the cause of the thrombocytopenia. General threshold for transfusion is counts < 20,000–50,000/mm^3 and unexpected excessive bleeding.

- Platelets recommended when patients undergoing major surgery have counts < 50,000/mm^3 and evidence of microvascular bleeding (e.g., ecchymosis).
- Platelets recommended in patients undergoing cardiopulmonary bypass (which can destroy platelets and render them dysfunctional) with counts < 100,000/mm^3 and major unexplained bleeding.
- Neurologic or ophthalmologic surgery may require counts near 100,000/mm^3
- Thrombotic thrombocytopenic purpura: platelets usually contraindicated.
- Idiopathic thrombocytopenic purpura: limit platelets to major surgery with excessive bleeding or life-threatening bleeding.

2. **Dosage**
   a. **1 unit of platelet (50 ml) increases the count by 5,000–10,000/mm^3.**
   b. Refractoriness to transfusion is a common occurrence in patients receiving frequent transfusion due to platelet-reactive and/or lymphocytotoxic antibodies. Such alloimmunized patients require platelets from HLA-matched and/or platelet cross-matched donors.

III. **Cryoprecipitate** is produced by freezing FFP (< –65°C), then allowing it to thaw 18 hr at 4°C. After centrifugation, cryoprecipitate proteins separate. Cryoprecipitate is a rich source for factors VIII and XIII and fibrinogen. FFP contains these factors, but it also contains plasminogen and therefore may theoretically increase the risk of bleeding. It is the agent of choice to reverse a thrombolytic state (e.g., when intracerebral hemorrhage complicates thrombolytic therapy). It is also used in the treatment of congenital deficiencies of VIIIc, vWF, and fibrinogen (e.g., when fibrinogen is < 60–100 mg/dl with bleeding or planned surgery). **Dose:** each bag = 30 ml; 4–6 bags (120–180 ml) are required to raise factor XIII by 3% and 12–16 bags (360–480 ml) to raise fibrinogen by 100 mg/dl (1 gm/L).

Key Reference: Development Task Force of the College of American Pathologists: Practice parameter for the use of fresh-frozen plasma, cryoprecipitate, and platelets. JAMA 271:777–781, 1994.

Disseminated Intravascular Coagulation

I. **Definition:** Disseminated intravascular coagulation (DIC) is a clotting disorder with secondary coagulation factor depletion, thrombocytopenia, and circulating fibrin degradation products. It is caused by activation of the extrinsic or intrinsic coagulation pathways by an underlying disease followed by secondary fibrinolysis. Clinically evident arterial or venous thrombosis is less commonly seen than bleeding.

II. **Causes**
   1. **Severe infections and endotoxemia:** bacterial (lipid A component of endotoxin activates factor XII [Hageman factor] and the intrinsic coagulation cascade), viral, fungal, parasitic, or rickettsial organisms.
   2. **Malignancy:** disseminated (mucin-secreting) adenocarcinoma, acute promyelocytic leukemia.
   3. **Obstetric complications:** abruptio placentae, amniotic fluid embolism, second-trimester abortion.
   4. **Endothelial damage:** aortic aneurysm, acute glomerulonephritis, fat embolism.
   5. **Tissue damage:** burns, frostbite, trauma.

III. **Clinical diagnosis**
   1. Blood oozing from surgical incisions, venipuncture sites, or catheter sites.
   2. Less commonly, there may be evidence of thrombosis with acrocyanosis and pregangrenous changes of the digits, genitalia, and nose.

IV. **Laboratory diagnosis**
   1. Fragmented red blood cells (schistocytes) on peripheral smear.
   2. Prolonged prothrombin time and partial thromboplastin time, thrombocytopenia, hypofibrinogenemia, and elevated levels of fibrin degradation products and D-dimers. In a retrospective study of 82 critically ill patients, the measurement of both D-dimer and fibrinogen/fibrin degradation products appears to be the most efficacious and cost-effective test to diagnose DIC. These tests, however, are not specific for DIC. A repeat of the tests a few hours or days later may indicate whether active consumption (a sign of DIC) is present.

V. **Treatment** (confusing and controversial; hematology consult recommended)
   1. Treat underlying disorder.
   2. Significant bleeding with [fibrinogen] < 100 mg/dl (< 1 gm/L) or platelet count < 50,000/μl (< 50 × 10^9/L): fresh frozen plasma and platelet concentrate transfusion. For patients who continue to bleed despite replacement of these products, consider adding IV heparin.
   3. Acrocyanosis, venous thromboembolism, or pregangrenous changes: IV heparin, generally 20,000–30,000 U/24 hr (higher dose) or 200 U/kg/day IV or subcutaneously (lower dose).

Key References: Bick RL: Disseminated intravascular coagulation. Semin Thromb Hemostasis 22:69–88, 1996; Yu M, Nardella A, Pechet L: Screening tests of disseminated intravascular coagulation: Guidelines for rapid and specific laboratory diagnosis. Crit Care Med 28:1777–1780, 2000.

Methemoglobinemia

I. Consider in any patient with **cyanosis.**
II. Methemoglobin (metHb) is formed when the Fe^{2+} in hemoglobin is oxidized to Fe^{3+}. MetHb is unable to bind O_2; in addition, metHb causes the oxygen dissociation curve to shift to the left with impaired unloading of oxygen to tissues.
III. Only 1.5–2 gm/dl (15–20 gm/L) of metHb (≈ 10% of total Hb) are needed to cause cyanosis. **MetHb ≈ 35%** → headache, weakness, breathlessness, changed mental status. **MetHb ≈ 50–60%** → acidosis, arrhythmias, and coma; often fatal.
IV. **Causes of methemoglobinemia are hereditary** (M hemoglobins, cytochrome b_5 reductase deficiency; rare) or **acquired** (usually due to drugs):
   1. **Nitrites and nitrates:** sodium nitrite, amyl nitrite, nitroglycerin, nitroprusside, silver nitrate, nitrate-contaminated well water
   2. **Aniline dyes**
   3. **Acetanilid, phenacetin, dapsone**—all aniline derivatives
   4. **Sulfonamides**
   5. Others: **lidocaine, benzocaine** (Hurricaine), **chlorate, phenazopyridine** (Pyridium), **quinones**
V. **Diagnosis**
   1. MetHb blood, when exposed to air, remains chocolate brown.
   2. Pulse oximetry (SpO_2) may either underestimate or overestimate the co-oximetry (SaO_2) in the presence of metHb; in a pulse oximeter, oxy-Hb absorbs more light at 940 nm than at 660 nm. Reduced Hb absorbs more light at 660 nm. MetHb absorbs light equally at both wavelengths. Thus, the higher the metHb level, the closer SpO_2 moves toward 85%.
   3. Direct methemoglobin measurement from arterial blood gas co-oximetry panel.
VI. **Treatment.** Methylene blue (co-factor for NADPH reductase, the enzyme that reduces Fe^{3+} to Fe^{2+}) increases rate of metHb reduction.
   1. For patients with very high levels (≥ 70% metHb), exchange transfusion or dialysis.
   2. For patients with high levels: **methylene blue, 1–2 mg/kg IV over 5–10 min**; repeat every 4 hr as needed (not to exceed 7 mg/kg); within 1 hr, the metHb is usually decreased by at least 50%.
   3. For less severe cases: oral methylene blue, 60 mg 3 or 4 times/day or vitamin C, 300–600 mg/day.
   4. In patients with G6PD deficiency, methylene blue may cause hemolysis.

Key Reference: Hall AH, Kulig KW, Rumack BH: Drug- and chemical-induced methaemoglobinemia: Clinical features and management. Med Toxicol 1:253–260, 1986.

Sulfhemoglobinemia

I. Sulfhemoglobinemia (sulfHb), like methemoglobinemia, also may result in cyanosis in the absence of any cardiopulmonary disorder. A mean capillary concentration of only 0.5 gm/dl (5 gm/L) of sulfHb is sufficient for detectable cyanosis. It is formed by the irreversible oxidation of the heme moiety of aniline dyes, acetanilid, phenacetin, nitrates, sulfonamides, metoclopramide (structurally similar to aniline dyes), flutamide, dapsone, dimethyl sulfoxide (DMSO) or by exposure to sulfurated chemicals. In the process, a sulfur atom is incorporated into the porphyrin ring. In rare instances, it has been hypothesized that the source of sulfur may be hydrogen sulfide released by intestinal organisms, particularly in patients who are constipated.

II. Sulfhemoglobin markedly reduces oxygen transport because the oxygen dissociation curve with sulfHb is shifted to the right. Thus, although oxygen binding is impaired, oxygen delivery in tissues is facilitated. Hence, unlike metHb, sulfHb has few adverse clinical consequences. However, because automated blood gas analysis using spectrophotometer does not accurately differentiate metHb and sulfHb, patients with sulfHb may be mistakenly treated for metHb.

III. There is no specific treatment for sulfHb. The concentration of sulfHb decreases as erythrocytes are destroyed and replaced.

Key References: Aravindhan N, Chisholm DG: Sulfhemoglobinemia presenting as pulse oximetry desaturation. Anesthesiology 93:883–884, 2000; Noor M, Beutler E: Acquired sulfhemoglobinemia: An underreported diagnosis? West J Med 169:386–389, 1998.

Tumor Lysis and Hyperleukocytic Syndromes

I. **Tumor lysis syndrome**

1. Most commonly seen in patients with acute lymphoblastic lymphoma, acute lymphocytic leukemia, Burkitt's lymphoma, and diffuse undifferentiated lymphoma in which rapid response (lysis) to chemotherapy is seen. Less common with small cell lung cancer and testicular carcinoma.
2. **Clinical manifestations: hyperuricemia** (urate nephropathy, acute renal failure), **hyperphosphatemia** (causing hypocalcemia), **hyperkalemia, lactic acidosis**, and **diffuse alveolar damage.**
3. Prior renal insufficiency and elevated lactate dehydrogenase increase the risk.
4. Onset usually occurs within 12–48 hr of chemotherapy.
5. Preventive measures with hydration, alkalinization (urinary pH > 7.5) of urine, and allopurinol, 300 mg 2 times/day, are more successful than treatment.

II. **Hyperleukocytic syndrome**

1. Syndrome in which various organ dysfunction results from intravascular occlusion of small arteries with white blood cells.
2. Occurs in patients with acute myeloblastic, chronic myelocytic, and acute lymphoblastic leukemia. Blood transfusion to correct anemia in a patient with high blast count may precipitate a hyperleukocytic syndrome, because previous anemia counteracts the hyperviscosity.
3. **Clinical presentation: diffuse interstitial infiltrates, adult respiratory distress syndrome (ARDS), cardiogenic pulmonary edema** (latter due to coronary artery occlusion), **neurologic abnormalities** (stupor, delirium, intracranial hemorrhage), and **vascular insufficiency**, all due to white cell thrombi.

4. **Pseudohypoxemia** is due to the consumption of oxygen dissolved in plasma. Immediate immersion of arterial blood sample in ice may delay drop in PaO_2, and addition of potassium cyanide inhibits cellular respiration. Measurement of SpO_2 by pulse oximeter may be more accurate assessment of oxygenation.
5. **Retinoic acid syndrome:** fever, dyspnea, interstitial infiltrates, pleural effusion, edema, episodic hypotension, renal insufficiency, and hyperbilirubinemia; occurs in ≈ 25% of patients with M3 AML (acute promyelocytic leukemia) treated with retinoic acid.
6. Treatment involves leukopheresis and chemotherapy. Treatment with leukopheresis before chemotherapy also may limit the development of tumor lysis syndrome.

Reference: Hess CE, Nichols AB, Hunt WB, et al: Pseudohypoxemia secondary to leukemia and thrombocytosis. N Engl J Med 301:361–363, 1979.

Acute Toxic Reactions to Chemotherapeutic Agents

Drug	Major Acute Toxicity
Doxorubicin	EKG changes (almost any type of arrhythmia) and sudden death, myocarditis, pericarditis, congestive heart failure
Vincristine	Neurotoxicity
Vinblastine	Myelosuppression
Mitomycin C	Microangiopathic hemolytic anemia
5-Fluorouracil	Myocardial ischemia
Cisplatin	Nephrotoxicity Hypomagnesemia Anaphylactoid reactions
Methotrexate	Myelosuppression, nephrotoxicity
Cyclosporine	Nephrotoxicity
All-trans retinoic acid	Retinoic acid syndrome (capillary leak)
Paclitaxel and other Cremophor-containing agents	Hypersensitivity reaction
Ara-C (arabinoside C)	Capillary leak syndrome causing noncardiogenic pulmonary edema and fluid loss through gastrointestinal tract
Cyclophosphamide	Myelosuppression, hemorrhagic cystitis

Key Reference: Santomauro E, Groeger JS: Managing severe—but reversible—complications in cancer patients. J Crit Illness 10:399–406, 1995.

Bleeding Diathesis Due to Uremia

I. Uremia itself causes an intrinsic platelet dysfunction and alters platelet-vessel wall interaction. Anemia also decreases platelet adhesion to the endothelium.

II. **Treatments to correct bleeding time:** transfusion of platelets causes only transfused platelets to become dysfunctional and therefore is **not** generally an option.

1. **Correction of anemia** to hematocrit ≥ 30% may normalize bleeding time.
2. **Cryoprecipitate:** effect is maximal at 4–8 hr and undetectable after 24 hr.
3. **Desmopressin (DDAVP)** releases factor VIII from storage sites into plasma. Dose of 0.3 μg/kg IV decreases bleeding time within 1 hr and lasts 6–8 hr.
4. **Conjugated estrogens** may be useful for treating mucosal bleeding from gastrointestinal angiodysplastic lesions. **Dose** of 0.6 mg/kg/day decreases bleeding time with 2–9 days of treatment.

Key Reference: Manucci PM, Remuzzi G, Pusineri F, et al: Deamino-8-D-arginine vasopressin shortens the bleeding time in uremia. N Engl J Med 308:8–12, 1983.

Thrombotic Thrombocytopenic Purpura

I. **Thrombotic thrombocytopenic purpura (TTP)** is a disorder characterized by a clinical spectrum in which platelet aggregation produces fluctuating ischemia or infarction in various organs. It is related to **hemolytic uremic syndrome (HUS)**, although generally the thrombocytopenia and hemolysis are less severe in HUS. Most patients who develop TTP have been previously healthy. In adults, HUS may complicate treatment with mitomycin, cyclosporine, and other chemotherapeutic agents; in children, HUS may be precipitated by gastroenteritis associated with verotoxin-producing serotype of *Escherichia coli* (0157:H7) or *Shigella* sp.

II. **Five major criteria:**
1. **Microangiopathic hemolytic anemia.** This test is most useful immediately; it reveals striking RBC fragmentation with burr cells, helmet cells, and schistocytes, polychromatophilia, basophilic stippling, microspherocytes, and nucleated RBCs.
2. **Renal insufficiency**
3. **Thrombocytopenia**
4. **Neurologic abnormalities**
5. **Fever**

III. Myocarditis and myocardial hemorrhage have been described as manifestations or complications of TTP.

IV. Platelet transfusion may exacerbate the disease process and is **contraindicated**.

V. **Treatment**
1. **Plasma exchange** (i.e., plasmapheresis + platelet-poor fresh frozen plasma) is the best therapy currently available for severe cases. Plasma infusion alone is not as effective as plasma exchange but may be tried in less severe cases or if plasmapheresis is not immediately available. Plasma infusion is also beneficial as prophylaxis in patients with frequently relapsing TTP. One recommended dose: **65–140 ml platelet-poor FFP/kg/exchange.** For plasma infusion alone, one recommended dose: **30 ml/kg over the first 24 hr, then 15 ml/kg/day thereafter.**
2. **Corticosteroid** (e.g., prednisone, 4 mg/kg/day up to 200 mg/day) is an effective adjunctive treatment and has been associated with the disappearance of the unusually large von Willebrand factor forms that have been implicated as one of the major platelet-aggregating substances in TTP.

Key References: Bell WR, Braine HG, Ness PM, Kickler TS: Improved survival in thrombotic thrombocytopenic purpura-hemolytic-uremia syndrome. N Engl J Med 325: 398–403, 1991; Rock GA, Shumak KH, Buskard NA, et al: Comparison of plasma exchange with plasma infusion in the treatment of thrombotic thrombocytopenic purpura. N Engl J Med 325:393–397, 1991.

Heparin-induced Thrombocytopenia

I. Roughly 10–20% of patients treated with heparin develop a mild thrombocytopenia secondary to a direct interaction between heparin and platelets. This condition is relatively benign and resolves spontaneously. The incidence of the potentially life-threatening heparin-induced thrombocytopenia (HIT) ranges from 1–5%. It may be an asymptomatic laboratory abnormality or associated with arterial or venous thromboses.

II. **Pathogenesis** of HIT involves an IgG (> IgA, IgM) antibody that is directed against the platelet factor 4 (PF4)–heparin complex. PF4 is a heparin-binding protein normally found in the alpha granules of platelets. HIT may occur with both low-molecular-weight heparin (LMWH) and unfractionated heparin, although the incidence appears be less with LMWH. However, once HIT has occurred, LMWH will perpetuate the condition.

II. **Clinical manifestations**

1. HIT most commonly occurs **within 5–12 days of therapy** and is more common with **bovine** (2.9%) than with porcine (1.1%) heparin. Although reported in patients given low-dose subcutaneous heparin, development of HIT is usually dose-related.
2. Thrombocytopenia, typically < 50,000
3. Thrombus formation ("white clot syndrome") may affect the arterial and/or venous circulation.
4. Other manifestations include bleeding complications, heparin resistance, and skin necrosis.

III. **Diagnosis**

1. Clinically, HIT should be considered in anyone who develops thrombocytopenia 5–10 days into heparin therapy.
2. A confirmatory test is the ^{14}C-labeled serotonin release assay (almost 100% specific but only 60–80% sensitive), a platelet aggregation assay (exposing donor platelets to patient serum + heparin and observing for platelet aggregation), and/or a PF4 ELISA. The serotonin release assay is time consuming and only a few centers in the U.S. perform this test. The platelet aggregation assay is highly specific, but the sensitivity is only 30–50%.

IV. **Prevention and treatment**

1. Ninety percent of HIT cases can be avoided by starting oral anticoagulation concurrently with heparin to limit the duration of heparin therapy. However, the duration of heparin therapy for venous thromboembolism should never be less than 5 days.
2. Heparin should be discontinued immediately. Platelet counts typically return to normal after several days. LMWH is **not** a suitable alternative in this setting. Warfarin is **contraindicated** in a patient with active HIT because of the significant risk of venous limb gangrene.
3. If anticoagulation is still required, initiate one of the two approved alternate anticoagulants, the thrombin inhibitors **argatroban** or **hirudin** (lepirudin), until platelet count recovers. If long-term anticoagulation is necessary, warfarin may be begun **after** platelet count recovers.
   a. **Lepirudin (Refludan)**. **Dosing**: 0.4 mg/kg slow bolus followed by a drip rate of 0.15 mg/kg/hr. Then adjust to achieve a PTT of 1.5–2.5 × control. **For renal failure**, the bolus dose should be 0.2 mg/kg. Adjust drip rate to creatinine clearance: for clearance of 45–60, 50% of original dose; for clearance of 30–44, 30% of original dose; for clearance of 15–29, 15% of original dose; and for clearance of < 15, no infusion. Side effects include bleeding, allergic reactions, and bronchospasm.

b. **Argatroban (Novastan).** Because argatroban is hepatically metabolized, it may be a better option for patients with renal insufficiency. A disadvantage is that there is no reversing agent for bleeding complications related to its use.

c. **Danaparoid (Orgaran)** is a combination of heparan sulfate, dermatan sulfate, and chondroitin sulfate. It works via anti-factor Xa activity, without much antithrombin activity. In vivo, it cross-reacts with HIT-antibody ~ 5%.

4. HIT is associated with a high rate of amputation (about 20%) and mortality (about 30%).

Key References: Greinacher A: Treatment of heparin-induced thrombocytopenia. Thromb Haemost 82:457–467, 1999; Warkentin TE: Heparin-induced thrombocytopenia: A clinicopathologic syndrome. Thrombosis & Haemostasis 82:439-447, 1999.

Red Blood Cell Morphology

I. Examination of the red blood cell morphology may be a rapid method to suggest a possible cause of anemia. In some instances, such as the presence of schistocytes, the mechanism of the anemia may be determined. It also may to help secure a systemic diagnosis such as thrombotic thrombocytopenic purpura.

II. Common abnormal red blood cell morphology include:

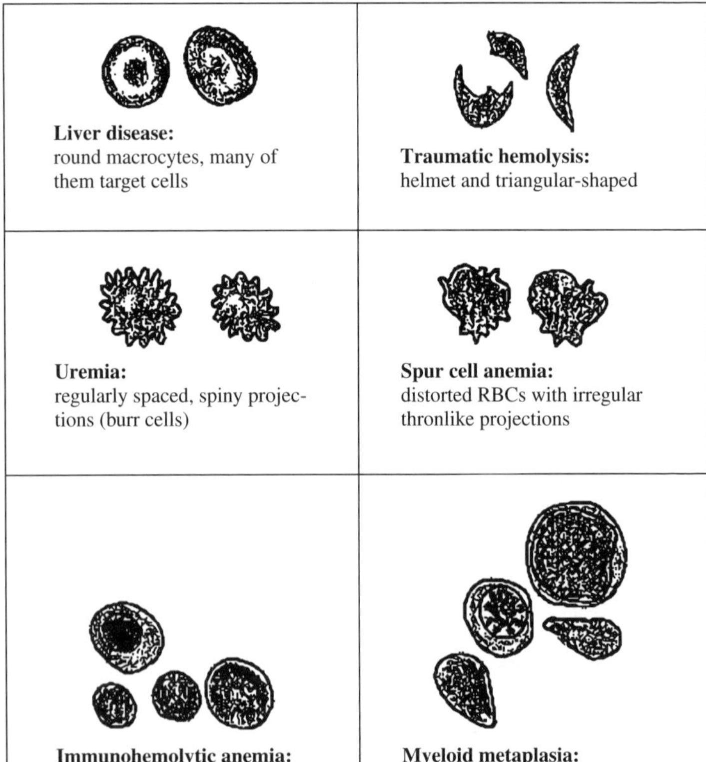

Liver disease:
round macrocytes, many of them target cells
Traumatic hemolysis:
helmet and triangular-shaped
Uremia:
regularly spaced, spiny projections (burr cells)
Spur cell anemia:
distorted RBCs with irregular thronlike projections
Immunohemolytic anemia:
microspherocytes, macrocytes with polychromasia, nRBC
Myeloid metaplasia:
tear-drop shaped RBC, nRBC, immature myeloid cells

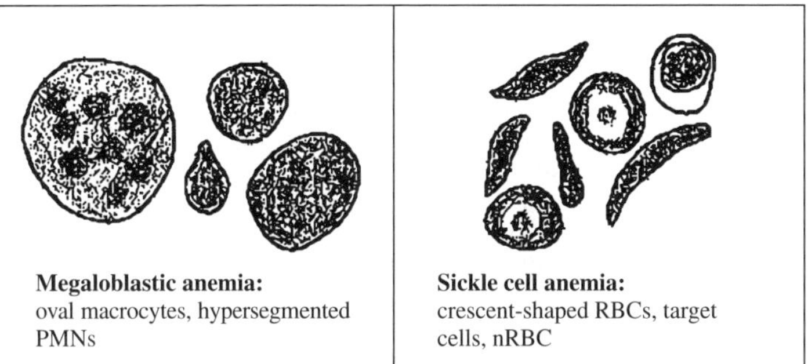

Megaloblastic anemia: oval macrocytes, hypersegmented PMNs

Sickle cell anemia: crescent-shaped RBCs, target cells, nRBC

Adapted from Isselbacher KJ, Braunwald E, Wilson JD, et al (eds): Harrison's Principles of Internal Medicine, 13th ed. New York, McGraw-Hill, 1994.

Hemostatic Drugs

I. **Nontransfusional hemostatic drugs** may be indicated in patients with life-threatening hemorrhage who refuse blood-products and prophylactically in patients undergoin surgical procedures associated with large blood losses.

II. **Antifibrinolytic agents** (ε-aminocaproic acid, tranexamic acid)
   1. **Mechanism of action**: by binding to plasminogen, antifibrinolytic agents block the binding of plasminogen to fibrin and its activation and transformation to plasmin. Thus, they inhibit fibrinolysis and consequent stabilization of clots. Tranexamic acid is significantly more potent and has a longer half-life than aminocaproic acid.
   2. **Primary menorrhagia**: in recalcitrant cases, tranexamic acid, 10–15 mg/kg every 8 hr, was effective in a randomized trial.
   3. **Gastrointestinal bleeding**: rarely used because effective pharmacologic and endoscopic treatments are available.
   4. **Urinary tract bleeding**: uncommonly, tranexamic acid is used to control prostatectamy bleeding. It is contraindicated in patients with *upper* urinary tract bleeding because of the risk of ureteral clots.
   5. **Oral bleeding** (e.g., dental extraction) in patients with congenital or acquired coagulation disorder (e.g., hemophilia or those on oral anticoagulants). Mouth washes containing tranexamic acid are also available.
   6. **Cardiac surgery**
      a. Aminocaproic acid: 150 mg/kg before surgery, then 15 mg/kg/hr infusion during surgery.
      b. Tranexamic acid: 10 mg/kg before surgery, then 1 mg/kg/hr infusion during surgery.
   7. **Adverse effects**: nausea, vomiting, abdominal pain, diarrhea, thrombosis (exact risk is unknown).

III. **Aprotinin**
   1. **Mechanism of action**: inhibits serine proteases (trypsin, chymotrypsin, plasmin, and tissue and plasma kallikrein). By inhibiting kallikrein, aprotinin indirectly inhibits the formation of activated factor XII. Thus, aprotinin inhibits both coagulation and fibrinolysis induced by the contact of blood with a foreign surface.
   2. Aprotinin is given **prophylactically** in cardiac surgery and orthotopic liver transplantation to reduce blood loss. The amount of aprotinin given is measured in kallikrein inactivation units (KIU).

3. **Adverse effects**
   a. Hypersensitivity reaction: skin flushing to shock, particularly after repeated exposure.
   b. Venous and arterial thrombosis: more of a theoretical risk as there does not appear to be an increase incidence of graft thrombosis.

IV. **D-arginine vasopressin (desmopressin)**
1. **Mechanism of action**: both factor VIII and von Willebrand factor can be increased for a short time by dDAVP.
2. **von Willebrand disease or hemophilia**
   a. The evidence for efficacy in patients with these two disorders who have spontaneous bleeding or who are scheduled for surgery is very clear.
   b. **Dosage**: 0.3 μg/kg IV or SQ or 300 μg intranasally every 12–24 hr, although tachyphylaxis may occur after 3–4 doses.
3. **Uremia**: dDAVP may shorten bleeding time and may be useful prior to invasive procedures.
4. **Cirrhosis**: although cirrhotics have high plasma factor VIII and vWF concentrations, they have prolonged bleeding time that is shortened by intravenous dDAVP. It may be useful prior to invasive procedures.
5. **Drug-induced bleeding** (e.g., aspirin, ticlopidine): as in uremia and cirrhosis, efficacy is shown by case series but no well-controlled studies.
6. **Adverse effects**: water retention with hyponatremia, facial flushing, headache, and theoretical risk for thrombosis.

Key Reference: Mannucci PM: Hemostatic drugs. N Engl J Med 339:245–253, 1998.

Cardiology

Cardiac Auscultation

I. A **ventricular gallop (S_3)** occurs in the rapid filling phase of the ventricles. A right ventricular (RV) S_3 is best heard over the anterior precordium and increases in intensity with inspiration. A left ventricular (LV) S_3 is best heard at the cardiac apex and becomes fainter or does not change in intensity with inspiration. S_3 may be heard in patients with high cardiac output or ventricular failure, atrioventricular (AV) valve regurgitation (mitral/tricuspid regurgitation), or other conditions that increase the rate or volume of ventricular filling. Left-sided S_3: bell piece of stethoscope at the LV apex during expiration and in left lateral decubitus position. Right-sided S_3: left sternal border or beneath the xiphoid; increases with inspiration. The differential diagnosis of a **third heart sound** (during diastole) includes (1) loud and delayed P_2 (e.g., pulmonary hypertension, atrial septal defect, right ventricular dysfunction); (2) S_3 gallop; (3) opening snap of mitral stenosis; (3) pericardial knock; and (5) tumor plop of atrial myxoma.

II. **S_4** occurs during LV filling during active atrial contraction (thus it is absent in atrial fibrillation). S_4 is associated with decreased LV compliance (e.g., systemic hypertension, aortic stenosis, hypertrophic cardiomyopathy, acute myocardial infarction/coronary artery disease, acute mitral regurgitation) or normal compliance associated with increased ventricular filling (e.g., severe anemia, thyrotoxicosis, or peripheral AV fistula).

III. **Pulsus alternans** is a reliable sign of LV dysfunction; it is seen only when the rhythm is normal (e.g., absent in atrial fibrillation).

IV. **Paradoxical splitting of S_2.** A2–P2 widens with expiration and shortens with inspiration (opposite of normal); caused by conditions that delay A2 (aortic insufficiency, aortic stenosis, hypertrophic cardiomyopathy, myocardial ischemia, left bundle-branch block, RV pacemaker).

V. A **short A2–OS (opening snap) interval** is a reliable indicator of severe mitral stenosis because it signifies high left atrial pressure.

Advanced Cardiac Life Support

I. **Ventricular fibrillation (VF) or pulseless ventricular tachycardia (VT)**
   1. **Condensed treatment algorithm** (check pulse between each attempt)
      a. **200 J, desynchronized**
      b. **300 J, desynchronized**
      c. **360 J, desynchronized**
      d. **Vasopressin 40 units IV × one dose only; epinephrine, 1 mg IV or ET every 5 min if no response to vasopressin, 360 J every 5 min**
   2. **Adjunctive therapy**
      a. Lidocaine, 1.5 mg/kg (≈ 100 mg) every 5 min to total of 3 mg/kg (≈ 200 mg).
      b. Amiodarone
         - IV amiodarone may be quite effective in patients with VF or destabilizing or incessant VT unresponsive to other agents.
         - The most common side effects are hypotension (~ 15–20%) and bradycardia/AV block (~ 5%). Other adverse effects include hepatic dysfunction

(fatal hepatocellular necrosis has been reported), QT prolongation, proarrhythmic effects, adult respiratory distress syndrome, and worsening congestive heart failure.

- **Dosage.** First 24 hr: 150 mg in a glucose solution (without electrolyte) IV over 10 min, then 1 mg/min for 6 hr (360 mg); maintenance dose of 0.5 mg/min for 18 hr (540 mg). Supplemental infusions of 150 mg over 10 min may be given for recurrent VT/VF. The usual duration of therapy is 2–4 days, but maintenance infusion can be continued for 2–3 weeks.

Reference: Intravenous amiodarone. Med Lett 37:114–115, 1995.

c. Bretylium, 5 mg/kg (≈ 300 mg) push; may repeat 10 mg/kg (≈ 600 mg) in 5 min.

d. Magnesium sulfate, 1–2 gm in torsades or refractory VF

e. Procainamide, 20 mg/min (≈ 200 mg/10 min), maximum of 17 mg/kg (≈ 1000 mg).

II. **Asystole**

1. Consider immediate transcutaneous pacing.
2. **Epinephrine, 1 mg IV or ET every 5 min** (IV preferred).
3. **Atropine, 1 mg IV or ET every 5 min for 2 doses** (IV preferred).

III. **Electrical mechanical dissociation (EMD) or pulseless electrical activity (PEA)**

1. **Causes:** consider hypovolemia, hypoxia, cardiac tamponade, tension pneumothorax, hypothermia, massive pulmonary embolism, hyperkalemia, acidosis, drug overdose (tricyclic antidepressants, digitalis, β-blockers, calcium channel blockers). One caveat is that although hyperkalemia may produce a severe hypotension, it occurs in the setting of a sine wave and not a sinus tachycardia. Thus, EMD and sinus rhythm are not due to hyperkalemia.
2. **Treatment algorithm**
   a. IV saline; give volume.
   b. **Epinephrine, 1 mg IV or ET every 5 min** (IV preferred).
   c. Atropine, 1 mg every 5 min for 3 doses if heart rate < 60 beats/min.
   d. Assess for tension pneumothorax, and consider pericardial aspiration if clinical setting warrants.
   e. Ensure that hypothermia is not present.

IV. **Ventricular tachycardia with pulse (unstable)**

1. **Treatment algorithm** (check BP and pulse between each attempt)
   a. 50 J, synchronized
   b. 100 J, synchronized
   c. 200 J, synchronized
   d. 360 J, synchronized
2. **If recurrent**, add lidocaine; cardiovert at previously successful energy level; then procainamide or bretylium if still recurrent (see above for dosages).

V. **Ventricular tachycardia with pulse (stable)**

1. Lidocaine, 1 mg/kg IV.
2. Lidocaine, 0.5 mg/kg every 8 min until VT resolves or up to 3 mg/kg.
3. Procainamide, 20 mg/min till VT resolves or up to 1000 mg.
4. Cardiovert as in unstable patient.

VI. **Drugs that may be given endotracheally during advanced cardiac life support**

Drug	Dosage
Epinephrine	0.5–1.0 mg IV or ET every 5 min
Lidocaine	1.0 mg/kg IV or ET; repeat 0.5 mg/kg every 5 min for total of 3 mg/kg

(Table continued on next page.)

Drug	Dosage
Atropine	1.0 mg IV or ET for 2 doses for asystole 0.3–1.0 mg IV or ET as needed for bradyarrhythmia
Bretylium tosylate	5 mg/kg IV or ET; may repeat 10 mg/kg every 15 min for total dose of 30 mg/kg

VII. **Cardiopulmonary resuscitation:** although the protocol of airways, breathing, and circulation (ABCs) is traditionally taught, increasing evidence suggests that the highest priority of CPR is **D (for early defibrillation) followed by C (for precordial compression)**. If cardiac arrest is due to asphyxia, airway and breathing take precedence over cardiac compression.

Reference: Weil MH, Tang W: Science challenges the dogmas of CPR. Chest 109: 597–598, 1996.)

Key Reference: American Heart Association: Textbook of Advanced Cardiac Life Support. Dallas, American Heart Association, 1988.

Electrocardiographic Pearls

I. **Electrical alternans:** cardiac tamponade, constrictive pericarditis, tension pneumothorax, myocardial infarction (MI), severe myocardial dysfunction.

II. **Pseudoinfarction patterns on EKG**

1. Left or right ventricular hypertrophy
2. Left bundle-branch block
3. Wolff-Parkinson-White syndrome
4. Hypertrophic cardiomyopathy
5. Hyperkalemia
6. Early repolarization
7. Cardiac sarcoid or amyloid
8. Intracerebral hemorrhage
9. Leftward axis with anterior pseudo-Qw's

III. **Estes criteria for left ventricular hypertrophy (LVH)**

	Points
1. R or S in limb lead (20 mm or more) *or* S in V_1, V_2, or V_3 (25 mm or more) *or* R in V_4, V_5, or V_6 (25 mm or more)	3
2. Any ST shift (without digitalis)	3
Typical "strain" ST T wave (with digitalis)	1
3. Left axial deviation of –15° or more	2
4. QRS interval of 0.09 sec or more	1
5. Intrinsicoid deflection in V_{5-6} of 0.04 sec or more	1
6. P terminal force in $V_1 > 0.04$	3
7. Total: 5 = LVH; 4 = probable LVH	

IV. **Right ventricular hypertrophy (RVH):** right axis deviation, tall R in V_1 (R, qR, or Rs), and rS in V_{5-6} (or rS across precordium from R to L); T-wave inversion in V1; associated right atrial enlargement.

V. **Left anterior hemiblock (LAHB):** left axis deviation (more than –45°), small Q in I,L; small R in 2,3,F; increased QRS voltage in limb leads. LAHB may **mimic** anterior MI, lateral MI, or LVH and may **mask** anterior MI, inferior MI, LVH, or right bundle-branch block.

VI. **Left posterior hemiblock (LPHB):** right axis deviation (usually +120°), small R in I,L; small Q in 2,3,F; increased QRS in limb leads, no evidence of RVH. The axis may be within normal limits, yet there is a rightward axis shift due to LPHB compared with older EKGs. LPHB may mimic or mask anterior MI.

VII. **Right bundle-branch block (RBBB):** QRS ≥ 0.12 sec. Terminal broad S wave in lead I. RSR complex in V1.

VIII. **Left bundle-branch block (LBBB):** QRS ≥ 0.12 sec. ST depression and T wave inversion, especially in lead I, L, V5, V6.

IX. **Morphologies**

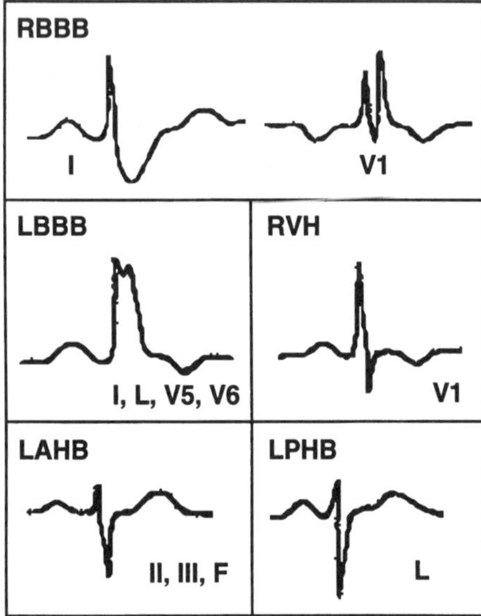

X. **Atrioventricular blocks**

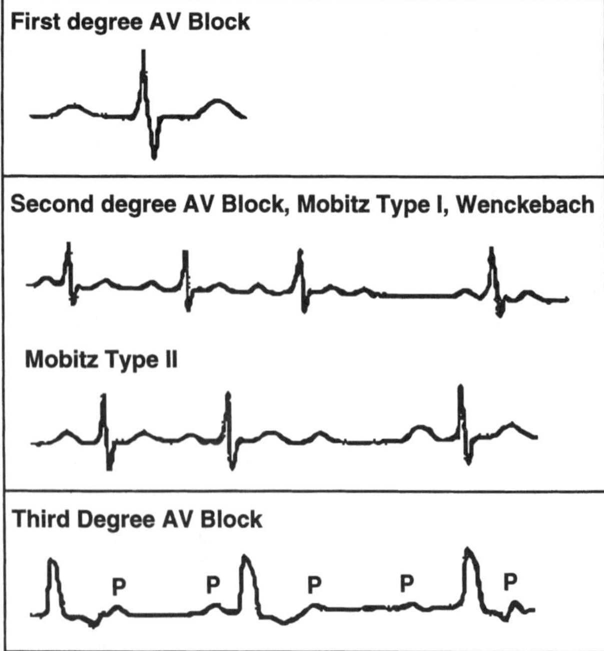

XI. **Supraventricular tachycardias**

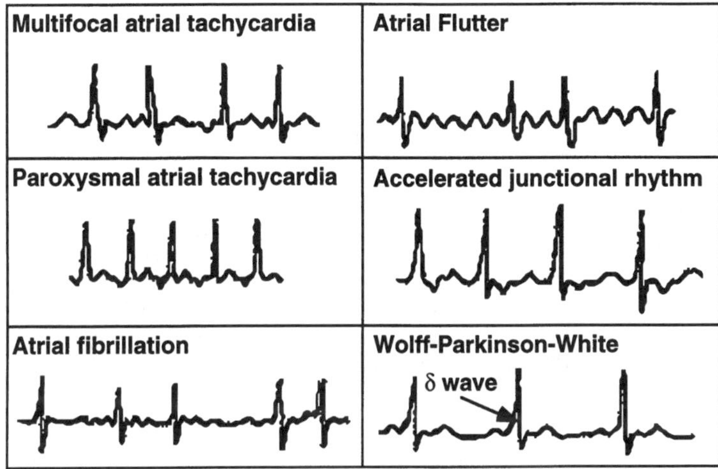

Differential Diagnosis of Wide-complex Tachycardia

I. The distinction between supraventricular tachycardia (SVT) with aberrancy and ventricular tachycardia (VT) is not important in patients with significant hypotension and shock. In such patients, direct current cardioversion is required.

II. **Physical exam**

1. **Variability in S_1 intensity is suggestive of VT** because it is a sign of atrioventricular (AV) dissociation: the intensity of S_1 depends on the position of the tricuspid valve (TV) and mitral valve (MV). In VT with AV dissociation, atrial systole occurs independently of ventricular systole. If atrial systole occurs just before ventricular systole, the MV and TV are wide open, and ventricular contraction results in a loud S_1. If atrial systole occurs earlier, the valves have had time to drift close and with ventricular systole, S_1 is soft.
2. **Cannon A waves in jugular vein pulse (JVP) is also suggestive of VT** (due to AV dissociation) because atrial systole occurs against a closed tricuspid valve during (simultaneous) ventricular systole.

III. **Electrocardiogram**

	Ventricular	**SVT with aberrancy**
Fusion beats	+	–
Capture beats	+	–
AV dissociation	+	–
Similar QRS with NSR	–	+
Positive concordance in V1–V6	+	–
LBBB + right axis	+	–
P waves	–	+
RSR' in V1	–	+

(Table continued on next page.)

	Ventricular	SVT with aberrancy
Slowing by increased vagal tone	–	+
RBBB + QRS > 0.14 sec	–	+
LBBB + QRS > 0.16 sec	+	–

IV. **History**

	Ventricular	SVT with aberrancy
MI	+	–
Ventricular aneurysm	+	–

V. The absence of an RS complex in all precordial leads is easily recognizable and highly specific for the diagnosis of VT. When an RS complex is present in one or more precordial leads, an RS interval of more than 100 msec is highly specific for VT.

Key References: Brugada P, et al: A new approach to the differential diagnosis of a regular tachycardia with a wide QRS complex. Circulation 83:1649–1659, 1991; Miles WM, Prystowsky EN, Heger JJ, et al: Evaluation of the patient with wide complex QRS tachycardia. Med Clin North Am 68:1015–1038, 1984.

Torsades de Pointes

I. Torsades de pointes is a **polymorphic variant of ventricular tachycardia** associated with oscillation of the axis and magnitude of the QRS complex between positive and negative deflections. Torsades may progress to ventricular fibrillation or terminate with sinus arrest. It occurs in association with prolonged QT interval (QT > 0.44 sec).

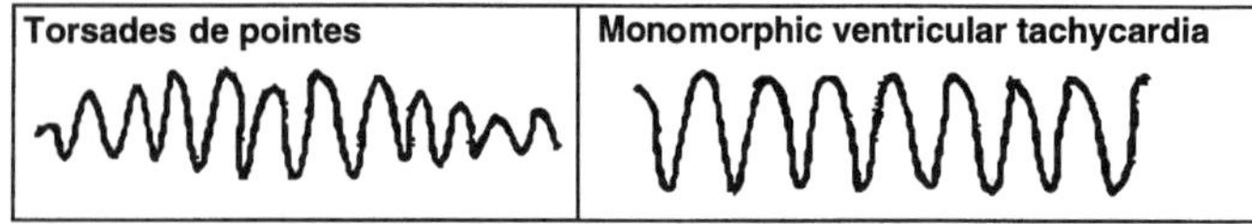

II. **Causes of prolonged QT:** Class IA antiarrhythmics (quinidine, procainamide, disopyramide), class III antiarrhythmics (amidarone), congenital prolongation, hypokalemia, hypocalcemia, hypomagnesemia, phenothiazines, tricyclic antidepressants, pentamidine, liquid protein diets, intracranial events, and bradyarrhythmias (especially third-degree atrioventricular block).

III. **Presentation:** lightheadedness, syncope, and sudden death.

IV. **Treatment**

1. For hemodynamically unstable patients: cardiovert with synchronized direct current
2. Congenital QT prolongation: beta blockers
3. Acquired
   a. Discontinue offending agent.
   b. Correct electrolyte abnormalities.
   c. **Magnesium sulfate, 1–2 gm IV over 3 min (10 ml of 20% solution), followed by 3–20 mg/min infusion.**
   d. Acceleration of sinus rate by cardiac pacing or with isoproterenol (isoproterenol is contraindicated in the setting of ischemic heart disease and, if given mistakenly for monomorphic ventricular tachycardia, will be detrimental).

Key Reference: Tzivoni D, Banai S, Schuger S, et al: Treatment of torsade de pointes with magnesium sulfate. Circulation 77:392–397, 1988.

Treatment of Unstable Angina

I. Clinically, unstable angina is defined as an increase in the frequency and severity of baseline angina due to coronary artery disease. New-onset angina could also be classified as unstable angina. The obvious concern of unstable angina is its progression to myocardial infarction. In fact, both unstable angina and the closely-related condition non-ST-segment elevation myocardial infarction (NSTEMI) are common manifestations of coronary artery disease.

II. **Early risk stratification**

1. In addition to a 12-lead ECG, biomarkers for cardiac injury, such as cardiac-specific troponin, should be obtained. In patients with negative cardiac markers within 6 hr of the onset of pain, another sample should be drawn in the 6–12 hr time frame.
2. If the repeat ECG and cardiac enzymes are negative, a stress test to provoke ischemia may be performed. Low-risk patients with a negative stress test can be managed as outpatients.

II. **Treatment**

1. **Aspirin**, 160–325 mg oral chewable. A thienopyridine (clopidogrel or ticlopidine) may be used for patients allergic or intolerant to aspirin.
2. **Heparin**, 5000–10,000 U IV bolus, then 10–15 U/kg/hr infusion, keeping partial thromboplastin time 1.5–2.5 times control.
3. A platelet **GP IIb/IIIa receptor antagonist** (eptifibatide or tirofiban) should be administered, in addition to aspirin and unfractionated heparin, to patients with continuing ischemia, to patients in whom a percutaneous coronary intervention is planned, and to patients with high-risk features such as accelerating tempo of ischemic symptoms, prolonged chest pain, pulmonary edema secondary to ischemia, age > 75 years, angina at rest, new bundle-branch block, sustained ventricular tachycardia, or elevated troponin. Abciximab can also be used for 12–24 hr in patients with unstable angina or NSTEMI in whom percutaneous coronary intervention is planned within the next 24 hrs.
4. **Nitroglycerin IV:** begin at 5 μg/min, then increase by increments of 5–20 μg/min every 5 min, titrating to relieve symptoms and target blood pressure (or until BP drops more than 10%).
5. **Beta blockers:** metoprolol, 5 mg IV bolus every 5 min times 3; if it is tolerated, then 50 mg orally every 6 hr for 48 hr, then 100 mg orally 2 times/day.
6. Consider a nondihydropyridine **calcium channel blocker** (e.g., verapamil or diltiazem) in nonresponders in the absence of severe left ventricular dysfunction or other contraindication. Avoid monotherapy with nifedipine, which may cause reflex tachycardia and worsening angina.
7. Consider an **angiotensin-converting enzyme inhibitor** (ACEI) when hypertension persists despite treatment with nitroglycerin and beta blockers in patients with left-ventricular systolic dysfunction or congestive heart failure and in acute coronary syndrome patients with diabetes mellitus.
8. Consider **angioplasty or bypass surgery** for patients refractory to medical therapy.

Key Reference: Braunwald E, et al: ACC/AHA guidelines for the management of patients with unstable angina and non-ST-segment elevation myocardial infarction: Executive summary and recommendations. Circulation 102:1193–1209, 2000.

Cocaine-induced Myocardial ischemia

I. The mechanisms of cocaine-induced myocardial ischemia include increased oxygen demand, vasoconstriction, in-situ thrombus formation, premature atherosclerosis, and left ventricular hypertrophy.

II. Therapy
   1. **Oxygen, benzodiazepines, aspirin, and nitroglycerin** are the mainstays of therapy.
   2. Phentolamine and calcium antagonists (verapamil) are second-line agents.
   3. Consider angioplasty or thrombolytics if myocardial infarction persists after above therapy.
   4. For ventricular arrhythmias immediately after cocaine use, $NaHCO_3$ may be a safer alternative than lidocaine (the proarrhythmic and proconvulsive effects of both lidocaine and cocaine are mediated through sodium-channel blockade). **Beta blockers are contraindicated** in this setting because they enhance cocaine-induced coronary vasoconstriction, increase blood pressure, fail to control heart rate, increase likelihood of seizures, and decrease survival.

   Reference: Hollander JE: The management of cocaine-associated myocardial ischemia. N Engl J Med 333:1267–1272, 1995.

Thrombolytic and Adjunctive Therapy in Acute Myocardial Infarction

I. In treating patients with acute myocardial infarction (MI), ensure comfort and relief of pain with narcotics, and offer reassurance to limit endogenous catecholamine output. Prophylaxis for deep venous thrombosis (patients are often already anticoagulated for the MI) and oxygen (as needed) are recommended.

II. **Original indications for thrombolytics:** chest pain consistent with acute MI, > 1 mm ST-segment elevation in at least two contiguous EKG leads, presentation within 12 hr of symptom onset, no contraindications to thrombolytic therapy.

III. **Expanded indications for thrombolytics:** no absolute contraindication on the basis of age, controllable hypertension and initial systolic blood pressure < 180 mmHg, new right or left bundle-branch block of unknown duration, cardiopulmonary resuscitation of < 5 min without known trauma.

IV. **Contraindications for thrombolytics:** recent or ongoing serious bleeding or bleeding tendency, major trauma, surgery, or delivery of baby within 10 days, uncontrolled hypertension, traumatic CPR, arterial vascular puncture at a noncompressible site, previous use (< 1 yr ago) of streptokinase or antistreplase (APSAC). For patients with contraindications to thrombolysis, timely measures to perform an emergent angioplasty should be taken.

V. **Aspirin**, 325 mg orally. All patients with acute MI should receive aspirin whether or not they receive thrombolytics (unless the patient has a severe allergy to aspirin).

VI. **Thrombolytic dosages**
   1. **Streptokinase (SK)**, 1.5 million U over 60 min (severe hypotension in < 5%)

      or
   2. **Tissue plasminogen activator (tPA)**, 10 mg bolus, 50 mg over first hr, 20 mg over each hour for 2 hr

      or

3. **Anisoylated plasminogen-streptokinase activator complex (APSAC)**, 30 mg over 5 min.

VII. **Heparinization.** Heparin use in patients given thrombolytics is controversial because of the increased risk of major bleeding. One recommendation is to start heparin concurrently with tPA for 5–7 days to decrease reocclusion rates. Keep PTT ~ 2–2.5 times control. For tPA, give heparin bolus of 100 U/kg, then 1000–1300 U/hr, and adjust as needed. For streptokinase or APSAC use, check PTT 2–3 hr after thrombolysis, and give maintenance heparin (without bolus) as needed to keep PTT ~ 2–2.5 times control, or give heparin. 5000–10,000 units every 12 hr subcutaneously.

VIII. **Analgesia: morphine** (4–8 mg IV every 5–30 min as needed for pain). **Meperidine** (25–50 mg IV) may cause less vagal stimulation, especially in patients with inferior wall MI.

IX. **Intravenous nitroglycerin:** begin at 5 μg/min, increase by 5 μg/min till pain is relieved or blood pressure drops more than 10%.

X. **Beta blockers: metoprolol** should be begun for all patients with no contraindications: 5 mg IV every 5 min times 3, then 25 mg orally every 8 hr, then 50 mg orally every 8 hr or 100 mg orally 2 times/day.

XI. **Management of bleeding complications from thrombolysis.** Major bleeding typically occurs with gastrointestinal or intracranial bleeds. Development of any focal neurologic deficit should be presumed to be an intracranial hemorrhage and treated empirically before obtaining diagnostic tests.

1. **Protamine sulfate** (antagonizes heparin), **50 mg slow IV over 1–3 min** (see also Administration of Protamine Sulfate in Pulmonology Section).
2. **Cryoprecipitate, 10 units IV** (may be repeated as needed), if fibrinogen is suspected to be low (typically within 6–8 hr after tPA, 30 hr after SK, and 36 hr after APSAC).
3. For continuing bleeding, give **2 units of fresh frozen plasma**.

Key Reference: Belli G, Topol EJ: Reperfusion and thrombolytic strategies for acute myocardial infarction. Contemp Intern Med 7:31–45, 1995.

Complications of Myocardial Infarction

I. **Ventricular septal rupture**

1. Occurs in ~4% of all MIs (⅔ occur with anterior wall MI and ⅓ occur with inferior wall MI), usually occurs 2–5 days after MI.
2. **Diagnosis**
   a. Holosystolic murmur, significant increase in left ventricular failure
   b. Oxygen saturation step-up from right atrium to right ventricle: (Qp/Qs) = shunt ratio = (SaO_2 – RA sat) / (SaO_2 – PA sat), where Qp = pulmonary blood flow, Qs = systemic blood flow, SaO_2 = oxygen saturation in arterial blood, RA sat = oxygen saturation in right atrium (proximal port), and PA sat = oxygen saturation in pulmonary artery (distal port).
   c. Large *v* wave in pulmonary capillary wedge pressure because of increased left atrium filling.
3. **Treatment.** Stabilizing measures include nitroprusside (0.3–10 μg/kg/min) and intraaortic balloon pump, followed by surgical correction. Medical therapy alone has a high (~ 90%) mortality rate. Surgical mortality is greater (70%) for rupture associated with inferior wall MI than with anterior wall MI (30%) for technical reasons.

II. **Right ventricular (RV) infarction**

1. **Complicates ~ 40% of inferior wall MI**, although not all RV infarcts are clinically significant.
2. **Presentation:** shock with isolated signs of RV failure such as jugular venous distention with few or no rales. Marked hypotensive response to nitrates in a patient with inferior wall MI suggests RV infarction. If severe hypoxemia that is refractory to 100% oxygen therapy occurs in the setting of a RV infarction, consider a right-to-left shunt through a patent foramen ovale (due to acute rise in right atrial pressure).
3. **Diagnosis**
   a. Clinical signs of shock, right ventricular failure in the setting of inferior wall MI.
   b. EKG: ST elevation in precordial right ventricular leads (e.g., in RV_1 and RV_2 leads).
   c. Echocardiogram: poorly contractile right ventricle.
   d. Right heart catheterization: increased RA pressure, steep y descent of the RA pressure tracing, narrowed PA pulse pressure, modest increase in LV filling pressure.
4. **Treatment**
   a. **Volume expansion** to increase RV filling (RA pressure > 20 mmHg) and thus augment LV filling.
   b. **Dobutamine** (5–20 μg/kg/min) often required because volume administration alone may increase RV distention to such an extent that LV filling is decreased.
   c. Dopamine (5–20 μg/kg/min) for refractory hypotension; use cautiously because it may increase pulmonary vascular resistance.

Reference: Ferguson JJ, et al: Significance of nitroglycerin-induced hypotension with inferior wall acute myocardial infarction. Am J Cardiol 64:311–314, 1989.

III. **Conduction blocks** in anterior wall MI, which may require temporary ventricular pacemaker

1. Alternating right bundle-branch block (RBBB) or left bundle-branch block (LBBB)
2. LBBB
3. RBBB with left axis deviation
4. RBBB with right axis deviation
5. Complete heart block
6. Mobitz type II second-degree block

IV. **Papillary muscle rupture with acute mitral regurgitation**

1. **Incidence is ~ 1%**, mainly with inferior wall MIs, due to rupture of posteromedial papillary muscle.
2. Patients present with **acute pulmonary edema** within 1 week after MI with holosystolic murmur at the apex that radiates to the axilla.
3. **Treatment**
   a. Nitroprusside, 0.3–10 μg/kg/min
   b. Dobutamine, 5–20 μg/kg/min
   c. Mitral valve repair or replacement

V. **Postinfarction angina**

1. Continue or resume IV heparin.
2. Add or increase beta blockade as tolerated.
3. Consider angioplasty or bypass graft surgery.

VI. **Cardiogenic shock** is the leading cause of death for patients hospitalized with acute myocardial infarction, and the mortality remains high during the following year. For patients with acute myocardial infarction with cardiogenic shock, early revascularization (percutaneous coronary angioplasty [PTCA] or coronary artery bypass graft [CABG]) at 6 hrs or less from onset of symptoms results in improved 6-month and 1-year survival rates compared with initial medical stabilization strategy of thrombolysis and intra-aortic balloon counterpulsation, with subsequent PTCA or CABG as required. Arrangements should be made for emergent cardiac catheterization and angioplasty as soon as possible.

1. Aspirin, 325 mg oral chewable
2. Heparin, 10,000 U bolus, then 1000 U/hr
3. Dopamine, 5–20 μg/kg/min
4. Dobutamine, 5–20 μg/kg/min
5. Nitroprusside, 0.3–10 μg/kg/min
6. Angioplasty with or without intraaortic balloon pump
7. For left main artery, severe three-vessel disease, or failed angioplasty, bypass surgery is needed.

Key References: Freed M Grines C: Essentials of Cardiovascular Medicine. Birmingham, MI, Physicians' Press, 1994, pp 60–62; Hochman JS, et al: Early revascularization in acute myocardial infarction complicated by cardiogenic shock. N Engl J Med 341:625–634, 1999; Hochman JS, et al. One-year survival following early revascularization for cardiogenic shock. JAMA 285:190–192, 2001.

Agents Used in Therapy for Shock

Agent	Dose	Receptor	HR/Contractility	Vasoconstriction	Vasodilation	Pearls
Dopamine (DA)	1–4 μg/kg/min 4–20 μg/kg/min	Dopami--nergic $\beta_1 \rightarrow \alpha_1$	2+/2+	0 2–3+	2+ 2–3+	DA also releases NE
Norepinephrine (NE)	1–50 μg/min	$\alpha_1, \alpha_2, \beta_1$	2+/2+	4+	0	
Epinephrine	0.5–1 mg IV/ET 0.3–0.5 mg IV/SC 1–8 μg/min	$\alpha_1, \alpha_2, \beta_1, \beta_2$	4+/4+			
Dobutamine	2.5–15 μg/kg/min	β_1	1+/4+	1+	2+	Less tachycardic than NE; contraindicated in IHSS
Phenylephrine (PE; Neosynephrine)	20–200 μg/min	α_1	0/0	4+	0	Hypotensive emergencies with spinal anesthesia*

IHSS = idiopathic hypertrophic subaortic stenosis.

* Useful when pressors such as DA or NE precipitate tachyarrhythmia because PE has purely alpha-adrenergic effects.

General Classification of Shock Syndromes

I. **Cardiogenic shock**
   1. Myopathic: acute MI, cardiomyopathy, myocardial depression of sepsis
   2. Mechanical: mitral regurgitation, ventricular septal defect, ventricular aneurysm, LV outflow obstruction (aortic stenosis, IHSS)
   3. Arrhythmic

II. **Extracardiac obstructive shock**
   1. Pericardial tamponade
   2. Constrictive pericarditis
   3. Massive pulmonary embolism
   4. Severe pulmonary hypertension
   5. Coarctation of the aorta

III. **Oligemic shock**
   1. Hemorrhage
   2. Fluid depletion

IV. **Distributive shock**
   1. Septic shock
   2. Overdose
   3. Anaphylaxis
   4. Neurogenic shock
   5. Endocrinologic shock

Key Reference: Parillo JE, Ayres SM (eds): Major Issues in Critical Care Medicine. Baltimore, Williams & Wilkins, 1984.

Anaphylaxis

I. An acute allergic reaction following exposure to an antigen that is recognized by IgE and involves release of mediators (mainly histamines and leukotrienes) from mast cells and basophils.

II. **Causes of anaphylaxis**

Immunologic mechanisms	Nonimmunologic mechanisms	Other disorders associated with increased histamine release
IgE-mediated: medications (e.g., penicillin, insulin), horse serum, foods, *Hymenoptera* stings, IgA-deficient recipient receiving IVIG (patients develop antibodies to IgA), allergen immunotherapy, seminal fluid, latex	**Direct activation of mast cells:** opiates, dextran, radiocontrast media, antibiotics (e.g., vancomycin, aminoglycosides)	Exercise-induced anaphylaxis; food-dependent, exercise-induced anaphylaxis; systemic cold-induced urticaria; systemic mastocytosis; sulfites; angiotensin-converting enzyme inhibitor; solar urticaria, idiopathic
Complement activation: blood and blood products, dialysis membranes	**Modulation of arachidonic acid metabolism:** NSAIDs, aspirin	

III. **Manifestations:** apprehension, disorientation, pruritus, urticaria, angioedema, and hypotension. GI symptoms include abdominal distention, vomiting, and diarrhea due to hyperperistalsis effects of histamine. Respiratory compromise caused by laryngeal edema, laryngospasm, bronchorrhea, and bronchospasm. Shock due to hypoxia, vasodilation, and hypovolemia from capillary leakage.

IV. **Diagnosis:** on clinical grounds. Mast cell tryptase is a useful test to obtain for retrospective diagnosis but is not available on an emergency basis. Histamine is evanescent in the blood and is hard to measure.

V. **Treatment**
   1. Stop offending antigen (e.g., stop medication, remove insect parts). Epinephrine, 0.2–0.3 ml of 1:1000 solution, around the sting site may delay absorption of more antigen. Tourniquet proximal to the injection site may delay systemic absorption of antigen.
   2. **Epinephrine**
      a. For life-threatening reactions (hypotension): **0.5 mg (5 ml of a 1:10,000 solution) IV every 5–10 min as needed** (also may be given sublingually or via endotracheal tube). An IV drip at 0.5–5 μg/min (1 ml of 1:1000 [1 mg] in 500 ml D_5W IV at 0.25–2.5 ml/min) may be required.
      b. For less severe reactions: **0.3–0.5 mg (0.3 ml–0.5 ml of 1:1000 solution) SQ every 20–30 min as needed for up to 3 doses.**
      c. Epinephrine dosages in self-injection kits
         - **Epipen or Ana-Kit:** 0.3 ml of a 1:1000 epinephrine solution (0.3 mg)
         - **Epipen Jr:** 0.15 mg
   3. **Maintain airway patency**
   4. **Beta agonists** (albuterol, 0.5 ml of 0.5% solution in 2 ml sterile saline, via nebulizer every 15–30 min) with or without aminophylline (load: 5–6 mg/kg) over 30 min. Maintenance of aminophylline: 0.2–0.9 mg/kg/hr to maintain serum level ~ 10–15 μg/dl [~ 55.5–83.25 μmol/L]) for treatment of bronchospasm.
   5. **Volume expansion** with normal saline with or without vasopressor.
   6. **Hydrocortisone**, 5 mg/kg IV every 6 hr (peak effect occurs in 6–12 hr), or methylprednisolone, 1 mg/kg IV every 6 hr for 24 hr.
   7. **Diphenhydramine**, 25–50 mg IV (IM or PO) every 6 hr, *or* **hydroxyzine (Atarax)**, 50–100 mg (IM or PO) every 6 hr.
   8. **Cimetidine**, 300 mg IV every 6 hr.

Key Reference: Bocher B, Lichtenstein L: Anaphylaxis. N Engl J Med 324:785–790, 1991.

Hypertensive Emergencies

I. **Causes:** abrupt increase in blood pressure (BP) in a patient with chronic hypertension (most common), renovascular hypertension, parenchymal renal disease, scleroderma or other collagen-vascular disease, drug ingestion (tricyclic antidepressants, sympathomimetic agents such as cocaine, amphetamines, phencyclidine, LSD, and diet pills), withdrawal from antihypertensive drugs (clonidine, beta blockers), preeclampsia/eclampsia, pheochromocytoma, acute glomerulonephritis, head injury, ingestion of tyramine with monoamine oxidase inhibitor, renin-secreting tumor, vasculitis, autonomic hyperactivity with Guillain-Barré or other spinal cord syndromes.

II. **Definition** of malignant/accelerated hypertension (HTN)
   1. Marked blood pressure elevation (diastolic BP > 130 mmHg)
   2. Neuroretinopathy → necrotizing arteriolitis
      a. Accelerated HTN: flame-shaped hemorrhages, cotton-wool (soft) exudates
      b. Malignant HTN: accelerated HTN + papilledema

III. **Clinical syndromes** associated with malignant hypertension: renal disease, hypertensive encephalopathy (mental status changes, seizures, focal neurologic deficits), neuroretinopathy, pulmonary edema, disseminated intravascular coagulation, weight loss, pancreatitis, gastrointestinal bleeding.

IV. **Types of hypertensive emergencies and treatment recommendations.** In general reduce BP by 20% (e.g., diastolic BP 150 → 120). If patient tolerates it, reduce diastolic BP by 10% every 2–4 hr until diastolic BP ~ 90 mmHg.

Type of Hypertensive Emergency	Recommended Treatment	Drugs to Avoid
Hypertensive encephalopathy	Nitroprusside, labetalol, diazoxide	Beta blockers, methyldopa, clonidine
Cerebral infarction	No treatment, nitroprusside, labetalol	Same as above
Intracerebral or sub-arachnoid hemorrhage	Same as above	Same as above
Myocardial ischemia/infarction	Nitroglycerin, labetalol, calcium blockers, nitroprusside	Hydralazine, diazoxide, minoxidil
Acute pulmonary edema	Nitroprusside + furosemide Nitroglycerin + furosemide	Hydralazine, diazoxide, beta blockers, labetalol
Aortic dissection	Nitroprusside + beta blockers Trimethaphan + beta blockers Labetalol	Hydralazine, diazoxide, minoxidil
Eclampsia	Hydralazine, diazoxide, labetalol, calcium blockers, nitroprusside	Trimethaphan, diuretics, beta blockers
Acute renal insufficiency	Nitroprusside, labetalol, calcium blockers	Beta blockers, trimethaphan
Grade II or IV Keith-Wagener funduscopy	Same as above	Beta blockers, clonidine, methyldopa
Microangiopathic hemolytic anemia	Same as above	Beta blockers

V. **Parenteral Medications**

Drug	Mode	Onset	Duration	Dosage	Adverse effects
Nitroprusside	IV infusion	Immediate	2–3 min	0.5–10 μg/kg/min	Thiocyanate and cyanide toxicity
Diazoxide	IV bolus IV infusion	1–5 min	6–12 hr	50–100 mg every 5–10 min, up to 600 mg; 15–30 mg/min	May worsen cardiac ischemia CHF Dissection
Labetalol	IV bolus IV infusion	5–10 min	3–6 hr	20–80 mg every 5–10 min, up to 300 mg; 0.5–2 mg/min	CHF Bronchospasm Paradoxical HTN
Nitroglycerin	IV infusion	1–2 min	3–5 min	5–100 μg/min	Headache Nausea and vomiting
Phentolamine	IV bolus	1–2 min	3–10 min	5–10 mg; repeat as necessary	Angina- Headache- Paradoxical HTN
Trimethaphan	IV infusion	1–5 min	10 min	0.5–5 mg/min	Ileus Urinary retention Respiratory arrest Mydriasis Dry mouth

(Table continued on next page.)

Drug	Mode	Onset	Duration	Dosage	Adverse effects
Hydralazine (eclampsia)	IV bolus	10–20 min	3–6 hr	5–10 mg; repeat every 20 min as needed	Fetal distress Thrombo-phlebitis
Diltiazem	IV infusion			Load 0.25 mg/kg over 2 min, then 5 mg/hr infusion. Increase as tolerated and needed to 15 mg/hr	
Nicardipine	IV infusion	1–5 min	3–6 hr	5 mg/hr; increase by 1–2.5 mg/hr every 15 min, up to 15 mg/hr	Headache Tachycardia, Nausea and vomiting

CHF = congestive heart failure.

VI. Reduced cerebral perfusion is a concern when patients with malignant hypertension are treated too aggressively. Normally the cerebral blood flow remains constant between mean blood pressure of 60–160 mmHg. However, in patients with chronic uncontrolled hypertension, the autoregulatory range is higher; therefore, with BP reduction, cerebral ischemia may develop.

Key Reference: Calhoun DA, Oparil S: Treatment of hypertensive crisis. N Engl J Med 323: 1177–1183, 1990 (source of table).

Nitroprusside

I. **Dose: 0.3–10 μg/kg/min**

II. **Uses**
 1. Combined with beta blockers to decrease LV pressure rise (dp/dt) in aortic dissection.
 2. Malignant hypertension.
 3. Afterload reducing agent in patients with congestive heart failure.

III. **Metabolism:** by sulfhydryl groups in red blood cells to **cyanogen** (cyanide radical). Cyanogen is metabolized in the liver by thiosulfate sulfurtransferase (rhodanase) to **thiocyanate**. The second step depends on the availability of sulfur donors; e.g., thiosulfate and cysteine.

IV. **Contraindication:** patients with compensatory hypertension (e.g., arteriovenous shunts or coarctation of the aorta).

V. **Warnings**
 1. Rates > 2 μg/kg/min may generate cyanogen in amounts greater than methemoglobin can effectively buffer.
 2. May increase intracranial pressure; use with caution in patients with decreased glomerular filtration rate, hepatic insufficiency, hypothyroidism, and hyponatremia.

VI. **Toxicity**
 1. The toxic effects of cyanogen may be rapid and fatal, manifested by **venous hypoxemia** (secondary to the inability of tissues to extract O_2 from RBCs), **lactic acidosis, dyspnea, vomiting, dizziness, ataxia, confusion, and death.**
 2. Metabolic acidosis is one of the most reliable signs of cyanogen toxicity.
 3. May result in sequestration of hemoglobin or methemoglobin when cyanogen combines with methemoglobin to form cyanmethemoglobin. Suspect

methemoglobinemia in patients who exhibit signs of impaired oxygen delivery despite adequate cardiac output and PaO_2.

VII. **Treatment of toxicity**

1. Rationale: cyanogen-cytochrome oxidase complex is converted to cyanomethemoglobin-cytochrome oxidase complex (nontoxic) by **nitrites**. Cyanogen gradually dissociates from cyanomethemoglobin and is converted to thiocyanate by **thiosulfate** therapy.
2. **Amyl nitrite inhalation** while sodium nitrite is prepared.
3. **3% sodium nitrite** (4–6 mg/kg = 0.2 ml/kg of 3% = 14 ml in a 70-kg person) IV over 4 min (which produces about 10% methemoglobinemia and may cause vasodilatation and hypotension).
4. **10% or 25% solution of sodium thiosulfate** in a dose of 150–200 mg/kg (e.g., 50 cc of 25% solution).
5. May repeat 3 and 4 at one-half the initial doses after 2 hr.
6. Hemodialysis removes thiocyanate but not cyanogen.

Cardiac Tamponade

I. **Pathophysiology.** When the intrapericardial pressure exceeds right atrial (RA) and right ventricular (RV) diastolic pressures, the transmural pressure distending these chambers becomes close to zero, and tamponade results. Further accumulation of fluid causes both the intrapericardial and RV diastolic pressure to rise to the level of the left ventricular diastolic pressure, which also rises. The result is a marked decrease in the diastolic volumes of both ventricles and a fall in stroke volume. Reduced tissue perfusion, including the myocardium, occurs. Occurrence of tamponade depends on the **volume** of the effusion and the **rapidity** with which the fluid accumulates. In cardiac trauma, tamponade may occur with only 50–100 ml of blood.

II. **Causes. Tamponade** most often results from bleeding into the pericardial space after cardiac surgery (postpericardiotomy syndrome), **trauma, malignancy** (lung, breast, lymphoma), myocardial infarction (in patients receiving heparin), tuberculosis, myxedema, systemic lupus erythematosus, aortic dissection, pericarditis (idiopathic, viral, postirradiation, uremic, anticoagulant-precipitated). Although cardiac involvement occurs in only 2% of patients with thoracic actinomycosis, the most common sites of involvement are the pericardium (50% tamponade, 40% constrictive pericarditis), myocardium (50%), and endocardium (35%).

III. **Diagnosis**

1. Severe, acute tamponade may result in the classic finding of hypotension, increased venous pressure, and faint heart sounds. For most other cases, signs resemble heart failure.
2. **Pulsus paradoxus.**
   a. Defined as a > 10 mmHg inspiratory decrease in systolic arterial pressure. In normal patients, there is an inspiratory decline of LV stroke volume by ~ 7% and systemic arterial pressure by ~3%. It is believed to occur secondary to differential filling of the two ventricles during inspiration. Normally inspiration enhances RV filling, causing a shift of the interventricular septum toward the LV, reducing the LV dimensions, and thereby reducing systemic cardiac output and blood pressure. The presence of a tamponade exaggerates this process. Thus, pulsus paradox in tamponade is critically dependent on the inspiratory augmentation of systemic venous return and RV filling.
   b. Pulsus paradoxus may be detected by an inspiratory decrease in the amplitude of the palpated pulse in the femoral or carotid arteries. Total paradox

(complete disappearance of the palpated pulse during inspiration) occurs with severe tamponade or tamponade with hypovolemia. Alternatively, inflate cuff 20 mmHg above systolic pressure and slowly deflate until the Korotkoff sounds are heard only during expiration. The cuff is then deflated to the point at which the Korotkoff sounds are heard equally well in inspiration and expiration. The difference between these pressures is the estimated magnitude of the pulsus paradoxus.

c. Paradox may also be seen in restrictive cardiomyopathy, constrictive pericarditis (occurs in about one-third of such patients), massive pulmonary embolism, hypovolemic shock (absent jugular vein pulse [JVP]), and severe obstructive lung disease. Pulsus paradox may be absent in cardiac tamponade when (1) left ventricular hypertrophy (LVH) or heart failure causes a marked elevation of LV diastolic pressure so that the LV resists the inspiratory effects of increased RV filling, (2) pulmonary hypertension and right ventricular hypertrophy (RVH) impede the inspiratory increase in RV filling, or (3) atrial or ventricular septal defect is present.

3. **Chest x-ray.** In acute hemopericardium, the cardiac silhouette may be normal in size. Large effusion results in a water-bottle configuration. Tension pneumopericardium results in air between the myocardium and pericardium.
4. **Echocardiogram** (not 100% specific or sensitive)
   a. Pericardial effusion should be present (exception is the postoperative cardiac patient in whom loculated fluid or thrombus may cause compression).
   b. Pulsus paradox: sudden leftward motion of the septum during inspiration and an exaggerated increase in RV size with reciprocal decrease in LV size.
   c. Diastolic RA and RV collapse (RV collapse may be absent in RVH).
5. **EKG.** Decreased QRS amplitude, electrical alternans of the P, **QRS**, and T waves (reflects pendular swinging of the heart in the pericardial space).
6. **Equalization of intracardiac pressures** (i.e., pulmonary capillary wedge pressure $\approx P_{RA,\ diast} \approx P_{RV,\ diast} \approx P_{PA,\ diast}$)

IV. **Treatment:** needle pericardiocentesis (see Procedure Section), surgical pericardiotomy.

Key Reference: Lorell BH, Braunwald E: Pericardial disease. In Braunwald E (ed): Heart Disease, 4th ed. Philadelphia, W.B. Saunders, 1992.

Valvular Heart Disease

I. **Aortic stenosis (AS)**

1. **Causes:** rheumatic disease (almost always with concomitant mitral valve disease), degenerative calcification of aortic cusps (especially of bicuspid AV)
2. **Pathophysiology.** All based on obstruction to left ventricular (LV) outflow. Systolic pressure gradient between LV and aorta > 50 mmHg or aortic orifice < 0.5 cm^2 / body surface area (m^2) is considered critical. LV dilatation; left ventricular hypertrophy (LVH) is compensatory. Increased LV end-diastolic pressure (LVEDP) due to LV failure or LVH; ischemia due to (1) increased demand from LVH and (2) excessive myocardial compression of the coronaries that may exceed coronary perfusion pressure. Aortic stenosis intensifies mitral regurgitation.
3. **Presentation.** Severe AS may be asymptomatic for years because of compensatory LVH.
   a. Exertional dyspnea: due to increased LVEDP from LVH or heart failure
   b. Angina pectoris: usually the initial clinical manifestation.

c. Exertional syncope: precipitated by peripheral vasodilatation in the presence of a fixed cardiac output or by arrhythmia.
d. Late: congestive heart failure

4. **Auscultation/examination**
   a. Systolic crescendo-descrendo ejection murmur, low-pitched, and loudest at the 2nd right intercostal space (ICS) → to the jugular notch and along carotids.
   b. Single S_2 or paradoxical splitting of S_2 (P_2 preceding A_2) due to prolongation of LV systole.
   c. S_4 due to LVH, S_3 with heart failure.
   d. Blood pressure may fall and pulse pressure narrows with severe AS.
   e. Delayed carotid upstroke.
   f. Increased right atrial *a* wave (increased jugular vein pressure) due to bulging of the hypertrophied interventricular septum into the right ventricle.
   g. Point of maximal impulse (PMI) displaced inferiorly and laterally due to LVH. Systolic thrill at base of the heart, in the jugular notch, and along carotids (accentuated by expiration with the patient leaning forward).
5. **Chest radiograph.** LVH: rounding of the cardiac apex, poststenotic dilatation of the ascending aorta, aortic calcification (absence of calcification in an adult essentially rules out severe AS). Late: cardiac enlargement with dilatation.
6. **EKG.** LVH with strain pattern, atrioventricular or intraventricular conduction defects due to calcification / fibrosis of involved myocardium, left atrial abnormality with associated mitral valve disease.
7. **Treatment.** Avoidance of exertion, volume depletion, and vasodilator therapy. Digitalis for heart failure. Aortic valve replacement in symptomatic patients before development of heart failure. Balloon valvuloplasty for temporizing relief of symptoms or as a bridge to valve replacement in the very ill.

II. **Aortic regurgitation (AR)**

1. **Causes:** rheumatic disease, infective endocarditis, congenital bicuspid valve, aortic dilatation (syphilis, ankylosing spondylitis, Marfan's syndrome), aortic dissection, myxomatous transformation of the leaflets.
2. **Pathophysiology:** increased stroke volume and increased systolic blood pressure (BP) due to the regurgitant volume. LV dilatation is compensatory to accommodate the increased LVEDV. Heart failure due to increased LV systolic tension (wall tension = intracavitary pressure times radius); myocardial ischemia due to decreased diastolic BP, Venturi effect, decreased coronary reserve, and increased requirement due to wall thickening and dilatation. In acute AR, the compensatory mechanisms are absent, and patients present with markedly elevated LVEDP, low ejection fraction, and marked tachycardia.
3. **Presentation** may remain asymptomatic for many years in chronic AR. In contrast, acute AR may present dramatically with:
   a. **Signs of heart failure** when compensatory mechanisms are overcome
   b. **Myocardial ischemia**
4. **Auscultation/examination.** High-pitched, blowing **descrendo diastolic murmur**, heard best in third left intercostal space (left ICS in primary AR, right ICS in AR due to aortic dilatation) with the diaphragm of the stethoscope with the patient sitting up, leaning forward, and breath held in forced expiration. The murmur may become holosystolic with severe AR. A **loud systolic ejection murmur** from base of heart to the jugular notch and carotids. **Austin Flint murmur:** a soft low-pitched rumbling middiastolic or presystolic bruit (due to displacement of the mitral valve by the regurgitant stream). $\mathbf{S_3}$ with or without $\mathbf{S_4}$. **Corrigan's pulse** (water-hammer pulse felt in femoral arteries), **Quincke's pulse** (visible capillary pulsations in nail beds), **Duroziez's sign** (diastolic and systolic murmur heard in femoral artery with with compression),

de Musset's sign (head bobbing with each systole), **Traube's sign** (pistol-shot sounds over the femoral artery), **Müller's sign** (systolic pulsation of uvula), widened pulse pressure due to elevated systolic pressure and lowered diastolic pressure, **PMI displaced laterally and inferiorly, hyperdynamic precordium, systolic thrill** along jugular notch and carotids due to increased blood flow, **diastolic thrill** along left sternal border. Many of these peripheral pulse signs are absent in patients with acute AR.

5. **Chest radiograph.** LV enlargement in chronic AR, with or without aortic dilatation. Patients with acute AR may have normal-sized myocardium with pulmonary edema, and patients with chronic AR may have enlarged heart and clear lung fields.
6. **EKG:** LVH with strain in chronic AR; sinus tachycardia with acute AR.
7. **Treatment**
   a. For **acute AR**, afterload reduction with nitroprusside (beta blockade first if due to aortic dissection). Urgent valve replacement is the mainstay of therapy although patients with infective endocarditis may be treated with antibiotics for several days before surgery. Intraaortic balloon pump is contraindicated.
   b. For **chronic AR**, medical therapy consists of digitalis, afterload reduction (e.g., hydralazine, captopril, or nifedipine), and diuretics for congestive symptoms. Unlike aortic stenosis, patients with chronic AR may not experience improvement in heart failure following valve replacement. Thus valve replacement is timed to symptomatic patients who have deteriorating but **not** severe LV dysfunction.

III. **Mitral stenosis (MS)**

1. **Causes:** rheumatic disease, congenital condition, malignant carcinoid, systemic lupus erythematosus, rheumatoid arthritis, amyloid deposits, methysergide therapy, mitral annulus calcification.
2. **Pathophysiology:** critical MS is defined as $\leq 1\ cm^2$ of mitral valve (MV) opening. Increased left atrial pressure, increased pulmonary venous, capillary, and arterial pressures leading to right heart failure. Tachycardia and atrial fibrillation increase the transmitral valvular pressure gradient and thus the left atrial pressure (doubling the flow rate quadruples the pressure gradient).
3. **Presentation**
   a. Shortness of breath precipitated by physical exertion, infection, or atrial fibrillation
   b. Hemoptysis
   c. Chest pain
   d. Systemic thromboembolism due to left atrial thrombus: cerebral, coronary, renal
   e. Infective endocarditis
4. **Auscultation/examination:** Opening snap (occurs during diastole due to sudden tensing of the valve leaflets), diastolic murmur of MS is low-pitched, rumbling, best heard at the apex with the bell of the stethoscope, and follows the opening snap. The duration, not the intensity, of the murmur correlates with the severity of the stenosis. A short A_2–opening snap interval is a reliable indicator of severe MS. Auscultation is facilitated in a left lateral decubitus position.
5. **Chest radiograph:** left atrial enlargement, pulmonary hypertension right ventricular enlargement, signs of congestive heart failure, pulmonary hemosiderosis.
6. **EKG:** left atrial abnormality (p terminal force in $V_1 > 0.04$ sec). RVH: QRS axis $> 80°$ and R:S ratio in $V1 > 1$.
7. **Treatment:** endocarditis prophylaxis, anticoagulation, prophylaxis with digitalis or beta blockers against rapid atrial fibrillation, balloon valvuloplasty, surgery with commissurotomy or valve replacement.

IV. **Mitral regurgitation (MR)**

1. **Causes:** rheumatic disease, myxomatous degeneration, infective endocarditis, ruptured chordae tendinae, congenital condition.
2. **Pathophysiology:** increased LVEDV in chronic MR; in acute MR, there is no time for a compensatory increase in LA and LV compliance. Thus, pulmonary venous congestion occurs, leading to acute pulmonary edema and right heart failure.
3. **Presentation.** Chronic MR may be asymptomatic for many years with slow progression of LV dysfunction; in acute MR, because of acute diastolic overload in the uncompensated LV, there is acute pulmonary edema and hypotension.
4. **Auscultation/examination:** apical holosystolic murmur, enlarged PMI.
5. **Chest radiograph:** enlarged LV and LA, pulmonary edema, calcification of leaflets (rheumatic disease), and calcification of annulus (degenerative).
6. **EKG:** left atrial abnormality, ± atrial fibrillation.
7. **Treatment.** For chronic MR, patients should be considered for mitral valve replacement or repair when ejection fraction (EF) approaches 50–55% because once EF falls significantly, marked LV dysfunction has already occurred. The treatment for acute MR consists of afterload reduction with nitroprusside, furosemide, intraaortic balloon pump, and surgery.

V. **Tricuspid regurgitation (TR)**

1. **Causes:** rheumatic disease, endocarditis, RV infarction, cardiomyopathies, carcinoid syndrome, pulmonary hypertension of any cause.
2. **Pathophysiology:** elevation of mean RA pressure due to the regurgitant volume.
3. **Presentation:** predominantly right heart failure with ascites, peripheral edema, bowel edema.
4. **Auscultation/examination:** prominent CV (regurgitant) wave in the RA.
5. **Chest radiograph/EKG:** RV enlargement, right atrial enlargement, RV strain, pulmonary hypertension pattern, atrial fibrillation.
6. **Treatment.** Treat underlying disorder (e.g., pulmonary hypertension), nitrates, angiotensin-converting enzyme inhibitors, and for severe refractory TR, consider tricuspid valve repair or valve replacement.

VI. **Tricuspid stenosis (TS)**

1. **Causes:** rheumatic disease (often occurs with mitral or aortic valve disease); isolated TS may be seen with carcinoid syndrome and systemic lupus erythematosus.
2. **Pathophysiology:** decreased diastolic flow across valve, elevated right atrial pressure, and decreased cardiac output.
3. **Presentation:** chronic right heart failure (or biventricular failure with aortic or mitral valve involvement), dyspnea.
4. **Auscultation/examination:** prominent *a* wave, diastolic rumble best heard at left lower sternal border and accentuated during inspiration.
5. **Chest radiograph/EKG:** large P wave of right atrial enlargement in absence of RV hypertrophy; enlarged RA without significant enlargement of pulmonary arteries.
6. **Treatment:** diuretics, venodilators (nitrates). Consider balloon valvuloplasty.

VII. **Idiopathic Hypertrophic Subaortic Stenosis**

1. **Pathophysiology:** the anterior leaflet of MV plays an active role in the obstruction.
2. **Presentation:** angina, syncope, congestive heart failure.
3. **Auscultation/examination:** dehydration or Valsalva maneuver increases obstruction, increasing systolic ejection murmur; in contrast, squatting decreases obstruction and murmur. Carotid upstroke has a spike and dome pattern.

4. **Chest radiograph, EKG, and echocardiography** reveal increased septal thickness, systolic anterior motion, LVH.
5. **Treatment:** increase intravascular volume to increase LV cavity and decrease obstruction, beta blockers, calcium blockers, phenylephrine (0.02–0.18 mg/min IV to increase systemic vascular resistance and decrease outflow obstruction) myomectomy. **Avoid** digitalis or diuretics.

Key Reference: Carabello BA, Crawford FA: Valvular heart disease. N Engl J Med 337:32–41, 1997.

Cardioversion

I. **Indications**
   1. Supraventricular tachycardias (SVTs) that are unstable (emergent) or stable (elective).
   2. Ventricular tachycardia with pulse: rapid or unstable (asynchronous cardioversion) or slow rate and stable (treat medically first, then synchronous cardioversion if still present).

II. **Conditions with relative refractoriness**
   1. Long-standing atrial fibrillation (AF) or atria > 4.5 cm.
   2. Torsades de pointes: consider cardioversion for hemodynamic instability, but effect may be temporary until cause of the torsade (e.g., hypokalemia) is corrected.
   3. Ventricular tachycardia or fibrillation associated with amiodarone.

III. **Relative contraindications**
   1. Digitalis intoxication: cardioversion may result in profound bradycardia or degeneration into ventricular tachycardia or fibrillation.
   2. Stable AF of unknown duration because patients may require period of prior anticoagulation

IV. **Technique**
   1. **Informed consent** if feasible.
   2. **Premedication** (all should be given slowly)
      a. Etomidate, 0.3 mg/kg IV over 30–60 sec *or*
      b. Midazolam, 1–2 mg IV, repeat if needed every 2–5 min
   3. Consider **prophylactic endotracheal intubation** in patients whose oxygenation and mental status are marginal and may worsen with sedation.
   4. **Adjuvant medical therapy**
      a. **Ventricular tachycardia:** lidocaine
      b. **SVT:** verapamil, esmolol, adenosine
      c. **AF:** quinidine or procainamide may help to prevent reversion into AF.
   5. **Synchronous cardioversion** may be attempted if the operator agrees with the monitor that the highlighted segment is the R wave. The synchronous mode is used for SVT and stable ventricular tachycardia. If there is disagreement or the defibrillator does not recognize a QRS complex, use the **asynchronous mode**.
   6. **Energy**
      a. Atrial flutter: 5–50 joules (J)
      b. AF or SVT: 50–360 J, typically 200 J for AF and 100 J for SVT
      c. Stable ventricular tachycardia: < 100 J
      d. Guide for incremental increase: 10 J for the first 50 J, then 25–50 J for > 50 J

V. **Adverse sequelae**
   1. Elevations of isoenzymes of creatine kinase containing MM and MB subunits are common but are mostly clinically insignificant.

2. **Postshock arrhythmias**
   a. Postshock supraventricular or ventricular tachyarrhythmias may occur (dilated cardiomyopathy may increase risk).
   b. Bradycardia and atrioventricular block: risk factors include remote or recent myocardial infarction, digitalis intoxication, sick sinus syndrome, and concurrent antiarrhythmics (e.g., beta blockers)
3. **Systemic embolization:** anticoagulation is recommended for 2–3 weeks before elective cardioversion and for 3–4 weeks after cardioversion for AF of unknown duration. Absence of thrombi on transesophageal echocardiography obviates the need for anticoagulation before cardioversion.
4. **Atrial electrical-mechanical dissociation.** Related issues include:
   a. Need for anticoagulation for several weeks after cardioversion of AF
   b. Risk for pulmonary edema because right atrial activity frequently returns before left atrial activity after cardioversion.

Key Reference: Rogove HJ, Hughes CM: Defibrillation and cardioversion. Crit Care Clin 8:839–863, 1992.

Myocardial Injury in the Critically Ill

Myocardial injury in critically ill patients is a frequent occurrence of critical illness that often goes unrecognized and is associated with increased morbidity and mortality. Myocardial injury was detected in 15% (32) of 209 patients admitted to a respiratory/medical ICU over an 8-week period by an elevation of cardiac troponin I. Using measurements of creatine kinase isoenzyme with M and B subunits (CK-MB) and EKG, acute infarction (injury) was detected in only 12 (38%) of the 32 patients. Patients with myocardial injury were more likely to be hypotensive (75% vs. 50%), require vasopressors (53% vs. 24%), have congestive heart failure (35% vs. 14%), experience arrhythmias (44% vs. 17%), and require mechanical ventilation (66% vs. 27%) than patients without injury. Overall mortality was 19% vs. 41% in patients with elevated troponin I levels. In most instances, the complications followed the myocardial injury.

Reference: Guest TM, et al: Myocardial injury in critically ill patients: A frequently unrecognized complication. JAMA 273:1945–1949, 1995.

Acute Pericarditis

I. It is extremely important to distinguish acute pericarditis from acute myocardial infarction because pericarditis is a major contraindication to lytic therapy.

	Pericarditis	**Myocardial infarction**
Reciprocal segment depression	Absent	Present
Echocardiography	Pericardial effusion	Regional wall motion abnormality
Pain quality	Pleuritic	Pressure, visceral

II. **Causes:** idiopathic, myocardial infarction, infection (tuberculosis, viral), uremia, connective tissue disorder, irradiation, drugs, and thoracic surgery.

III. **Purulent pericarditis** with or without tamponade. Consider in anyone with refractory hypotension due to bacteremic sepsis, especially with staphylococcal infections and, less commonly, gram-negative bacilli. Patients who recently had thoracic surgery are also at increased risk as are patients with preexisting pericardial effusion (e.g., uremic pericarditis), burns, and immunosuppression (leukemia, lymphoma, AIDS). Pericarditis may result from contiguous spread of infection from a pleural, mediastinal, or pulmonary focus. High fevers, chills, and dyspnea are the most common signs and symptoms. Unlike viral pericarditis, pericardial chest pain is often absent in bacterial pericarditis. Mortality is high because of low index of suspicion.

IV. **Treatment.** In the case of viral or immunologic pericarditis, antiinflammatory agents such as NSAIDs, aspirin, and prednisone are recommended. In the case of purulent pericarditis, treatment consists of prolonged antibiotic therapy (4–6 weeks) and aggressive drainage of the pericardium. Subxiphoid pericardiotomy is usually required, and pericardiectomy is occasionally required.

Key Reference: Rubin RH, Moellering RC: Clinical, microbiologic and therapeutic aspects of purulent pericarditis. Am J Med 59:68–78, 1975.

Constrictive Pericarditis

I. **Common causes** of constrictive pericarditis are neoplasm, radiation, infection (tuberculosis), idiopathic disease, and trauma.

II. **Clinical manifestations**

1. Insidious symptoms include those due to **low cardiac output** (fatigue, tachycardia, relative hypertension) and **right-sided heart failure** (jugular vein distention, hepatomegaly, ascites, edema). Jugular vein pressure is increased with **steep y** (and x) **descent** and a pericardial knock. **Kussmaul's sign:** an inspiratory increase in systemic **venous** pressure, common in chronic constrictive pericarditis but rare in tamponade.
2. A normal-appearing pericardium on CT or MRI argues against the diagnosis. There is a < 5 mmHg difference between the mean right atrial pressure, right ventricular diastolic pressure, left ventricular diastolic pressure, and pulmonary artery wedge pressure. **A dip-and-plateau (square root sign) configuration is seen in the ventricular waveform.**

III. **Cardiac tamponade and constrictive pericarditis** share important features, including impaired diastolic filling. However, in constrictive pericarditis, ventricular filling is unimpeded during early diastole but reduced abruptly when the elastic limit of the pericardium is reached. In cardiac tamponade, ventricular filling is impeded throughout diastole. In both, systemic and pulmonary venous pressures are increased, cardiac output is decreased, and left and right ventricular diastolic pressures are equalized. Tamponade involves a dominant x descent, whereas constrictive pericarditis involves a rapid y descent. Kussmaul's sign (increased right atrial pressure with inspiration) occurs in constrictive pericarditis, whereas pulsus paradoxus occurs in tamponade.

Aortic Dissection

I. Occurs when blood disrupts the aorta by dissecting between the intima and the media.

II. **Predisposing conditions:** presence of cystic medial necrosis (normal aging process, Marfan's syndrome, long-standing, poorly-controlled hypertension), Ehlers-Danlos syndrome, Turner's syndrome, coarctation of aorta, and pregnancy.

III. **Proximal dissection:** arising in the ascending aorta. **Distal dissection:** arising in the descending aorta distal to the left subclavian artery. Prognosis depends on whether the ascending aorta is involved.

IV. **Presentation.** Patients appear shocklike but with elevated blood pressure.
1. Severe chest pain (tearing) that may radiate to the back
2. Myocardial infarction
3. Strokes
4. Aortic insufficiency
5. Cardiac tamponade
6. Unequal pulses, peripheral limb ischemia
7. Horner's syndrome, pleural effusions

V. **Chest radiograph** may be normal or display a widened cardiac shadow or separation of mural calcification from the edge of the aorta (calcium sign).

VI. **Diagnosis:** for patients who are hemodynamically compromised, transesophageal echocardiography; for stable patients, MRI.

Test	Comments
Transesophageal echocardiogram	Sensitivity ~ 99% Specificity ~ 75–98%
Transthoracic echocardiogram	May show an aortic dissection if it is within 2–3 cm from the aortic valve
CT scan	As good as angiography and may even show dissection when angiography is considered normal. CT scan is the second procedure of choice following transesophageal echocardiogram
Angiogram	Vast experience required; a normal study does not rule out dissection
MRI	High sensitivity and highest specificity. However, it is often not available and not appropriate for the unstable patient.

VII. **Treatment.** Monotherapy with vasodilators may increase shear forces and extend the dissection.
1. Beta blockers (metoprolol, 5 mg IV every 5 min × 3, then 50 mg orally every 6 hr) + nitroprusside (0.5–10 μg/kg/min).
2. Distal dissection: medical therapy, then surgery if progression.
3. Proximal dissection: surgery.

Key Reference: Nienaber CA, von Kodolitsch Y, Nicolas V, et al: The diagnosis of thoracic aortic dissection by noninvasive imaging procedures. N Engl J Med 328:1–9, 1993.

Congestive Heart Failure with Normal Systolic Function

I. Patients present with signs and symptoms of congestive heart failure in which the pulmonary artery catheter may reveal an increased pulmonary artery wedge pressure and normal or elevated ejection fraction.

II. **Differential diagnosis**
1. **Volume overload** (e.g., iatrogenic or in the setting of oliguric renal failure).
2. **Regurgitant valvular lesion** results in the overestimation of the forward flow during systole.
3. **Diastolic dysfunction:** in the setting of hypertension, ischemic heart disease, idiopathic hypertrophic subaortic stenosis, hypertrophic cardiomyopathy, and aortic stenosis. In these disorders, congestive heart failure is due to increased resistance to filling and accounts for ~ 20% of all heart failure episodes.

4. **High-output heart failure:** hyperthyroidism, anemia, pregnancy, arteriovenous fistulas, beri beri (thiamine deficiency), and Paget's disease.

III. In patients with diastolic dysfunction, treatment with inotropic agents, diuretics, and vasodilators may be detrimental.

IV. **Treatment**

1. **Correction of underlying disorder** (e.g., blood transfusion for anemia, thiamine for beri beri) may result in dramatic improvement in cardiogenic shock, and diuretics or dialysis for volume overload.
2. **Maintain adequate intravascular volume** in the case of diastolic dysfunction. Careful titration of diuretics and venodilators (e.g., nitroglycerin) may be required to relieve congestive symptoms, although excessive amounts may result in worsening symptoms because of further decreased filling.
3. In patients with hypertension and left ventricular hypertrophy, **negative inotropes** such as a calcium channel blocker or beta blocker may decrease the resistance to filling in patients with diastolic dysfunction.
4. **Treat atrial tachyarrhythmia** aggressively with a calcium-channel blocker or beta blocker to control the rate because tachycardia only worsens the already compromised cardiac filling in diastolic dysfunction.

Key Reference: Freed M, Grines C: Essentials of Cardiovascular Medicine. Birmingham, MI, Physicians' Press, 1994, pp 112–113.

Cardiac Enzymes

I. Enzymes measured include **creatine kinase (CK)-MB, lactate dehydrogenase (LDH), and cardiac troponin.**

II. **CK-MB fractions**

1. In **myocardial infarction (MI)**, elevation occurs within 4–6 hr of chest pain, peaks at ~ 12–20 hr, and returns to baseline at 36–48 hr. The normal total CK varies slightly with the laboratory but is ~ 24–195 mg/dl (55–170 U/L for males, 30–135 U/L for females). CK-MB > 10 mg/dl and the relative index (CK-MB/total MB) > 5% are highly suggestive of MI.
2. **Other causes of elevated CK-MB** include cardiac resuscitation with high energy defibrillation, myocarditis, cardiac surgery, small bowel infarction, renal infarction, esophageal ischemia, rhabdomyolysis, polymyositis, and muscular dystrophy, hypothyroidism, prostatic or bronchogenic carcinomas.

III. **LDH measurements.** Increased LDH is detectable in the serum 12 hr after onset of MI, peaks in 24–48 hr, and may remain elevated 10–14 days after MI. Normally the **LDH1/LDH2** ratio is less than 1. **A ratio > 1.0 is evidence for a myocardial source.**

IV. **Troponin measurements.** Cardiac troponin I (cTnI) is a highly specific protein for the heart and a measure for cardiac injury. Its specificity is ~ 98–99% vs. ~ 85% for CK-MB. cTnI is elevated within 6 hr of onset of MI, peaks in 12 hr, and remains elevated for at least 6 days after onset of symptoms. Recommended times for obtaining samples (from onset of chest pain): 0, 6, 12, and 24 hr.

1. ≤ 0.5 ng/ml: normal
2. 0.6–1.4 ng/ml: subtle changes
3. ≥ 1.5 ng/ml: positive for MI or myocardial source

Key References: Antman EM, Tanasijevic MJ, Thompson B, et al: Cardiac-specific troponin I levels to predict the risk of mortality in patients with acute coronary syndromes. N Engl J Med 335:1342–1349, 1996; Dunagan WC, Ridner ML: Manual of Medical Therapeutics, 26th ed. Boston, Little, Brown, 1989.

Common Intravenous Cardiac Drug Dosages

Drug	Indications	Dosage
Adenosine	Supraventricular tachycardia	6 mg IV bolus over 1–2 sec, then 12 mg IV every 1–2 min × 2 as needed
Amrinone	Congestive heart failure	Initial dose: 0.75 mg/kg IV bolus over 2–3 min, then 5–10 μg/kg/min Maximal dose is 10 mg/kg/day
Bretyllium tosylate	Ventricular tachyarrhythmia	**Load:** 5–10 mg/kg IV every 15–30 min to total dose of 30 mg/kg **Maintenance:** 0.5–2.0 mg/min
Digoxin	Atrial tachyarrhythmia, inotropic support	**Load:** 0.5 mg IV , then 0.25 mg every 4 hr to 1.25 mg total load
Diltiazem	Atrial tachyarrhythmias	**Load:** 0.25 mg/kg (~20 mg) over 2 min (repeat load at 0.35 mg/kg [~ 25 mg] over 2 min in 15 min as needed) **Infusion:** 5 mg/hr; increase as tolerated and needed to 15 mg/hr
Dobutamine	Inotropic support	2.5–20 μg/kg/min. Maximal rate is 40 μg/kg/min.
Dopamine	Shock	2.5–10 μg/kg/min Maximal rate is 20–50 μg/kg/min For renal perfusion 0.5–5 μg/kg/min
Epinephrine	Bradycardia (not cardiac arrest)	2–10 μg/min
Esmolol	Supraventricular tachyarrhythmia	Loading: 500 μg/kg/min × 1 min, then 50 μg/kg/min × 4 min May repeat loading as needed and increase infusion by 50 μg/kg/min every 4 min as needed to a maintenance of 50–200 μg/kg/min
Labetalol	Hypertension Aortic dissection	20 mg IV over 2 min, then 40–80 mg IV every 10 min as needed and as tolerated
Lidocaine	Symptomatic ventricular tachyarrhythmia	Bolus: 50–100 mg IV over 2–4 min May repeat bolus; then 1–4 mg/min
Metoprolol	Acute MI, unstable angina	5 mg IV every 5 min times 3 If tolerated, 50 mg orally every 6 hr (15 min after last IV dose), then 100 mg orally 2 times/day
Nitroglycerin	Hypertension, acute MI, unstable angina	Start at 5 μg/min, increase infusion by 5–20 μg/min every 5 min to relief of symptoms, target blood pressure, or blood pressure drops by > 10%
Nitroprusside	Hypertension, cardiogenic shock	0.3–10 μg/kg/min
Norepinephrine	Hypotension, shock	Initial dose at 8–12 μg/min; titrate to blood pressure
Phenylephrine	Shock	0.1–0.18 mg/min, adjust to desired blood pressure (typical dosage is 0.04–0.06 mg/min)

(Table continued on next page.)

Drug	Indications	Dosage
Procainamide	Atrial tachyarrhythmia	**Load:** 15–20 mg/kg (max 1000 mg) over 30 min (≤ 20 mg/min) **Maintenance:** 1–6 mg/min
Verapamil	Supraventricular tachycardia	5–10 mg IV over 2 min; repeat 10 mg in 30 min if needed

Key Reference: Freed M, Grines C: Essentials of Cardiovascular Medicine. Birmingham, MI, Physicians' Press, 1994.

Gastroenterology

Fulminant Hepatic Failure

I. **Definition:** acute liver failure associated with encephalopathy and coagulopathy within 8 weeks of symptom onset.

II. **Causes:** hepatitis A virus, hepatitis B with or without hepatitis D virus, hepatitis E virus, herpes simplex virus, **acetaminophen**, halothane (especially in obese, atopic, middle-aged women), *Amanita phalloides* poisoning, phosphorus, CCl_4, fatty liver of pregnancy, Reyes' syndrome, Wilson's disease, hyperthermia, autoimmune hepatitis, iron overload, alpha-1 antitrypsin deficiency, and **septic shock**. Survival is better in young patients and in fulminant hepatic failure (FHF) due to acetaminophen.

III. **Encephalopathy.** Encephalopathy is due to **cerebral edema > ammoniagenesis**. Grade correlates with other complications and mortality. Withdrawal of dietary protein and administration of lactulose may offer more benefit during early than late stages of encephalopathy. **Encephalopathy may progress precipitously; therefore, early endotracheal intubation is recommended.**

1. **Grade 1:** altered sleep habits, altered affect (euphoria or belligerence), loss of spatial orientation
2. **Grade 2:** drowsy but responsive to simple commands; asterixis present
3. **Grade 3:** stuporous, responsive only to painful stimuli
4. **Grade 4:** unresponsive to painful stimuli

IV. **Cerebral edema with intracranial hypertension** (major cause of death)

1. Develops in 75–80% of patients with grade 4 encephalopathy; both vasogenic and cytotoxic types of edema are seen.
2. **Features:** increased blood pressure, decerebrate posturing with increased muscle tone, hyperventilation, abnormal pupillary reflexes, and impaired brainstem reflexes. **Papilledema is unusual** in FHF.
3. **Intracranial pressure monitoring** (see also Neurology section)
   a. **Normal intracranial pressure (ICP)** is 10–15 mmHg.
   b. **Cerebral perfusion pressure (CPP) = MAP – ICP**, where MAP = mean arterial pressure.
   c. Goals are to keep ICP < 20 mmHg and CPP > 50 mmHg. If **ICP > 20–25 mmHg, give mannitol, 0.5–1.0 gm/kg every 4 hr as needed** as long as osmolarity < 320 (in patients with renal failure, combine mannitol with ultrafiltration). Diurese, and keep sodium infusion to a minimum.
   d. **Monitors**
      - Although intraventricular pressure monitoring is most accurate, the compression of the ventricles by the swollen brain makes them difficult to catheterize and involves increased risk of infection and bleeding. In general, bleeding risk far outweighs any benefits.
      - Subdural ICP monitoring may be helpful in identifying patients with prolonged increase ICP who would no longer be a liver transplant candidate due to permanent neurologic injury.
      - Subarachnoid bolt: less risk of infection and bleeding, but focal seizures and hematoma may result.
4. If resistant to mannitol, try **pentobarbital, 5–10 mg/kg load** as tolerated by blood pressure and CPP; **maintenance: 2–5 mg/kg** as needed to maintain ICP.

5. Hyperventilation to induce alkalosis may be beneficial in acute events, but **sustained hyperventilation is not useful**. Chronic hyperventilation may theoretically decrease resistance in splanchnic bed and portal blood flow, further compromising hepatic function.
6. Keep head elevated at 30°, still, and midline.
7. Lidocaine, 1 mg/kg IV, before intubation may blunt rise in ICP.
8. Treat hyperthermia (common with FHF); increased temperature increases ICP by increasing cerebral blood flow.

V. **Renal failure** occurs in ≈ 75% of patients with grade 4 encephalopathy with acetaminophen overdose.

VI. **Hypoglycemia** needs close monitoring because encephalopathy masks symptoms.

VII. **Metabolic acidosis** is a marker of high mortality in acetaminophen overdose, independent of renal failure.

VIII. Increased risk of **infection, gastrointestinal hemorrhage, and respiratory and circulatory failure**.

IX. **Prognostication and consideration for orthotopic liver transplantation.** The following patient selection criteria should be considered for orthotopic liver transplantation because the likelihood of survival without transplant is < 20%:

1. **Acetaminophen:** (1) **pH < 7.30** independent of encephalopathy stage *or* (2) stage 3 or 4 encephalopathy, prothrombin time (PT) > 100 sec (INR > 6.5), and serum creatinine > 3.5 mg/dl (> 300 μmol/L), which are associated with a poor prognosis (~ 5% chance of survival with medical therapy alone).
2. **Other causes:** (1) **PT > 100 sec** (INR > 6.5) independent of encephalopathy stage *or* (2) **3 of the following 5 variables** also associated with poor prognosis with medical therapy alone:
   a. Age < 10 or > 40 years
   b. Indeterminate cause, halothane, or drugs other than acetaminophen
   c. INR > 3.5
   d. Bilirubin > 17.5 mg/dl (> 100 μmol/L)
   e. Duration of jaundice before onset of encephalopathy > 7 days
3. If intracranial hypertension resolves, patients usually survive even without liver transplantation.
4. Persistent CPP < 50 mmHg is associated with poor neurologic prognosis, even with liver transplantation.

Key Reference: Lee WM: Acute liver failure. N Engl J Med 16:1862–1872, 1993.

Liver Disease Associated with Pregnancy

I. **Liver disease associated with pregnancy** usually occurs in the third trimester and often in association with preeclampsia or eclampsia.

II. **Differential diagnosis**:

1. **Acute fatty liver of pregnancy** (hypoglycemia, increase in prothrombin time, increase in bilirubin, modest increase in alanine aminotransferase [SGPT] and aspartate aminotransferase [SGOT], microvesicular steatosis of the liver).
2. **HELPP syndrome** (**h**emolysis, **e**levated liver function tests, **l**ow platelets; resembles disseminated intravascular coagulation of sepsis but with hypertension and **p**roteinuria)

3. **Hepatic rupture** (sudden abdominal pain with bloody paracentesis fluid); (4) **hepatic infarction** (high fever, signs of preeclampsia or eclampsia, right upper quadrant pain, extreme increase in SGOT and SGPT).

III. **Treatment** is supportive, with delivery of the fetus.

Hepatic Encephalopathy

I. **Causes:** cirrhosis, hepatic artery occlusion, Budd-Chiari syndrome, and venoocclusive disease of the liver. The hepatic encephalopathy (HE) due to FHF is due mainly to cerebral edema and has a worse prognosis than HE due to chronic liver disease.

II. **Precipitating causes:** upper GI bleeding, infections (consider occult sepsis, spontaneous bacterial peritonitis), renal insufficiency (e.g., diuretics, sepsis), hypokalemic metabolic alkalosis and other electrolyte and acid–base disturbances, vomiting, diarrhea, constipation, diuretic therapy, noncompliance with medications (e.g., lactulose), increased protein intake, sedatives (benzodiazepines, morphine, barbiturates), hypoglycemia, trauma, surgery.

III. **Diagnosis.** Although essentially a diagnosis of exclusion in a patient with cirrhosis or FHF, hepatic encephalopathy (HE) should be treated empirically and aggressively.

1. Signs of chronic liver disease may be present but by themselves do not validate the diagnosis of HE because other causes of encephalopathies may occur simultaneously.
2. Electroencephalogram (EEG) may help to differentiate HE from focal brain abnormalities and seizure activities. Paroxysmal triphasic waves, which appear in later stages of HE, are characteristic but not specific for HE.
3. Fetor hepaticus: subjective and not necessarily specific for liver disease.

IV. **Treatment**

1. Treat any precipitating factors; in cases of FHF, monitor meticulously for hypoglycemia.
2. **Lactulose**
   a. Lactulose not only serves as an osmotic cathartic but also acidifies the colon (after it is metabolized by colonic bacteria to lactic acid), which may serve to trap low-molecular-weight nitrogenous substances in the colon. Lactitol may be preferable in the outpatient setting because it is significantly less sweet.
   b. **Oral dose:** for rapid catharsis during initial treatment of HE, 30–45 ml orally every 1 hr until stooling, then 15–45 ml orally 2–4 times/day. Adjust maintenance dose to 2–3 soft stools/day.
   c. **Enemas:** 300 ml lactulose + 700 ml tap water via retention enema with the patient on left side in Trendelenburg position.
3. **Neomycin**, 1 gm orally every 4 hr, or **metronidazole**, 250 mg orally every 8 hr. Consider combination therapy with lactulose and neomycin in refractory cases, although nephrotoxicity from neomycin is possible.
4. **Flumazenil** may be useful as an adjunct in the diagnosis of HE. A dose of 0.2–0.5 mg over 30 sec may be tried, but infusion appears not to be cost-effective.
5. Consider **branch-chain amino acid feedings** because patients may be able to tolerate higher protein loads.
6. **Experimental drugs** to promote hepatic regeneration: insulin and glucagon, cytosolic extracts from regenerating liver.

7. **For patients with FHF**, treat cerebral edema as noted in previous section and monitor for hypoglycemia. Consider liver transplantation for stage 3 or 4 HE + FHF; hepatic cell infusion.

Key Reference: Gammal SH, Jones EA: Hepatic encephalopathy. Med Clin North Am 73:793–813, 1989.

Hepatorenal Syndrome

I. **Definition:** hepatorenal syndrome (HRS) is a complication of advanced liver disease in which renal failure occurs in the absence of intrinsic or anatomic renal dysfunction. Occasionally, HRS may complicate fulminant hepatic failure. It is occasionally precipitated in cirrhotics by large volume paracentesis performed without albumin replacement. When there is rapid reaccumulation of ascites, the effective plasma volume is decreased, resulting in increase renin activity, decrease cardiac output, and increase systemic vascular resistance. These events result in decrease perfusion pressure to the kidneys.

II. **Major criteria:** (1) low glomerular filtration rate (serum creatinine > 1.5 or 24 hr urine creatinine clearance < 40 ml/min); (2) absence of shock, ongoing bacterial infection, fluid losses, and current treatment with nephrotoxic drugs; (3) no substantial improvement in renal function following diuretic withdrawal and/or expansion of plasma volume; (4) proteinuria < 500 mg/dl (< 5 gm/L), and (5) no ultrasound evidence of obstructive uropathy.

III. **Additional criteria:** (1) urine volume < 500 ml/day; (2) urine sodium < 10 mmol/L; (3) urine osmolality > plasma osmolality; (4) urine red blood cell < 50 per high power field; and (5) plasma sodium < 130 mmol/L.

IV. **Treatment** is usually unsuccessful. Every effort should be made to prevent or treat concomitant renal dysfunction, such as cautious use of nephrotoxic drugs, treating infections, and ensuring that the patient is not intravascularly depleted. Because prerenal azotemia mimics HRS, a cautious trial of fluid resuscitation may be tried. Transjugular intrahepatic portosystemic shunt (TIPSS) may help in some cases.

V. **Median survival** for hepatorenal syndrome is ~ 2 weeks, although recovery of renal function may occur with recovery of hepatic function.

Management of Acute Bleeding Esophageal Varices

I. **Volume resuscitation** with saline, packed red blood cells, and fresh frozen plasma to reverse any coagulopathy.

II. Consider **endotracheal intubation** for airway protection.

III. **Lavage patient for endoscopy** to confirm diagnosis and possible endoscopic variceal ligation ("banding") or sclerotherapy.

IV. Consider one of the following **vasoconstrictor regimens**, although a meta-analysis has found that somatostatin is more likely to achieve initial control of bleeding than vasopressin. Thus the somatostatin analogs are considered the agents of choice. These agents should be begun as soon as possible, even before patients enter the ICU.

   Reference: Imperiale TF, et al: A meta-analysis of somatostatin versus vasopressin in the management of acute esophageal variceal hemorrhage. Gastroenterology 109:1289–1294, 1995.

1. **Somatostatin** acts more selectively at the mesenteric circulation.
   a. Mechanism is reduction in splanchnic blood flow by inhibiting the release of vasodilatory gastrointestinal peptides such as glucagon, vasoactive intestinal peptide, and substance P.
   b. Dosage is 250 μg bolus, then 250 μg/hr.
2. **Octreotide** is a long-acting somatostatin analog with strong antisecretory and antimotility effects.
   a. Intracellular inhibition of adenylate cyclase with accumulation of cyclic adenosine monophosphate decreases intracellular calcium and secretion. It decreases splanchnic blood flow, thereby lowering variceal pressures. Half-life is 90–155 min.
   b. **Dose for bleeding esophageal varices:** 50–100 μg IV bolus, then 25–50 μg/hr for 48 hr

   Reference: Lamberts SWJ, et al: Octreotide. N Engl J Med 334:246–254, 1996.
3. **Vasopressin** (Pitressin)
   a. 20 U load IV, then 0.1–0.9 U/min IV (typically **0.2–0.4 U/min**).
   b. **Adverse effects:** cardiac and gastrointestinal ischemia and increased afterload due to potent vasoconstriction; cardiac arrhythmias and decreased contractility; nausea, belching, and cramps due to increased gut motility from smooth muscle stimulation, acute renal failure, and hyponatremia.
4. **Vasopressin and vasodilators**
   a. Nitroglycerin dilates peripheral arteries and enhances vasopressin by further reducing portocollateral resistance by venodilation.
   b. **Dose of nitroglycerin:** 40–400 μg/min IV; keep systemic blood pressure > 100 mmHg.
5. **Terlipressin**, a synthetic analog of vasopressin, has long duration of action. Pharmacologic effect may last 6 hr after a single (2-mg) bolus IV.

V. **Endoscopic variceal ligation** ("banding") is considered the preferred treatment over sclerotherapy because of its lower complication rates (e.g., less bacteremia, strictures, and perforation).

VI. **Endoscopic sclerotherapy.** Injection sclerotherapy is 90–95% effective in controlling variceal hemorrhage and seems to be superior to balloon tamponade or pharmacologic therapy alone. **Combined pharmacologic and endoscopic therapy** (e.g., somatostatin + sclerotherapy) appears to be more effective than either alone. Complications include perforation (1–3%), aspiration (5–7%), pyrexia, and pain. Several agents can be used for sclerosis:
1. **Sodium morrhuate:** a mixture of sodium salts of the fatty acids present in cod liver oil.
   a. On venous injection, it causes inflammation of the intima, which may cause thrombus formation.
   b. **Side effects:** hypersensitivity reaction, fever, chest pain, mucosal ulceration. Acute respiratory distress syndrome (ARDS) is rare (if it occurs at all) because only 20% of the injected morrhuate reaches the lung and causes no change in diffusing capacity.
2. **Sodium tetradecyl sulfate:** no impairment of pulmonary function.
3. **Ethanolamine oleate:** side effects include pleural effusion, pulmonary edema, pneumonia, anaphylactic reactions, acute renal failure, pyrexia, and retrosternal discomfort.

VII. **Pulmonary complications of sclerotherapy**
1. Pleural effusions (common): typically exudative with normal pH, glucose, and amylase; unilateral or bilateral.
2. Pneumonia and empyema due to aspiration or perforation.

3. Retrocardiac or mediastinal densities due to paraesophageal/contiguous mediastinal inflammation.
4. Perforation: avoid barium in suspected cases of esophagopleural fistula; avoid water-soluble contrast in cases suspected of esophagobronchial fistula; in uncertain cases, use water-soluble contrast for diagnosis because the former fistula is more common.
5. Atelectasis
6. Rarely ARDS (probably due to underlying disease and not to sclerosant).

VIII. **Sengstaken-Blakemore tube**

1. After the tube is inserted into the stomach, the gastric ballon is inflated with 100 ml of air, then 400 ml of air, and pulled back into the cardia of the stomach. If bleeding does not stop, the esophageal balloon is inflated for additional tamponade.
2. Great care must be taken with dilation of the esophageal balloon because of possible rupture or necrosis. Intermittent suction from proximal port or a proximal nasogastric tube is required to prevent aspiration.

IX. **Percutaneous transjugular intrahepatic portosystemic shunt (TIPSS)** has been shown to be an effective salvage therapy for patients who fail pharmacologic and/or endoscopic therapy (e.g., bleeding continues or re-bleeding in 48 hrs). TIPSS is generally considered to be a "bridge" to transplant and reserved for transplant candidates. It is performed in the angiography suite.

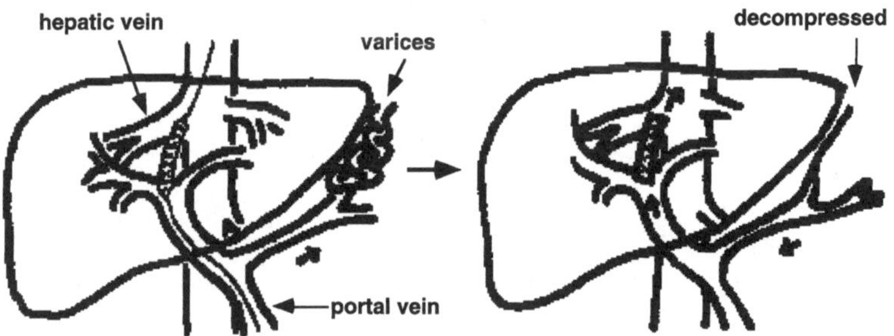

1. First, the hepatic vein is cannulated. Second, the needle is passed through the liver parenchyma into an intrahepatic branch of the portal vein, as confirmed angiographically by retrograde flow of dye. Third, an expandable metallic stent is placed, connecting the hepatic vein with the portal vein.
2. **Gastric varices**: patients with isolated gastric varices bleeding may have an underlying splenic vein thrombosis, an entity best treated with splenectomy. Sclerotherapy with the standard agents are significantly less effective in bleeding gastric varices from portal hypertension. TIPSS may be the best option in preliminary studies.
3. **Beneficial aspects** include: (1) effective control of acute bleeding and often prevents further variceal bleeding when TIPSS patency maintained, (2) increase sodium excretion and decrease ascites due to decrease activity of antinatriuretic system, (3) improved renal function in patients with hepatorenal syndrome.
4. **Complications** include (1) shunt occlusion, (2) increased incidence of encephalopathy (25%), (3) intraabdominal bleeding into the liver capsule, biliary tree, or peritoneum, (4) acute renal failure, (5) bacteremia, and (6) right-sided heart failure.

X. **Portosystemic surgical shunts** are used as a last resort; mortality rate is ~ 50%.

1. **Nonselective shunts:** end-to-side or side-to-side portocaval shunt (essentially a surgical TIPSS) and proximal splenorenal shunt; decompresses the entire portal system and more likely to cause hepatic encephalopathy.

2. **Selective (distal splenorenal) shunt:** decompresses only the varices while maintaining blood flow into the liver itself. The distal end of the splenic vein (receiving blood from the portal circulation in the cirrhotic patient via collaterals) is anastomosed to the left renal vein (which drains into the inferior vena cava).

XI. **Role of prophylactic antibiotics**
1. Cirrhotic patients with acute gastrointestinal hemorrhage have a high risk of developing bacterial infections, which are associated with poor outcome and failure to control the hemorrhage.
2. A meta-analysis has shown that patients who are treated with prophylactic antibiotics had fewer episodes of bacterial infection, bacteremia, and spontaneous bacterial peritonitis, and had better survival compared to untreated patients. Regimens included oral or combinations of intravenous and oral agents that included fluoroquinolones, amoxicillin + clavulinic acid, oral aminoglycosides, vancomycin, nystatin, and colistin for 4–10 days.
3. A reasonable regimen is ciprofloxacin iv during active bleeding, followed by oral administration for at least 3 days after cessation of bleeding.

XII. **Recalcitrant or repeated bleeding** may also be an indication for liver transplant.

Key References: DeSimone JA, et al: Sustained bacteremia associated with transjugular intrahepatic portosystemic shunt (TIPS). Clin Infect Dis 30:384-386, 2000; Navarro V, Guadalupe GT: Variceal hemorrhage. Crit Care Clin 11:391–414, 1995; Pratt DS, Epstein SK: Recent advances in critical care gastroenterology. Am J Respir Crit Care Med 161:1417–1420, 2000.

Portal Vein Thrombosis

I. Portal vein thrombosis should be considered in patients with evidence of portal hypertension (e.g., variceal hemorrhage) but no evidence of liver disease. However, it also may be seen in patients with cirrhosis and hepatoma. There may be associated splenomegaly. In contrast, acute occlusion is associated with acute ascites.

II. **Causes**
1. Pancreatic cancer, hepatocellular cancer
2. Pancreatitis, diverticulitis, hepatic abscess, septicemia
3. Myeloproliferative disorder, other hypercoagulable state
4. Liver transplantation
5. Splenectomy
6. Cirrhosis: in some series, up to 25% will be found

III. Typically occurs in middle-aged adults with evidence of portal hypertension. Splenomegaly may be massive. Bleeding from variceal hemorrhage is the most frequent reason for seeking medical attention. Small bowel infarction may occur due to thrombus extension into superior mesenteric vein.

IV. A good screening test is **ultrasonography with dopplers**, provided all pertinent structures are seen. Accuracy is enhanced by addition of Doppler techniques.

V. **Treatment** for portal vein thrombosis is uniformly poor. Treat underlying disorder (e.g., myeloproliferative disorder) or its complications (e.g., esophageal varices). Treatment for portal vein thrombosis itself is limited. Chronic anticoagulation and thrombolysis are generally ineffective or contraindicated. Depending on the location and extent of the thrombosis, a portosystemic shunt procedure may be tried.

Key Reference: Cohen J, Edelman RR, Chopra S: Portal vein thrombosis: A review. Am J Med 92:173–182, 1992.

Acute Cholecystitis

I. Gallstones impacted in the cystic duct are the major cause of acute cholecystitis. In the critical setting, however, one should also consider **acalculous cholecystitis (ACC)**, which accounts for ~ 2–10% of all cholecystitis. The pathogenesis of ACC is not known, but bile stasis is believed to be a major factor.

II. **Risk factors for ACC** include postoperative period (nonbiliary), severe trauma, burns, total parenteral nutrition, multiorgan failure, and immunocompromise (AIDS, cancer, chemotherapy, leukemia, lymphoma, uremia, advanced age).

III. **Signs and symptoms** include epigastric pain radiating to the right upper quadrant, nausea, vomiting, referred pain to the right shoulder or scapula, fever, and chills. Jaundice suggests cholangitis. Murphy's sign: inspiratory arrest when the patient takes a deep breath while the examiner's fingers are held under the liver border. However, patients with ACC usually not symptomatic because many are critically ill, intubated and sedated.

IV. **Diagnostic tests**

1. In diagnosing acute cholecystitis by **real-time ultrasonography**, the following findings may be noted:
   a. **Major criterion:** Gallstones or nonvisualized gallbladder
   b. **Minor criteria:** Gallbladder wall > 5 mm
      Tenderness of the gallbladder with ultrasound probe
      Gallbladder > 5 cm in any dimension
      Pericholecystic fluid
2. **^{99m}Technetium-labeled derivatives of iminodiacetic acid (e.g., HIDA) scans** are a sensitive way to diagnose acute cholecystitis in which a positive scan is nonvisualization of the gallbladder. False-positive scans may occur with total parenteral nutrition, alcoholism, and prolonged fast. False-negative scans (visualization of the gallbladder in the presence of cholecystitis) may occur with ACC.

V. **Causative organisms** include gram-negative rods (*Escherichia coli, Klebsiella, Enterobacter* and *Proteus* spp., *Streptococcus faecalis, Bacteroides fragilis,* and *Clostridia* and *Fusobacterium* spp.

VI. **Sepsis and septic shock** are potential complications of untreated cholecystitis. Other infectious complications include empyema, emphysematous cholecystitis (more common in diabetics, higher mortality rate, greater association with *Clostridia* sp.), pericholecystic abscess, intraperitoneal abscess, peritonitis, cholangitis (inflammation and infection of the hepatic and common bile ducts with Charcot's triad: biliary colic, jaundice, and fever [with rigors]; Raynold's pentad: Charcot's triad + hypotension and mental confusion), liver abscess, and perforation.

VII. **Treatment of cholecystitis or ACC**

1. Cholecystectomy
2. Percutaneous transhepatic cholecystostomy (contraindication: gallbladder perforation)

VIII. **Treatment of acute cholangitis**

1. IV hydration, antibiotics
2. Biliary decompression by endoscopic sphincterotomy and stone extraction or percutaneous transhepatic drainage are the treatment of choice
3. Cholecystectomy, common bile duct exploration + T-tube placement

Key Reference: Frazee RC, Nagorney DM, Mucha P: Acute acalculous cholecystitis. Mayo Clin Proc 64:163–167, 1989.

Diarrhea in Critically Ill Patients

I. The causes of diarrhea may be classified according to **five clinical syndromes:**
   1. **Cholera-like syndromes.** Small bowel involvement with watery diarrhea, dehydration, with or without nausea and vomiting, and no fecal leukocytes. Causes include *Vibrio cholerae*, enterotoxigenic *Escherichia coli* (ETEC, traveler's diarrhea), *Staphylococcus aureus, Giardia* sp., and initial phase of shigellosis.
   2. **Dysenteric syndromes.** Invasive/inflammatory colonic involvement with fever, bloody stool, abdominal cramping, tenesmus, and positive fecal leukocytes. Causes include *Shigella* sp., enteroinvasive *E. coli* (EIEC), enterohemorrhagic *E. coli* (EHEC, causes hemolytic uremic syndrome), *Clostridium difficile* (pseudomembranous colitis), *Campylobacter* sp., *Salmonella enteritidis,* and *Entamoeba histolytica.*
   3. **Diarrhea associated with systemic disorders.** May be due to organisms that cause a primary enteric illness, such as *Salmonella typhi* (typhoid) and *Salmonella paratyphi* (paratyphoid fevers), or nonenteric illnesses (e.g., *Legionella* sp., toxic shock syndrome, localized intraabdominal or pelvic infections such as diverticulitis, appendicitis, pelvic abscesses, ischemic colitis, mesenteric ischemia, intestinal vasculitis, toxic megacolon, and inflammatory bowel disease).
   4. **Nosocomial diarrhea**. Causes include enteral feeding (due to osmotic load), drugs (quinidine, colchicine, digitalis, magnesium-containing compounds, lactulose, antibiotics, chemotherapy, and sorbitol-containing compounds), nosocomial infections (enteric pathogens, *C. difficile, Candida* sp.)
   5. **Diarrhea in immunosuppressed patients.** Causes include:
      a. **Necrotizing enterocolitis** typically occurs in the setting of chemotherapy-induced neutropenia and is characterized by colonic inflammation caused by toxins from *Clostridium* sp. or gram-negative bacilli with fever, abdominal tenderness, thickened cecal wall with or without gas within the colonic wall, and mortality rate > 50%.
      b. **Hypogammaglobulinemia**, with spruelike syndrome of diarrhea, steatorrhea, protein-losing enteropathy, and malabsorption.
      c. **Radiation-induced diarrhea** may occur within the first or second week of therapy or not until years after treatment.
      d. **AIDS-associated diarrhea** may be due to traditional pathogens, such as *Shigella, Salmonella, Campylobacter,* and *Giardia* spp. and *E. histolytica,* but also to opportunistic pathogens such as *Cryptosporidium* sp., *Isospora* sp., *Mycobacterium avium*-complex, cytomegalovirus, and HIV itself.

II. **Laboratory tests**
   1. **Fecal leukocyte:** presence indicates nonspecific colonic inflammation; it is positive in cases of bacterial dysentery as well as pseudomembranous colitis. Its presence is an indication for obtaining stool culture.
   2. **Stool for ova and parasites** should be obtained for protracted diarrhea and in patients who have visited developing countries or day-care centers or are homosexual.
   3. **Stool for *C. difficile* toxin** in suspected cases of pseudomembranous colitis.

III. **Treatment**
   1. **Fluid and electrolyte replacement:** oral rehydration is recommended if there are no contraindications.
   2. **Empiric antibiotic therapy** is generally reserved for patients with evidence of bacterial dysentery.

a. **Industrial countries.** *Shigella* and *Campylobacter* spp., EIEC: norfloxacin, 400 mg 2 times/day, *or* ciprofloxacin, 500 mg 2 times/day, *or* ofloxacin, 200 mg 2 times/day, for 3–5 days.
b. **Severe watery diarrhea.** *Salmonella* sp. and ETEC: trimethoprim-sulfamethoxazole.
c. **Hemorrhagic colitis.** EHEC: antibiotics generally not indicated.

3. Antibiotic therapy includes (but is not limited to):
   a. ***Salmonella* sepsis and typhoid fever:** trimethoprim-sulfamethoxazole, 160–320 mg trimethoprim, 800–1600 mg sulfamethoxazole, 2 times/day, *or* ampicillin, 1.5 gm every 6 hr, *or* chloramphenicol, 1 gm orally or IV every 8 hr, *or* cefotaxime 2–12 gm/day or ceftriaxone 1–2 gm/day for 2 weeks.
   b. ***Campylobacter* sp:** erythromycin, 500 mg 4 times/day for 3–5 days.
   c. **Cholera:** tetracycline, 250–500 mg 4 times/day for 3–5 days.
   d. ***C. difficile* (pseudomembranous colitis):** metronidazole, 250 mg orally every 6 hr, *or* vancomycin, 125 mg orally 4 times/day for 10 days.
   e. **Necrotizing enterocolitis:** antibiotics effective against aerobic and anaerobic enteric pathogens are recommended.

Key Reference: Arduino RC, DuPont HL: Diarrhea in the critically ill: Causes and treatment in five clinical settings. J Crit Illness 7:170–191, 1992.

Acute Pancreatitis

I. **Causes:** gallstones, alcohol, ampullary or pancreatic tumors, pancreatic divisum with accessory duct obstruction, hypertensive Oddi's sphincter, scorpion venom, organophosphates, trauma, hypertriglyceridemia, hypercalcemia, viral (mumps, rubella, Coxsackie B, HIV, Epstein-Barr virus), bacteria (*Mycoplasma*, *Campylobacter* spp.) parasites (*Conorchis*, *Ascaris* spp.), vasculitis, atherosclerotic emboli, penetrating peptic ulcer, drugs (azathioprine, estrogens, valproic acid, pentamidine, dideoxyinosine [ddl], thiazides, furosemide, erythromycin, tetracycline, salicylates, H_2 blockers), biliary sludge, iatrogenic due to endoscopic retrograde cholangiopancreatography, cystic fibrosis, Crohn's disease, idiopathic.

II. **Clinical presentation:** (1) Sudden onset of epigastric pain radiating to the back; (2) intravascular depletion; (3) Cullen's sign (bruising of periumbilical region) and Grey-Turner's sign (bruising of flanks suggesting hemorrhagic pancreatitis); (4) respiratory complications: atelectasis, diaphragmatic splinting, pleural effusion, acute respiratory distress syndrome.

III. **Diagnosis**
   1. **Serum amylase:** generally higher in nonalcoholic than alcoholic pancreatitis; in rare patients with acute pancreatitis, it may be normal. On average, during uncomplicated cases, the serum amylase level starts rising from 2–12 hr after symptom onset and peaks at 12–72 hr. It usually returns to baseline after 1 week.
   2. **Serum lipase:** more sensitive and specific than amylase; particularly useful in patients who present several days after onset because it has longer serum half-life than amylase. Lipase levels rise within 4–8 hr after symptom onset and peak at ~ 24 hr. Levels decrease within 8–14 days.
   3. **Dipstick urinary trypsinogen-2:** excellent negative predictive value (i.e., a negative test essentially rules out acute pancreatitis). A positive test warrants further evaluation.

      Reference: Kemppainen EA et al. Rapid measurement of urinary trypsinogen-2 as a screening test for acute pancreatitis. N Engl J Med 336:1788–1793, 1997.

4. **Ultrasound:** helps in the detection of biliary stones as cause.
5. **CT scan:** useful in determining presence of local complications of acute pancreatitis (necrosis, pseudocyst, abscess); dynamic CT pancreatography (large doses of IV contrast with thin CT sections) may identify necrosis.
6. **Endoscopic retrograde cholangiopancreatography (ERCP):** useful in identifying less obvious (anatomic) causes of pancreatitis (e.g., small pancreatic tumors, divisum, and hypertensive sphincter of Oddi). This form of treatment is generally reserved for gallstone pancreatitis. It is often postponed to allow pancreatitis to subside unless clinical suspicion for persistent choledocholithiasis is high.

IV. **Prognostic indicators:** for Ranson's and Glasgow criteria, mortality rate is < 1% for 1–2 risk factors, 15% for 3–4 risk factors, and ~100% for 6–7 risk factors.

1. **Ranson's early prognostic criteria**

	Non-gallstone	**Gallstone pancreatitis**
On admission		
Age (yrs)	> 55	> 70
WBC (per mm^3) ($\times 10^9$/L)	> 16,000 (> 16)	> 18,000 (> 18)
Glucose (mg/dL) (mmol/L)	> 200 (< 11)	> 220 (> 11)
On admission		
LDH (U/L)	> 350	> 400
AST (U/L)	> 250	> 250
During initial 48 hrs		
Decrease in hematocrit	> 10	> 10
Increase in BUN (mg/dL) (mmol/L)	> 5 (> 1.79)	> 2 (> 0.714)
Calcium (mg/dL) (mmol/L)	< 8 (< 2)	< 8 (< 2)
PaO_2 (mmHg)	< 60	—
Base deficit (mmol/L)	> 4	> 5
Fluid sequestration (L)	> 6	> 4

2. **Modified Glasgow criteria (during initial 48 hr)**
   a. Age > 55 yr
   b. White blood cells > 15,000 mm^3 (> 15 $\times 10^9$/L)
   c. Glucose > 180 mg/dl (> 10 mmol/L)
   d. BUN > 45 mg/dl (> 16 mmol/L)
   e. LDH > 600 U/L
   f. Albumin < 3.3 gm/dl (< 33 gm/L)
   g. Calcium < 8 mg/dl (< 2 mmol/L)
   h. PaO_2 < 60 mmHg

V. **Complications**

1. **Local:** necrosis with or without infection, pseudocyst, abscess, necrotizing obstruction or fistulization of colon, gastrointestinal bleeding (stress ulcers, rupture or pseudoaneurysm formed by autodigestion of pancreatic blood vessels).
2. **Systemic:** circulatory shock, sepsis, coagulopathy, adult respiratory distress syndrome (release of phospholipase A_2 leads to surfactant degradation), acute tubular necrosis, hyperglycemia, hypertriglyceridemia, hypocalcemia, subcutaneous nodules due to extrapancreatic necrosis, psychosis.

VI. **Treatment**

1. **Largely supportive** with meticulous attention to fluid resuscitation, pain control with **meperidine**, nutritional support for protracted cases, and vigilance for local and systemic complications. Morphine may cause spasm of the sphincter of Oddi and worsen the pain.

2. **Nutrition in acute pancreatitis**: although it was previously thought that total parenteral nutrition is required for acute severe pancreatitis, more recent data suggest that TPN does not hasten pancreatic recovery and that enteral feeding is actually well-tolerated. Potential benefits of gut feeding include decreased gut permeability, prevention of bacterial translocation, less expense than TPN, and less incidence of catheter-related sepsis. Therefore, in the absence of severe ileus, patients with severe pancreatitis should have enteral feeding by a nasojejunal feeding tube.
3. **Gallstone pancreatitis:** most cases resolve spontaneously. However, if there is no improvement or deterioration at 48 hr, many advocate ERCP with sphincterotomy, **especially in patients with associated cholangitis.**
4. **Pseudocysts:** in general, pseudocysts can be left alone unless they are large (> 7 cm) and cause a mass effect. Many resolve spontaneously within 6 weeks. If drainage is required, percutaneous or endoscopic drainage may be tried first before resorting to operative debridement.
5. **Necrotizing pancreatitis:** The differentiation between non-necrotic and necrotic pancreatitis requires dynamic contrast enhanced CT scanning where **necrotic areas lack normal enhancement** because of disruption of the microcirculation. Patients with necrotizing or severe pancreatitis should be treated with prophylactic antibiotics since this has been shown to decrease pancreatic infection and mortality: e.g., imipenem (for 2–4 weeks) is the antibiotic with the best data to support its use in this setting. If a patient with necrotizing pancreatitis develops a fever, a pancreatic fine needle aspirate (FNA) should be considered and if infected, necrosectomy is indicated. If the necrosis is clinically sterile, management is controversial. Many advocate no surgical intervention; others still recommend necrosectomy, especially if the necrosis is extensive on CT scan (involving > 50% of pancreas). Necrotizing pancreatitis has a higher mortality rate than "interstitial" pancreatitis; mortality is even higher if the necrotic tissue becomes infected.
6. **Pancreatic abscesses** (infected pseudocysts) generally can be drained percutaneously (*Escherichia coli* and *Klebsiella, Proteus, Enterococcus,* and *Candida* spp.).
7. **Indications for surgical debridement:** infected pancreatic necrosis, because the infected material is thick and cannot be drained percutaneously.
8. **Antibiotics**: the role of antibiotics in the management of early acute pancreatitis is controversial. In general, antibiotics are recommended for patients with acute necrotizing pancreatic, especially with signs of infection (e.g., fever, leukocytosis). If the aspirate of the necrosis is positive for bacteria by Gram stain or culture, antibiotics are definitely indicated.

VII. **Nonpancreatic causes of high serum amylase and lipase levels**

1. **Elevated amylase**: alcohol intake, bile enteritis, biliary obstruction, bowel infarction, chemotherapy, cirrhosis, fat emboli, hepatic failure, hepatitis, intestinal obstruction, mumps, perforated ulcer, radiotherapy, renal failure.
2. **Elevated lipase**: bacterial gastroenteritis, bile duct obstruction, bowel obstruction, diarrhea, duodenitis, fallopian tube pathology, inflammatory bowel disease, opiate use, pyloric adenocarcinoma, renal failure, small bowel perforation, viral gastroenteritis.

Reference: Calleja GA, Barkin JS: Acute pancreatitis. Med Clin North Am 77:1037–1056, 1993.

Key References: Pratt DS, Epstein SK: Recent advances in critical care gastroenterology. Am J Respir Crit Care Med 161:1417–1420, 2000; Steinberg W, Tenner S: Acute pancreatitis. N Engl J Med 330:1198, 1994. (source of tables).

Ogilvie's Syndrome (Colonic Pseudo-obstruction)

I. **Definition**: acute megacolon in patients without obvious colonic disease or mechanical obstruction. Most cases are related to an underlying medical process such as trauma, orthopedic surgery, obstetric procedures, pelvic or abdominal surgery, metabolic imbalance (e.g., hypokalemia), congestive heart failure, mechanical ventilation, or a neurologic disorder. The pathogenesis is not precisely known, but dysfunction of the parasympathetic nerves supplying the colon/rectum (S2–S4) leads to atony or spasticity and functional obstruction.

II. **Clinical manifestation**: typically, Ogilvie's syndrome occurs in older patients who are recovering from a surgical or medical disorder and develop an acute-subacute onset of abdominal distention due to massive dilatation of the colon.

III. **Treatment**

1. Withhold oral feedings and start parenteral nutrition.
2. Consider discontinuation of incentive spirometry and intermittent positive pressure breathing, both of which may increase air swallowing.
3. A water-soluble contrast enema is used to exclude mechanical obstruction.
4. **Rectal decompression tube and enemas** often relieve symptoms and make the diagnosis.
5. Correct any electrolyte abnormalities.
6. Consider **cisapride**, 10 mg IV slow bolus every 4 hr for 4 doses, then 10 mg PO 3 times/day; **erythromycin**, 250 mg IV every 8 hr for 3 days; or **neostigmine** as medical therapy. Isolated reports have shown all three to be helpful.
7. Consider colonoscopic decompression or percutaneous cecostomy if the above measures fail.
8. Colonic resection may be necessary in rare instances, especially if the cecum is > 11 cm and remains refractory to medical treatment or if patient exhibits fever, leukocytosis, or peritoneal signs.

Key References: MacColl C, MacCannell KL, Baylis B, Lee SS: Treatment of acute colonic pseudoobstructio (Ogilvie's syndrome) with cisapride. Gastroenterology 98: 773–776, 1990; Vanek VW, Al-Salti M: Acute pseudo-obstruction of the colon (Ogilvie's syndrome): An analysis of 400 cases. Dis Colon Rectum 29:203–210, 1986.

Ischemic Necrosis of the Colon and Small Bowel

I. Ischemic necrosis of the intestine occurs in 1% of all patients with renal transplants. Potential causes include hypotension, immunosuppressives, irradiation, atherosclerosis, anemia, and uremia.

II. An association has been made between intestinal necrosis and the sorbitol added with Kayexalate enema.

III. Portal air may be seen in intestinal necrosis. The features favoring portal venous air over biliary air are (1) lack of previous biliary tract surgery and (2) the tendency of portal venous air to be more peripheral (biliary air is more central ["pruned tree"] in distribution).

Stress-related Erosive Syndrome

I. **Stress-related erosive syndrome (SRES)** is also known as stress ulcer, stress gastritis, and a number of other synonyms. The incidence of SRES appears to be decreasing probably due to improvement in supporting hemodynamics, tissue oxygenation, and, to a lesser extent, the use of gastrointestinal prophylaxis with H_2-blocker or proton-pump inhibitor.

II. **Risk factors**: mechanical ventilation and coagulopathy are the two most important risk factors. Others include sepsis, shock, acidosis, peritonitis, and multiorgan failure.

III. **Diagnosis**

1. When the criterion is at least a microscopic blood loss, SRES occurs in virtually all ICU patients.
2. Clinically significant hemorrhage due to SRES occurs in 1 to 30% of ICU patients.
3. Esophagogastroduodenoscopy (EGD) is the critical diagnostic test, showing diffuse shallow mucosal injury with oozing of blood.

IV. **Prophylaxis**

1. **Antacids** have been shown to be effective against SRES. The goal is to raise the intragastric pH > 4. Dose is 30–60 ml orally or by nasogastric tube every 1–2 hr.
2. **H_2 antagonists** are also effective. Continuous infusion may be more effective than boluses. In patients without renal insufficiency, the infusion rates are:
   a. Cimetidine, 37.5–100 mg/hr
   b. Ranitidine, 6.25–12.5 mg/hr
   c. Famotidine, 1.7–2.1 mg/hr
3. **Proton-pump inhibitors**. Although small studies have shown promise, these drugs are generally not recommended for prophylaxis because of the lack of evidence of significant benefit.
4. **Sucralfate**. Its role in preventing bleeding from SRES is controversial because of discordant results.

V. **Interventional therapy** for SRES may be required in recalcitrant cases, using endoscopic or angiographic techniques or surgery.

Key Reference: Beejay U, Wolfe MM: Acute gastrointestinal bleeding in the intensive care unit. Gastroenterol Clin North Am 29:309–336, 2000.

Nephrology

Assessing the Cause of Acute Renal Failure

I. **Definitions**

1. **Acute renal failure (ARF):** an increase in serum creatinine (Cr) ≥ 0.5 mg/dl (44 µmol/L) over the baseline value or an increase > 50% of the baseline value

   or

   a decrease in creatinine clearance of 50% or a decrease in renal function that results in the need for dialysis.
2. **Oliguric vs. nonoliguric ARF:** oliguric if urine volume is < 400 ml over 24 hr.
3. **Morbidity and mortality:** nonoliguric ARF has a better prognosis than oliguric ARF; 20–60% of patients with ARF require dialysis. Among the survivors, < 25% require long-term dialysis. ARF is important in the ICU because the mortality rate remains high (historically noted at ~ 60%).

II. **Causes of ARF.** Before diagnosing **acute tubular necrosis (ATN)**, one should exclude:

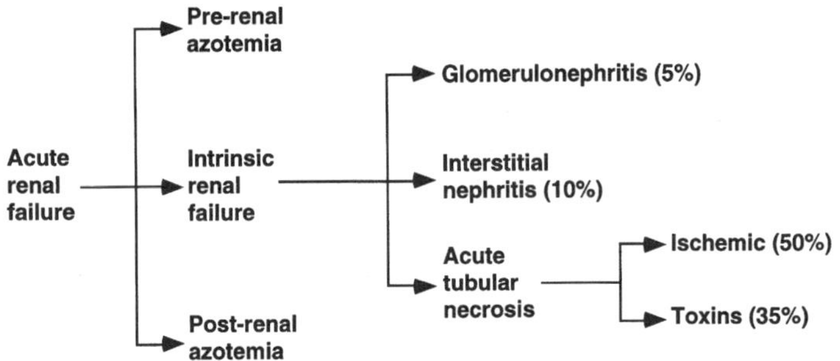

1. **Obstructive uropathy:** benign prostatic hypertrophy, bladder outlet obstruction, papillary necrosis that occurs in diabetes, sickle cell anemia, analgesic use, calculi, crystals due to uric acid, oxalic acid, methotrexate, sulfonamides.
2. **Prerenal azotemia:** probably the most common cause of elevated creatinine; a compromise in renal perfusion due to intravascular depletion or a decrease in effective circulatory volume (e.g., congestive heart failure).
3. **Acute renovascular disease:** renal artery thrombosis or embolism from thrombus or cholesterol, aortic aneurysm leading to dissection or thrombosis, renal artery dissection, and renal vein thrombosis.
4. **Acute interstitial nephritis:** the two most common causes are acute bacterial pyelonephritis and drug-induced hypersensitivity nephritis.
5. **Acute glomerulonephritis** (AGN): characterized by fever, skin rash, arthralgias, evidence of systemic disease or pulmonary involvement, high erythrocyte sedimentation rate, low complement levels, autoimmune antibodies, hematuria, and red blood cell casts.

III. **Prerenal azotemia**

1. **Causes:** intravascular volume depletion, reduced cardiac output, systemic vasodilation (anaphylaxis, sepsis, drug overdose), systemic or renal vasoconstriction (anesthesia, hepatorenal syndrome, α-adrenergic agonists).

2. **Laboratory findings:** hemoconcentration, blood urea nitrogen (BUN)/Cr > 20, urine specific gravity > 1.030, urine osmolality > 500 mOsm/kg (or mmol/kg), urinary sodium (U_{Na}) < 20 mmol/L, bland urinary sediment unless there is complicating acute tubular necrosis, and fractional excretion of sodium (FE_{Na}) < 1%.

$$FE_{Na} = [(U_{Na}/U_{Cr})/(P_{Na}/P_{Cr})] \times 100$$

   where U_{Cr} = urine creatinine, P_{Na} = plasma sodium, and P_{Cr} = plasma creatinine.
3. **Caveat:** in some patients with prerenal azotemia who are volume-depleted and oliguric, concomitant water reabsorption may result in U_{Na} > 20 mmol/L (in the absence of ATN). Thus the FE_{Na} is more specific for differentiating prerenal azotemia from ATN because it is not affected by water handling. Prerenal azotemia may lead to ATN if sustained.

IV. **Acute tubular necrosis (ATN)**

1. **Causes: hypoperfusion** that leads to ischemia, **nephrotoxins** (*endogenous:* myoglobin, hemoglobin, calcium phosphate precipitation, uric acid; *exogenous:* aminoglycosides, cephalosporins, tetracyclines, amphotericin B, pentamidine, radiocontrast media, heavy metals [e.g., mercury, lead, arsenic, bismuth], cisplatin, methotrexate, mitomycin, cyclosporine, ethylene glycol).
2. **Rhabdomyolytic ATN:** see Rhabdomyolysis/Myoglobinuria section.
3. **Aminoglycoside:** ATN is typically nonoliguric and may occur within the drug's therapeutic range. Nephrotoxicity correlates better with the total cumulative aminoglycoside dose than with plasma levels. Hypomagnesemia and hypokalemia may occur. Other risk factors: age, dehydration.
4. **Radiocontrast agents:** ATN due to radiocontrast agents is characterized by low FE_{Na} and high urine specific gravity. The nonionic agents appear to be less nephrotoxic. Risk factors include age, preexisting renal insufficiency, dehydration, diabetes, congestive heart failure, high-dose contrast, and concurrent use of nephrotoxins, such as nonsteroidal anti-inflammatory drugs (NSAIDs) or angiotensin-converting enzyme (ACE) inhibitors.
5. **Laboratory findings:** in the absence of recent diuretic therapy, FE_{Na} > 2%, urine osmolality < 350 mOsm/kg (or mmol/kg) H_2O, U_{Na} > 40 mmol/L. FE_{Na} < 2% may occur with ATN when associated with radiocontrast agents, sepsis, burns, liver failure, edematous states, interstitial nephritis, or acute obstruction and in acute poststreptococcal glomerulonephritis (see below).

V. **NSAID-induced renal failure** may cause renal insufficiency by a number of mechanisms:

1. Loss of renal vasodilators prostaglandin E and prostacyclin due to cyclooxygenase inhibition by NSAIDs, especially in the setting of low cardiac output, volume depletion, and sepsis.
2. ATN may develop if kidney hypoperfusion is severe enough.
3. Acute interstitial nephritis
4. Papillary necrosis
5. Minimal change or membranous glomerular disease

VI. **Acute (hypersensitivity) interstitial nephritis (AIN)**

1. Infiltration of the renal interstitium with edema, lymphocytes, monocytes, plasma cells, and eosinophils.
2. **Causes:** penicillin, cephalosporins, sulfonamides, thiazides, minocycline, allopurinol, NSAIDs, phenytoin, carbamazepine, ACE inhibitors, rifampin, furosemide.
3. Typically, fever is common. Rash and eosinophilia may also occur. However, in patients with NSAID-induced AIN, there may be renal insufficiency with few or no systemic signs and symptoms such as fever, rash, and eosinophilia.

4. **Eosinophiluria:** Hansel's stain is more sensitive than Wright's stain. The positive predictive value of eosinophiluria is not 100% because other disorders also may cause eosinophiluria. Other findings in the urine include red cells, white cells, and white cell casts. AIN should be suspected in cases of sterile pyuria.
5. Definitive diagnosis may require renal biopsy. Removal of offending agent typically results in return of creatinine to baseline. Treatment with corticosteroids may reverse the renal failure if creatinine does not improve with removal of the offending agent.

VII. **Drugs associated with ARF**

Mechanism	Drug
Reduction of intrarenal blood flow	NSAIDs, ACE inhibitor, cyclosporine, tacrolimus, radiocontrast, amphotericin B, interleukin-2
Direct tubular toxicity	Aminoglycosides, radiocontrast, cisplatin, cyclosporine, tacrolimus, amphotericin B, methotrexate, foscarnet, pentamidine, organic solvents, heavy metals, intravenous immunoglobulin
Heme-pigment–induced tubular toxicity (rhabdomyolysis)	Cocaine, ethanol, lovastatin
Intratubular obstruction by precipitation of the agent or its metabolite or byproducts	Acyclovir, sulfonamides, ethylene glycol (calcium oxalate crystals), chemotherapeutic agents (uric acid crystals—tumor lysis syndrome), methotrexate
Allergic interstitial nephritis	Penicillins, cephalosporins, sulfonamides, rifampin, ciprofloxacin, NSAIDs, thiazides, furosemide, cimetidine, phenytoin, allopurinol
Hemolytic-uremic syndrome	Cyclosporine, tacrolimus, mitomycin, cocaine, quinine, conjugated estrogens

Note: Heme-positive urine in the absence of erythrocytes suggests the presence of myoglobin.

VIII. **Urine findings in ARF**

	Prerenal	Intrinsic renal	Postrenal
Urine osmolality	> 500	**ATN:** < 350 **AGN:** > 500	< 350
Urine Na	< 20	> 40	> 40
FE_{Na}	< 1%	> 1% **AGN:** < 1%	>1 %
Urine dipstick	Trace or no protein	**ATN:** mild-to-moderate proteinuria **Nephrotoxins:** mild-to-moderate proteinuria **AIN:** mild-to-moderate proteinuria; hemoglobinuria, pyuria **AGN:** moderate-to-severe proteinuria; hemoglobinuria	Trace or no proteinuria; may have hemoglobinuria or pyuria
Urine sediment	Few hyaline casts	**ATN:** pigmented granular casts **Nephrotoxins:** pigmented granular casts **AIN:** white cells and white cell casts; eosinophils and eosinophil casts; red cells **AGN:** red cells and red cell casts; red cells may be dysmorphic	Crystals, red cells, and white cells possible

IX. **Differential diagnosis of renal failure using FE_{Na}**
   1. **Low FE_{Na} (< 1%):** prerenal azotemia, ATN superimposed on chronic prerenal disease such as cirrhosis and congestive heart failure, contrast-induced ATN, myoglobinuric ATN, glomerulonephritis, vasculitis, acute interstitial nephritis
   2. **High FE_{Na} (> 2%):** ATN (classic)

X. **Complications of ARF:** salt and water overload, hyperkalemia, hyperphosphatemia, hypocalcemia, hypermagnesemia, metabolic acidosis, hyperuricemia, anemia, qualitative defects in platelets, pericarditis, increased risk of infection, lethargy, confusion, anorexia, nausea.

XI. **Therapy for ARF**
   1. **Reverse any underlying cause** (e.g., bladder outlet obstruction) **and correct fluid and electrolyte imbalances.** Fluid management is critical because restoration of renal blood flow with volume resuscitation may limit damage if ATN has not yet occurred.
   2. No good evidence suggests that mannitol or loop diuretics improve renal outcome. Diuretics may convert early oliguric to nonoliguric renal failure. Nonoliguric renal failure is generally easier to manage before dialysis.
   3. **Discontinue any nephrotoxins.**
   4. **Treat hyperkalemia.** (see section on Hyperkalemia)
   5. **Adjust the dosages of medications eliminated by the kidney.**
   6. **Prevent and treat sepsis,** which is the most common cause of death in ARF.
   7. Low-dose dopamine does **not** offer significant renal protection in critically ill patients with early renal dysfunction.
      Reference: ANZICS Clinical Trial Group: Low-dose dopamine in patients with early renal dysfunction: A placebo controlled randomized trial. Lancet 356:2139–2143, 2000.
   8. **Renal replacement therapy**—see next section.

Key Reference: Thadhani R, et al: Acute renal failure. N Engl J Med 334:1448, 1996.

Renal Replacement Therapy

I. **Renal replacement therapy** consists of continuous renal replacement therapy (CRRT), intermittent hemodialysis, and peritoneal dialysis. CRRT uses convection, diffusion, or a combination of the two. It relies on a slow dialysate flow rate and is administered on a continual basis.
   1. **Advantages** of continuous renal replacement therapy (CRRT) over intermittent hemodialysis (IHD): more precise fluid and metabolic control, decreased hemodynamic instability, fewer cardiac arrhythmias, better respiratory gas exchange, better control of serum biochemical values, enhanced possibility of removing injurious cytokines (in sepsis or MODS), ability to administer unlimited nutritional support, and decreased stay in ICU.
   2. **Disadvantages** of CRRT vs. IHD: need for prolonged anticoagulation, need for constant surveillance, and more filter ruptures.

II. **Comparison of intermittent hemodialysis (IHD) and CRRT using typical settings**
   1. **IHD**
      a. Blood flow: 10–180 cc/min
      b. Dialysate flow: 1000 cc/hr
      c. Fluid removal: 1–4 L/hr
      d. Blood pressure: mean arterial pressure > 70 mmHg
      e. Duration: 4 hr

2. **CRRT**
   a. Blood flow: 200–400 cc/min
   b. Dialysate flow: 500–800 cc/hr when used
   c. Fluid removal: 1–4 L/day
   d. Blood pressure: mean arterial pressure < 70 mmHg
   e. Duration: 24 hr

III. **Indications for CRRT or IHD:** volume overload, hyperkalemia, metabolic acidosis, symptoms and signs of severe uremia (pericardial effusion, cardiac dysrhythmia).

IV. **Acute peritoneal dialysis** is also an option in unstable patients. Choosing one therapy over the other is often based on individual preferences, local resources, and hemodynamic stability of the patient.

V. **Choice of dialysis membrane:** synthetic membranes (e.g., polymethylmethacrylate, polyacrylonitrile, polysulfone) activate the alternate complement pathway less than cuprophane membranes and therefore cause less cellular activation, which may lead to improved recovery of renal function.

VI. **The timing of initiation of dialysis is still in debate.** Some evidence suggests that early initiation of dialysis improves survival, but other evidence suggests that early dialysis per se makes no difference.

VII. **Types of CRRT**
   1. **Slow continuous ultrafiltration (SCUF)**: CVVH without replacement fluid. No dialysate. Fluid removal is typically 50–100 cc/hr. Fluid removed (ultrafiltrate) has the same electrolyte composition as plasma. Minimal solute clearance.
   2. **Continuous venovenous hemofiltration (CVVH)**: SCUF with fluid replacement. Probably the most common form of CRRT because adequate fluid and solute removal can be achieved. No dialysate. Fluid removal (ultrafiltrate) is typically 1000 cc/hr. Replacement fluid is used (typically 900–950 cc/hr) to achieve a net loss of 50–100 cc/hr. Ultrafiltrate has the same composition as plasma. Adequate solute clearance. Hypokalemia, hypophosphatemia, and hypomagnesemia may occur.
   3. **Continuous venovenous hemodialysis (CVVHD)**: dialysate is used. Fluid removal is typically 50–100 cc/hr. No replacement fluid. Better solute clearance than CVVH.
   4. **Continuous venovenous hemodiafiltration (CVVHDF)**: dialysate is used, replacement fluid is used (typically 900–950 cc/hr) to achieve a net loss of 50–100 cc/hr. Fluid removal is typically 1000 cc/hr. Excellent solute removal by dialysis and loss of ultrafiltrate. Usually the added solute clearance of CVVHDF is not needed. CVVHDF should be used only when adequate clearances are not obtained because the addition of dialysate adds to the complexity and cost of the procedure.

VIII. Because the dialysis membranes allow passage of molecules up to 10–20 kDa, adjustment of many drugs is necessary in CRRT. Therefore, drug monitoring, when available, should be used. References for drug pharmacokinetics during CRRT are available.

References: Bressole F, et al: Clinical pharmacokinetics during continuous haemofiltration. Clin Pharmacokinet 26:457–471, 1994; Reetze-Bonorden P, Bohler J, Keller E: Drug dosage in patients during continuous renal replacement therapy. Clin Pharmacokinet 24:362–379, 1993.

Key References: McCarthy J: Renal replacement therapy in acute renal failure. Curr Opin Nephrol Hypertens 5:480, 1996; Meyer MM. Renal replacement therapies. Crit Care Clin 16:29–58, 2000.

Comparison of Dialysis and Hemofiltration Devices

Method	Principle	Advantages	Disadvantages	Complications
Hemodialysis (HD)	Double-lumen tube in large central vein; blood exposed to dialysate across semipermeable membrane Indications: symptomatic uremia, fluid overload, refractory hyperkalemia or metabolic acidosis	Technique for no-heparin dialysis with citrate regional anticoagulation; volume of blood dialysed over time results in more rapid removal of solutes and more rapid clearing of toxins and potassium	Disequilibrium syndrome: nausea, vomiting, muscle twitching, lethargy, confusion due to rapid removal of solutes from extracellular fluid, cerebrospinal fluid acidosis, and cerebral edema	Hypotension bleeding, hypoxemia, (white blood cell and platelet sequestration in pulmonary vascular bed)
Isolated ultrafiltration	Removes excess fluid only	Better tolerated than HD hemodynamically	Requires systemic anticoagulation	Hypotension with excess fluid removal
Continuous venovenous hemofiltration (CVVH) or continuous venovenous hemodialysis (CVVHD)	Double-lumen tube inserted in large vein and pump used to generate flow over semipermeable membrane. solute removed by convection across membrane highly permeable to water	Single catheter, not dependent on blood pressure, better tolerated than HD	Increased risk of air embolism Less circulatory compromise than CAVHD* because only vein is cannulated Requires blood pump and close supervision Requires some anticoagulation; higher incidence of clotting off kidney than in HD but less than in CAVHD	Complications of line insertion and indwelling catheter (i.e., higher incidence of infection than HD because it is always accessed)
Peritoneal dialysis (PD)	Continuous indwelling tube with 1–2 hr exchanges using 1–2 L of dialysate; efficacy is 1/5 of HD but since PD is performed 24 hr/day, inefficiency is not prohibitive; higher concentration of glucose in dialysate increases volume removed	Lower risk of hypotension No vascular access required No systemic anticoagulation required No rebound in solute concentration Less supervision and technical expertise required	Low solute clearance Produces protein losses May cause hyperglycemia or hypernatremia Risk of peritonitis Low ultrafiltration rate Weaning may be difficult because of peritoneal fluid load	Contraindications: peritoneal sclerosis, abdominal adhesions, fresh vascular grafts, recent abdominal surgery, peritonitis

* CA(arterial)VH or CAVHD is rarely used now because of arterial cannulation complications and the development of newer CVVH or CVVHD devices and pumps.

Key Reference: Bhatla B, Nolph KD, Khanna R: Choosing the right dialysis option for your critically ill patient. J Crit Illness 11:21–31, 1996.

Rhabdomyolysis and Myoglobinuria

I. **Causes:** alcohol, muscle compression (trauma, drug overdose), generalized seizures, medications (azathioprine, clofibrate, lovastatin with or without gemfibrozil, barbiturates, ε-amino caproic acid [Amicar], neuroleptics), toxins (staphylococci, tetanus, venomous snakes, toluene), and genetic enzyme deficiencies.

II. **Clinical features:** pain and swelling may or may not be present. Limb swelling after IV fluid administration suggests recent episode of rhabdomyolysis.

III. **Diagnostic tests**

1. **Gross "Coca-Cola" urine** suggests myoglobin concentration > 250 μg/ml.
2. **Positive orthotolidine dipstick:** heme proteins of myoglobin and hemoglobin can function as perioxidases and oxidize chromogens (orthotolidine) to form blue products. Orthotolidine does not distinguish between hemeglobinuria and myoglobinuria. Moreover, the absence of myoglobin by dipstick does not rule out rhabdomyolysis (sensitivity ~50% even in the absence of hematuria).
3. **Elevated serum creatine phosphokinase (CPK)**

IV. **Complications**

1. **Acute renal failure (ARF):** pathogenic mechanism includes tubular obstruction by precipitated myoglobin. Dehydration and urinary acidification appear crucial for rhabdomyolysis-induced ARF. One study developed a discriminant analysis for determining risk of ARF from admission laboratory values for potassium (K), creatinine (Cr), and albumin (AL):

$$\mathbf{R = 0.7\,[K, mmol/L] + 1.1\,[Cr, mg/dl] + 0.6\,[AL, gm/dl] - 6.6}$$

   a. If $R \geq 0.1$, high-risk group; if $R < 0.1$, low-risk group.
   b. This test has a low incidence of false negatives or a **high negative predictive value**, i.e., if $R < 0.1$, patients are truly at low risk. But it has a high incidence of false positives or a **low positive predictive value**, i.e., if $R \geq 0.1$, patient is at higher risk for ARF—but not always.

2. **Hyperkalemia**, especially with ARF
3. **Elevated anion gap** in patients with rhabdo-ARF: the anion gap is often significantly higher than with other causes of ARF.
4. **Hyperphosphatemia**
5. **Hyperuricemia**
6. **Hypocalcemia** (initially) due to calcium deposition in damaged muscle, followed by **hypercalcemia** due to calcium release and inappropriately normal or high levels of parathyroid hormone and 1,25-$(OH)_2D_3$ during recovery period.

V. **Prevention of renal failure**

1. Vigorous **hydration** with normal saline, 200–300 ml/hr
2. **Mannitol**, 12.5–25 gm IV
3. If urine flow is adequate, **$NaHCO_3$** 2–3 amps (e.g., 100–150 mEq) in 1 liter of D_5W to maintain urine pH > 6.5. One caveat is that in patients with metabolic acidosis (e.g., due to renal insufficiency) and hypocalcemia, HCO_3 administration may precipitate tetany due to decrease in ionized calcium.

Key Reference: Gabow PA, Kaehny WD, Kelleher SP: The spectrum of rhabdomyolysis. Medicine 61:141–152, 1982.

Postprostatectomy Syndrome

I. This unique syndrome, characterized by **circulatory** (initial hypertension, followed by hypotension and bradycardia) and **central nervous system disorders** (due to hyponatremia; symptoms include disorientation, blindness, coma, and seizures) is due to the systemic absorption of fluid used for bladder irrigation during transurethral resection of the prostate (TURP).

II. Fluid used for irrigation contains glycine, sorbitol, or mannitol. Pure water may lead to massive hemolysis if absorbed, whereas saline is electroconductive, rendering electrocautery dangerous.

III. **Types of irrigative solution**
1. **Mannitol** solution: osmolality remains normal; solute is excreted unchanged in urine.
2. **Sorbitol** solutions: nontoxic and metabolized to CO_2 and water.
3. **Glycine** solutions: toxic to the retina. As glycine is metabolized, it increases concentration of NH_3 and decreases plasma osmolality, resulting in cerebral edema.

IV. **Treatment**
1. Supportive therapy, including monitoring of oxygenation, central venous pressure, and urine output.
2. Specific treatment consists of producing a net loss of body water for the dilutional hyponatremia using diuretics (e.g., **furosemide, 40–100 mg IV**).
3. For neurologic crisis, hypertonic saline may need to be used.

Key Reference: Greene LF: Transurethral surgery. In Walsh PC, Gittes RF, Perlmutter AD, Stamey TA (eds): Campbell's Urology. Philadelphia, W.B. Saunders, 1986, p 2834.

Neurology

Management of Tonic-Clonic Status Epilepticus

I. **Definition:** Status epilepticus is a true medical emergency with a mortality rate of 10–12% and higher rates of brain damage. It is defined as a single episode of continuous seizure activity > 30 min *or* ≥ 2 seizures without recovery of baseline consciousness. Lactic acidosis, increased intracranial pressure, autonomic dysfunction (hyperthermia, excessive sweating), dysrhythmias, cerebral edema, pulmonary edema, aspiration pneumonitis, disseminated intravascular coagulation, and rhabdomyolysis are sequelae of prolonged convulsive status epilepticus.

II. **Causes:** noncompliance with anticonvulsants, hypoglycemia, hyperglycemia, alcohol, tricyclic antidepressants, cocaine, amphetamines, antihistamines, theophylline, isoniazid, lithium, carbon monoxide, and organophosphates. Other causes include traumatic or nontraumatic (e.g., infection, tumors) cerebral processes.

III. **Treatment**

1. Maintain airway and establish intravenous access with **normal saline** and **not** glucose because phenytoin precipitates in glucose solutions.
2. Obtain blood for glucose, calcium, magnesium, electrolytes, blood urea nitrogen, liver functions, anticonvulsant levels, complete blood count, and toxicology screen. Begin normal saline, give **100 mg thiamine and 50 ml of 50% glucose**. Monitor EKG, blood pressure, and, if possible electroencephalogram (EEG). Consider lumbar puncture to rule out meningitis.
3. **Diazepam** (Valium), **5 mg over 1–2 min every 5–10 min as needed**, up to 30 mg, *or* **lorazepam** (Ativan), **2–4 mg IV every 5–10 min as needed**, up to 10 mg.
4. **Phenytoin** (Dilantin), **18 mg/kg** (on average, **1000 mg IV over 30–40 min**). Slow the infusion rate with arrhythmia or hypotension; in general, give ≤ **50 mg/min**. **Fosphenytoin** is a water-soluble prodrug form of phenytoin. It can be administered up to 150 phenytoin equivalents / min.
5. If seizure persists, consider phenobarbital *or* diazepam drip: **phenobarbital, 50–100 mg/min until seizures stop or a max of 20 mg/kg; diazepam, 100 mg in 500 ml D_5W at 20–40 ml/hr (4–8 mg/hr).** Drip medications should always be administered in the ICU setting with EEG monitoring.
6. If seizure persists, an IV anesthetic agent should be administered in an ICU setting with EEG monitoring. The patient may require intubation if they are unable to maintain a patent airway.
   a. **Pentobarbital, 10–15 mg/kg IV as a loading dose** followed by 50 mg/min until burst suppression is achieved. The **maintenance dose is 0.5–1 mg/kg/hr.** Dopamine and fluids may be required to support the blood pressure. *or*
   b. **Midazolam, 0.2 mg/kg as a slow iv bolus** followed by a **maintenance dose of 0.75 to 10 μg/kg/min** *or*
   c. **Propofol, 1–2 mg/kg as a loading dose** followed by **2–10 mg/kg/hr,** titrating to spike suppression or burst suppression with 1 second interburst intervals.

Key References: Jagoda A, et al: Refractory status epilepticus in adults. Ann Emerg Med 22:1337–1348, 1993; Willmore JL: Epilepsy emergencies: The first seizure and status epilepticus. Neurology 51:S34–S38, 1998.

Malignant Hyperthermia

I. **Inherited disorders** characterized by a rapid increase in temperature in response to **inhalational anesthetics** or muscle relaxants (**succinylcholine**). Autosomal dominant form occurs in 1 in 40,000 adult surgical cases. More common in young adults.

II. **Pathogenesis:** the anesthetic releases calcium excessively from the abnormal sarcoplasmic reticulum, resulting in marked increases in myoplasmic calcium and contractions and markedly increased heat production.

III. **Manifestations**
1. Diminished relaxation during induction with anesthesia with or without **trismus**.
2. **Fever (a late sign)**, increased heart rate, arrhythmia, decreased blood pressure, **muscle rigidity**, decreased PaO_2 (cyanosis), and increased **$PaCO_2$ (end-tidal CO_2** is a useful early parameter to suggest malignant hyperthermia).
3. Respiratory and metabolic **acidosis (increased lactate)**, **hyperkalemia**, hypermagnesemia
4. Late signs: muscle swelling, pulmonary edema, disseminated intravascular coagulation, acute renal failure, cardiovascular collapse.

IV. **Treatment**
1. Stop anesthetic and change rubber tubing on anesthesia machine.
2. External cooling to 39° C (102.2° F).
3. 100% O_2; diuresis with fluids, with or without diuretics; $NaHCO_3$, 1–2 mEq/kg may be required.
4. **Dantrolene** inhibits calcium release from muscle storage sites, thereby reversing muscle rigidity.
   a. **Load:** 1–2 mg/kg IV infusion, then every 5–10 min until symptoms subside or up to total dose of 10 mg/kg.
   b. **Maintenance:** 2.5 mg/kg IV every 8 hr × 3 doses, then 4 mg/kg/day orally for 2–3 days.
5. Procainamide (prophylactic for ventricular fibrillation), 10–20 mg/kg IV at 40–50 mg/min, has been used in some patients.

Key Reference: Aiyer MK, et al: Recognizing hyperthermic syndromes in critically ill patients. J Crit Illness 10:630–640, 643–646, 1995.

Neuroleptic Malignant Syndrome

I. Most cases of neuroleptic malignant syndrome (NMS) occur with haloperidol, thiothixene, or piperazine phenothiazines, but metoclopramide (dopamine-depleting), various antidepressants (including tricyclic antidepressants and monoamine oxidase inhibitors), and **withdrawal** of amantadine or levodopa also may be implicated. A drug's potential for causing NMS depends on its antidopaminergic potential, i.e., ability to block the dopaminergic pathways in the basal ganglia and hypothalamus.

II. Most patients with NMS develop symptoms within 1–7 days of initiating the drug, but cases have followed dose escalation after long-term use. May last 5–10 days after neuroleptics are discontinued. Young males are most commonly affected.

III. **Clinical symptoms** may progress within hours, but there may be a prodromal period. Established cases are associated with frank **autonomic dysfunction** (tachycardia, labile blood pressure, diaphoresis, dyspnea, urinary incontinence, sialorrhea), **extrapyramidal dysfunction** (catatonia, dystonia, muscle rigidity, pseudoparkinsonism), **fever, fluctuation in consciousness** (from alertness to coma), **leukocytosis, increased creatine phosphokinase** (from myonecrosis), and **metabolic acidosis**. Onset is variable, but rigidity and involuntary movements always precede fever.

IV. Mortality approaches 20%. Fatalities may occur as late as 30 days after onset due to myoglobinuric renal failure, arrhythmia, pulmonary emboli, myocardial infarction, adult respiratory distress syndrome, or aspiration pneumonia.

V. **Differential diagnosis:** status epilepticus, CNS infection, classic heat stroke, toxic exposures to L-asparaginase or strychnine, salicylate overdose, malignant hyperthermia (anesthetics), succinylcholine, antidopaminergic drugs, withdrawal of L-dopa, and combination of lithium with neuroleptics or amphetamines with cocaine.

VI. **Treatment**
1. Stop neuroleptic, and initiate external cooling.
2. IV hydration with or without $NaHCO_3$ to prevent myoglobinuric renal failure.
3. **Bromocriptine** (postsynaptic dopamine agonist), **2.5–10 mg PO every 8 hr**; increase by 5 mg/day until improvement is seen. Total dose as high as 100 mg/day may be necessary. Continue bromocriptine for at least 10 days after the syndrome is controlled, then taper slowly.
4. **Levodopa/carbidopa**, 100 mg/10 mg orally 3 times/day in place of bromocriptine.
5. Dantrolene: use in NMS not well established. Major side effect of **hepatitis** is associated with long-term oral dantrolene use.
6. Amantadine (presynaptic dopamine agonist), 100 mg orally 2 times/day, may be substituted for bromocriptine.

Key Reference: Aiyer MK, et al: Recognizing hyperthermic syndromes in critically ill patients. J Crit Illness 10:630–640, 643–646, 1995.

Brain Death Guidelines

I. **General prerequisites**
1. Documentation of the **cause** of absent brain function (e.g., by CT scan or cerebrospinal fluid analysis) and demonstration of the **irreversibility of the loss**.
2. The reason for establishing the cause is that **mimics** of brain death may be present, such as **hypothermia** (at core body temperature < 89.6° F [32° C], brainstem reflexes are blunted), **drug intoxication or poisoning** (e.g., sedatives, aminoglycosides, tricyclic antidepressants, anticholinergics, antiepileptics, chemotherapeutics, or neuromuscular blocking agents), and **metabolic (electrolyte/acid–base) or endocrine** derangements. Such mimics confound the diagnosis of brain death.

II. **Diagnostic criteria**
1. **Coma:** cerebral motor responses to painful stimuli should be absent.
2. **Absence of brainstem reflexes:** no pupillary response, oculocephalics (i.e., no doll's eyes), corneal/jaw reflexes, or gag reflex; no cough reflex to suctioning.
3. **Apnea:** respiration is most likely to occur early during the apnea test; however, respiratory-like movements are most likely near the end of the test, when oxygenation is marginal.
4. **Apnea testing protocol**
   - Step 1: Ensure that apnea test prerequisites are present: core temperature ≥ 97.7° F (36.5° C), systolic blood pressure ≥ 90 mmHg, euvolemia, eucapnia, and normoxemia.
   - Step 2: Connect pulse oximeter; disconnect ventilator.
   - Step 3: Deliver 100% oxygen (6 L/min) into trachea.

Step 4: Check for respiratory movements.
Step 5: After 8 minutes, obtain blood for PaO_2, $PaCO_2$, and pH.
Step 6: Reconnect ventilator and immediately draw arterial blood gas if any of the following occurs during testing: systolic blood pressure < 90, marked decrease in SpO_2, or cardiac arrhythmias.

5. **Interpretation of test**
   a. Apnea if respiratory movements are absent and $PaCO_2 \geq 60$ mmHg.
   b. If respiratory movements are present or $PaCO_2$ is < 60 mmHg, test results are indeterminate. Repeat the apnea test; consider confirmatory laboratory test (see below).

III. **Potential pitfalls**
   1. In patients with severe facial trauma, preexisting pupillary abnormalities, drug intoxication, or prior lung or sleep disorder causing CO_2 retention, the diagnosis of brain death is difficult to make on clinical grounds.
   2. For **coma of undetermined origin**, the following are required in addition to the diagnostic criteria noted above: > 24 hr of observation, exclusion of confounding conditions, and lack of cerebral blood flow.
   3. Spontaneous motor responses (e.g., shoulder adduction, back arching) may occur during apnea testing, but they are of spinal (not brainstem) origin.

IV. **Laboratory tests:** not necessarily required. In order of decreasing sensitivity: nuclear brain perfusion scan, conventional angiography, EEG (no activity ≥ 30 min), transcranial Doppler ultrasound.

Key Reference: American Academy of Neurology: Practice parameters for determining brain death in adults. Neurology 45:1012–1014, 1995.

Guillain-Barré Syndrome

I. **Definition:** an acute demyelinating polyneuropathy that may have a fulminant course resulting in hypercarbic respiratory failure and prolonged weakness.

II. **Clinical manifestation: acute onset** (≈ 5 days to 3 weeks after viral upper respiratory infection or gastroenteritis or surgery) of **peripheral and cranial nerve dysfunction with progressive symmetric weakness, loss of deep tendon reflexes**, facial diplegia, oropharyngeal and respiratory paresis, and impaired sensation in hands/feet (although sensory exam may be normal, impaired joint position, vibration, pain, and temperature in a glove-stocking pattern may occur).

III. **Diagnosis**
   1. **Clinical diagnosis with elevated protein in cerebrospinal fluid**; one pearl to remember is that cerebrospinal fluid protein may be normal in the first week after onset; thus, a repeat lumbar puncture may be diagnostic. The spinal fluid should be acellular.
   2. **Nerve conduction studies**
      a. F-waves are absent or delayed. Nerve conduction velocities may be reduced due to demyelination and concomitant axonal loss.
      b. Clinical severity correlates poorly with the degree of slowing of nerve conduction velocities but well with the extent of electrophysiologically demonstrable nerve conduction block.
      c. Early electromyographic evidence of muscle denervation and axonal loss correlates with increased time to recovery and incomplete recovery.

IV. Death may be due to aspiration pneumonia, pulmonary emboli, intercurrent infection, or autonomic dysfunction (lethal dysrhythmias).

V. **Differential diagnosis: diphtheritic polyneuropathy** (long latent period between respiratory infection and onset of neuritis), **acute anterior poliomyelitis** (asymmetric paralysis with cerebrospinal fluid pleocytosis), **hypophosphatemia**-induced neural dysfunction (e.g., with prolonged total parenteral nutrition), and **botulism**.

VI. **Treatment**

1. **General supportive measures** such as **deep venous thrombosis prophylaxis, aspiration precaution**, and **telemetry monitoring** are vital in preventing or quickly diagnosing the complications of Guillain-Barré syndrome.
2. **Mechanical ventilation.** The need for intubation is best assessed by negative inspiratory force (NIF) and vital capacity (VC). Intubate with rapidly deteriorating levels or when NIF is ~ 20–25 cm H_2O or VC ~ 10 ml/kg. The absence of normal thoracic and abdominal muscle tone renders total static compliance (C_{stat}) higher than usual; therefore, patients require lower peak airway pressures. Patients prefer larger than normal tidal volume (~ 12–15 ml/kg), along with rapid inspiratory flow rates, because of diminished perception of lung-chest wall stretch with inspiration.
3. **Early plasmapheresis** accelerates recovery and decreases long-term neurologic disability.
4. Intravenous immunoglobulin (**IVIG**) has been shown to be as effective as plasma exchange.

Key References: Plasma Exchange/Sandoglobulin Guillain-Barré Syndrome Trial Group: Randomised trial of plasma exchange, intravenous immunoglobulin and combined treatments in Guillain-Barré syndrome. Lancet 349:225–230, 1997; Ropper AH: The Guillain-Barré syndrome. N Engl J Med 326:1130–1136, 1992.

Myasthenia Gravis

I. Myasthenia gravis (MG) results from antibody-directed destruction of muscle acetylcholine receptor sites. **Bimodal distribution:** third decade in women and sixth to seventh decade in men. Characterized by exercise-induced muscle fatigue, proximal weakness, ptosis, and diplopia.

II. **Myasthenic crisis** may occur spontaneously or be precipitated by an infection. Certain drugs, such as aminoglycoside or erythromycin, may precipitate a crisis. When forced vital capacity (FVC) drops below 15 ml/kg (or ≤ 1 liter), strongly consider mechanical ventilation. If an antibiotic is required, it is best to avoid those that may precipitate a myasthenic crisis (see below). Chronic therapy for MG consists of anitcholinesterase agents, prednisone, cytotoxics, and thymectomy.

III. **Cholinergic crisis.** Toxic doses of anticholinesterase (e.g., pyridostigmine) produce continuous depolarization of the postsynaptic membrane, leading to a depolarizing type of neuromuscular blockade with weakness, bronchoconstriction (nicotinic action), excessive respiratory secretions, blurred vision, abdominal cramps, and diarrhea (muscarinic action). Cholinergic crisis is extremely rare in the modern treatment of myasthenia gravis.

IV. **Myasthenic vs. cholinergic crisis.** Sometimes it is difficult to distinguish a myasthenic from a cholinergic crisis. In such instances, it is still paramount to monitor vital capacity and support respiratory failure. In regard to specific treatment, one recommendation is to stop all long-acting anticholinesterases and observe or measure objective response to edrophonium (a short-acting anticholinesterase).

V. **Use of edrophonium** to distinguish between myasthenic vs. cholinergic crisis
   1. **Do not undertake this test lightly**; if unsure, simply discontinue all anticholinesterases and observe.
   2. Many recommend that control ventilation be established in patients before the test.
   3. Edrophonium, 1 mg IV; repeat 1 mg IV in 1 min if no response. With myasthenic crisis, edrophonium improves respiration and weakness. With cholinergic crisis, weakness and oral secretions are increased. If no objective response, discontinue all anticholinesterases and give supportive therapy.

VI. **Prior to thymectomy**, the patient should have plasma exchange to optimize the state of their disease. The dose of anticholinesterase inhibitor should be reduced as much as possible to prevent cholinergic side effects.

VII. **Treatment**
   1. **Mechanical ventilation** when FVC approaches 15 ml/kg or patients are unable to handle secretions because of bulbar weakness.
   2. **Plasma exchange:** 50 ml/kg body weight is removed and replaced, providing an exchange of 60–70% of total plasma volume. Muscle strength usually improves within 48 hr.
   3. **Intravenous immunoglobulin** may result in improvement in cases where there has been minimal or no response to plasma exchange. However, randomized, controlled clinical data is not available to support the use of IVIG.

VIII. **Commonly used drugs that may exacerbate MG include but are not limited to:**
   1. Morphine, succinylcholine
   2. Aminoglycoside, tetracycline, mycin antibiotics (e.g., clindamycin)
   3. Quinidine, procainamide
   4. Lidocaine, propranolol
   5. Lithium, phenothiazines, phenytoin
   6. Thyroid hormone, corticosteroids (acutely)

Key References: Linton DM, Philcox D: Myasthenia gravis. Dis Month 36:593–637, 1990. Mayer SA: Intensive care of the myasthenic patient. Neurology 48:S70–S75, 1997.

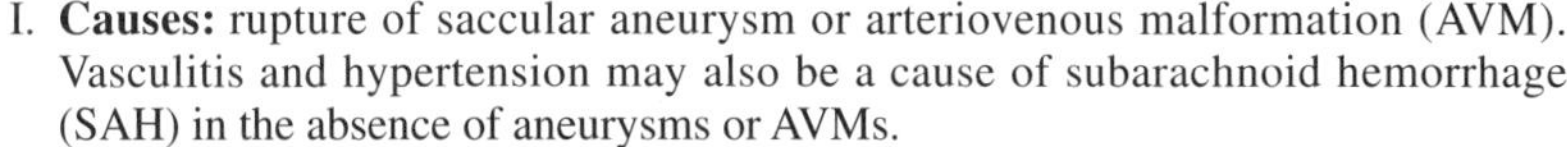

Subarachnoid Hemorrhage

I. **Causes:** rupture of saccular aneurysm or arteriovenous malformation (AVM). Vasculitis and hypertension may also be a cause of subarachnoid hemorrhage (SAH) in the absence of aneurysms or AVMs.

II. **Hunt-Hess clinical grading scale**
   - Grade 1: Asymptomatic or mild headache
   - Grade 2: Moderate to severe headache, nuchal rigidity with or without oculomotor palsy
   - Grade 3: Confusion, drowsiness, or mild focal signs
   - Grade 4: Stupor or hemiparesis
   - Grade 5: Coma, moribund, and/or extensor posturing

III. **Diagnosis**: a brain CT scan is the test of first choice although it may miss ~5% of SAH. A lumbar puncture may make the diagnosis in whom SAH is strongly suspected but has a normal or non-diagnostic CT scan. The first angiogram may not reveal the culprit aneurysm due to local vasospasm, and a second or third angiogram may be required to detect the aneurysm.

IV. **Complications and treatment**
   1. **Vasospasm** is the leading cause of morbidity and mortality. It is defined as the onset of confusion, decreasing mental status, or focal deficit in the absence of hematoma, rebleeding, hydrocephalus, or metabolic imbalance. Vasospasm

usually begins between the 4th and 9th day and **peaks around the 7th day**. **Treatment:** keep pulmonary artery wedge pressure (PAWP) around 14–18 mmHg; **nimodipine, 60 mg every 4 hr x 21 days**; maintain a hematocrit of at least 35%; allow blood pressure to increase to 140–160 mmHg.

2. **Rebleeding.** Risk is greatest within the first 48 hours. Mortality increases from 10–15% to 45% with rebleeding. **Treatment:** dark, quiet room; stool softeners, propranolol, 10 mg orally 4 times/day or 1 mg IV 4 times/day; phenobarbitol, 30–60 mg IV or orally 3 times/day for sedation.
3. **Hydrocephalus, intracranial hypertension, seizures:** due to impaired circulation of cerebrospinal fluid and mass effect if hematoma is present. **Treatment:** place ventricular catheter; drain if intracranial pressure (ICP) ≥ 15 mmHg; overdrainage may decrease ICP, causing an increase in transmural pressure (= arterial pressure – ICP) and an increased risk of rebleeding.
4. **Cardiac complications:** due to massive rise in catecholamines, which causes **ischemia and arrhythmias** (potentially malignant atrioventricular dissociation, idioventricular rhythm, or ventricular tachycardia occurs in 20–40%), **cardiogenic pulmonary edema** (ischemia or increased afterload).
5. **Pulmonary complications: pneumonitis and neurogenic pulmonary edema. Treatment:** keep PAWP around 12–15 mmHg; lower pressures may potentiate vasospasm.
6. **Hyponatremia:** due to combination of syndrome of inappropriate antidiuretic hormone (SIADH) and salt wasting due to atrial natriuretic factor (latter may lead to hypovolemia and vasospasm).

V. **Timing of surgery**

1. **Advantages of early surgery** (within 3 days of subarachnoid hemorrhage [SAH]) include (1) elimination of risk of rebleeding and (2) ability to remove SAH clot and thus decrease incidence and severity of vasospasm.
2. Early surgery for grades I and II and patients with an intracerebral hematoma whose condition is clinically deteriorating. Many even advocate early surgery for grades III and IV, although delayed surgery is often reserved for most grade III–IV patients whose condition is medically unstable.

Key References: Hongo K, Kobayashi S: Calcium antagonists for the treatment of vasospasm following subarachnoid hemorrhage. Neuro Res 15:218–224, 1993. Whiting DM, et al: Management of subarachnoid hemorrhage in the critical care unit. Cleve Clin J 56:775–785, 1989.

Intracranial Pressure Monitoring

I. Monitoring of intracranial pressure (ICP) is used mainly for severe head injury. Nontraumatic indications include intracerebral hemorrhage, Reye's syndrome, hepatic coma, encephalitis, stroke, normal pressure hydrocephalus, near-drowning, and subarachnoid hemorrhage. The Monro-Kellie doctrine states that $V_{brain} + V_{CSF} + V_{blood} + V_{mass}$ = constant, where V = volume and CSF = cerebrospinal fluid. Thus, as the V_{mass} increases, the ICP rises exponentially.

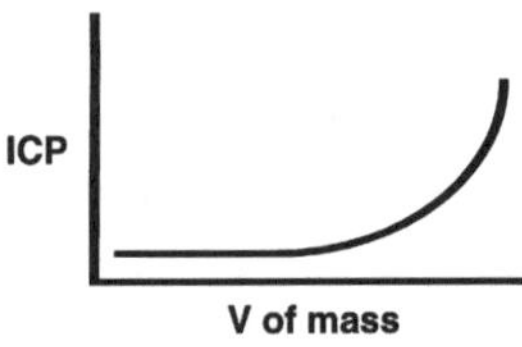

II. **Normal ICP = 10 mmHg** (136 mm H_2O); pressures > 20 mmHg are abnormal.

III. **Cerebral perfusion pressure (CPP) = mean arterial pressure (MAP) – ICP** (CPP < 80 mmHg is usually associated with poor outcome after injury).

IV. **Catheters** may be placed in the ventricle, parenchyma, or epidural, subdural, or subarachnoid space.

1. **Intraventricular catheter** is the gold standard of accuracy.
   a. **Advantages:** drainage of CSF for ICP control, CSF sampling, and monitoring for infection.
   b. **Disadvantages:** difficulty in cannulation, requires fluid-filled column that may be blocked by air bubbles or debris, and needs transducer repositioning with change in head position.
2. **Subarachnoid catheter (Richmond bolt)**
   a. **Advantages:** no invasion in the brain, lower infection rate.
   b. **Disadvantages:** blocking of port by swollen brain may artificially lower readings; needs repositioning after change in head position.
3. **Fiberoptic device**
   a. **Advantages:** can be placed subdurally, intraparenchymally, or intraventricularly; no need to reposition with change in head position.
   b. **Disadvantages:** inability to check calibration unless a ventriculostomy is used simultaneously.

V. Catheters may also be placed in jugular venous bulb (JVB).

1. Measures JVB saturation continuously; useful in head injury with increased ICP.
2. Saturation ≤ 50: need to increase cerebral blood flow by increasing blood pressure.

VI. **Complications: hematoma** (1%), **infection** (incidence of 6%, increase if left in place > 5 days; usually due to coagulase-negative staphylococci).

VII. **Positive end-expiratory pressure (PEEP) > 10 cm H_2O may increase ICP** (difficult to predict because it depends on what part of the Monro-Kellie curve the patient falls).

Delirium

I. **Characteristics:** agitation, lethargy, irritability, combativeness, confusion, disorientation, paranoia, hallucination, delusion, and autonomic system overactivity.

II. **Causes** are summarized by the mnemonic **I WATCH DEATH**:

I = Infection	Encephalitis, meningitis, syphilis
W = Withdrawal	Alcohol, barbiturates, sedatives-hypnotics
A = Acute metabolic disturbance	Acidosis, alkalosis, electrolytes, hepatic or renal failure
T = Trauma	Heat stroke, postoperative state, severe burns
C = Central nervous system pathology	Abscess, hemorrhage, normal-pressure hydrocephalus, seizures, stroke, tumor, vasculitis
H = Hypoxia	Anemia, carbon monoxide poisoning, hypotension, pulmonary or cardiac failure
D = Deficiencies	Vitamin B12, hypovitaminosis, niacin, thiamine
E = Endocrinopathies	Hyper- or hypoadrenocorticism, hyper- or hypoglycemia
A = Acute vascular disorder	Hypertensive encephalopathy, shock
T = Toxins/drugs	Medications, pesticides, solvents
H = Heavy metals	Lead, manganese, mercury

Other = psychiatric illness or patient on antipsychotics or sedatives; "ICU-itis"

III. **Use of intravenous haloperidol (Haldol) to control delirium and agitation**

1. Typical dose: 2–5 mg IV every 20–30 min until sedated; then adjust to maximum of 240 mg over 24 hr. (IV haloperidol is not FDA approved.)
2. Extrapyramidal symptoms may be controlled with benzodiazepines (lorazepam 0.5–10 mg IV) or 25–50 mg of diphenhydramine.
3. IV haloperidol has a half-life of ~ 14 hr, but because it is distributed extensively, it may remain in the body for prolonged periods.

Reference: Gelfand SB, et al: Using intravenous haloperidol to control delirium. Hosp Community Psychiatry 43:215, 1992.

Prolonged Paralysis

I. **Prolonged effects of neuromuscular blocking agents** (NMBs) may be neuropathic or myopathic. Pancuronium and vecuronium have active metabolites that may accumulate in patients with renal or liver insufficiency. Generally reversible but may be slow (weeks to months) to resolve. Risk factors include:

1. Hepatic or renal insufficiency due to drug accumulation
2. Metabolic acidosis
3. Female gender
4. Increased magnesium
5. Concomitant use of corticosteroids (causes mainly a myopathic process with proximal and distal weakness, decreased deep tendon reflexes, electrophysiologic evidence of muscle disease, and increased creatine phosphokinase). Steroidal NMBs (pancuronium and vecuronium) appear more likely to have this deleterious effect with corticosteroids than nonsteroidal NMB (atracurium).

II. **Critical illness polyneuropathy (CIP)**

1. Characterized by **distal motor weakness** (leg weakness > arm weakness), decreased deep tendon reflexes, sensory deficits, and electrophysiologic evidence of axonal degeneration involving both motor and sensory fibers.
2. Usually seen in the setting of systemic inflammatory response with multiorgan dysfunction syndrome after 2–4 weeks in ICU.
3. **Respiratory muscle dysfunction** may occur, resulting in inability to wean patient from the ventilator.
4. **Risk factors** include (1) hypoalbuminemia (may reflect either the severity of the illness or malnourished state), (2) hyperglycemia, and (3) prolonged ICU stay.
5. Diagnosis is established using nerve conduction studies and electromyography. Expected findings include **reduced sensory and motor amplitudes on nerve conduction studies** with relative preservation of normal conduction velocity. Evidence of **acute denervation may be observed on electromyography**.
6. **Recovery** may take weeks or months to years, with permanent neurologic deficits in some patients.

III. **Other causes**

1. **Primary neuromuscular disorders** (e.g., Guillain-Barré syndrome, myasthenia gravis)
2. **Neuromuscular disorder due to another primary disorder** (e.g., hypothyroidism)
3. **Electrolyte and metabolic causes** (e.g., hypophosphatemia)

Key Reference: Kelly B, Matthay M: Prevalence and severity of neurologic dysfunction in critically ill patients. Chest 104:1818, 1993.

Secondary Neurologic Dysfunction

I. **Common causes** of neurologic dysfunction in the ICU:
   1. Toxic and metabolic encephalopathies
   2. Seizures
   3. Stroke syndromes

II. **Metabolic encephalopathies**
   1. **Sepsis**
      a. The severity of encephalopathy is a predictor of mortality (~50% mortality in patients with severe cases).
      b. Electroencephalographic (EEG) abnormalities may occur before clinical signs and include diffuse or intermittent theta (4–7 Hz) or delta (0–3 Hz) frequency slowing, triphasic waves, or a burst-suppression pattern (the latter two indicate poor prognosis).
   2. **Hepatic dysfunction:** two major types of neurologic dysfunction may occur with liver disease.
      a. Patients with rapid onset of liver dysfunction (within 8 weeks) have **acute hepatic encephalopathy or fulminant hepatic failure** (when coma is present).
      b. **Chronic hepatic encephalopathy** has a better prognosis and occurs in patients with cirrhosis.
   3. **Renal disease**
      a. **Uremic encephalopathy:** asterixis, chorea, myoclonus, akathisia.
      b. **Dialysis disequilibrium syndrome:** an acute encephalopathy (headache, confusion, muscle cramps, seizure, coma) that develops during or shortly after dialysis.
      c. **Dialysis dementia syndrome:** a complication of prolonged dialysis manifested by personality changes, dysarthric speech, myoclonus, and seizures.
   4. **Hypoglycemia:** confusion, focal neurologic deficits (hemiparesis, isolated cranial nerve palsy, especially cranial nerve III), coma.
   5. **Hyperosmolar states**
      a. Occur in three principal settings: hyperglycemia, severe dehydration, and hypernatremia.
      b. The fluid deficit must be corrected cautiously to avoid brain swelling. Central pontine myelinosis (CPM), though associated with too-rapid correction of hyponatremia, may occur with correction of hypernatremia and in severe form may present as a "lock-in" state.
   6. **Malignant hypertension**
      a. Occurs with acute rise in blood pressure when normal autoregulation of cerebral blood flow is lost.
      b. Symptoms of headache, nausea, vomiting, papilledema, scotoma, seizures, stupor, and coma result from increased intracranial pressure due to increased permeability of blood–brain barrier.
   7. **Hypoxia-ischemia**
      a. Duration of coma is important in prognosis. Patients with coma < 12 hr usually recover completely, whereas patients with coma > 12 hr often have focal or multifocal deficits (amnesia, dementia, quadriparesis, visual agnosia, paraparesis, ataxia, seizures, myoclonus, extrapyramidal signs).
      b. In patients with no recovery of consciousness, there is global damage with persistent vegetative state or brain death.
   8. **Iatrogenic (drugs):** opiates, benzodiazepines, cimetidine, and corticosteroids are often implicated.

9. **Wernicke's disease**
   a. May occur not only in alcoholics but also in anyone with poor nutrition.
   b. May be precipitated in susceptible patients by glucose administration when thiamine prophylaxis is not given.
   c. Confusion, ophthalmoplegia, and ataxia are the classic triad, although there are many different presentations.
10. **Thyroid disease**
   a. **Hypothyroidism:** headache, depression, somnolence, confusion, muscle cramp, carpal tunnel syndrome, ataxia.
   b. **Hyperthyroidism:** anxiety, hyperreflexia, spasticity, chorea, proximal myopathy, seizures.

III. **Seizures**
1. Common underlying causes for seizures in the ICU include vascular abnormalities (arteriovenous malformations, vasculitis, intracerebral hemorrhage), infectious disorders (brain abscess, meningitis, toxoplasmosis), and metabolic disorders.
2. Electrolyte and glucose should be checked; lumbar puncture and head CT scan should be considered.
3. Prophylaxis against recurrent seizures with phenytoin should be strongly considered unless a reversible cause is apparent.

IV. **Stroke syndromes**
1. Cerebral infarction may complicate acute myocardial infarction in 1–2% of cases.
2. Underlying disorders that may predispose to an **ischemic stroke** are bacterial endocarditis, systemic lupus erythematosus, rheumatic heart disease, cardiomyopathies, thrombocytosis, thrombotic thrombocytopenic purpura, disseminated intravascular coagulation, sickle cell anemia, antiphospholipid antibody syndrome, and venous thromboembolism with paradoxical embolization.
3. Other **mimickers of ischemic strokes** are bacterial meningitis (due to septic thrombosis of cerebral veins) and brain abscess.

V. **Peripheral neuropathy**
1. Critical illness neuropathy: a sensorimotor axonal neuropathy that may make weaning very difficult.
2. Compression neuropathies: most commonly affect peroneal, ulnar, and median nerves.

VI. **Neuromuscular syndromes**
1. Prolonged neuromuscular blockade with nondepolarizing paralytics, even those that are short-acting.
2. Certain drugs also may cause or unmask neuromuscular disease; examples include aminoglycosides, certain tetracyclines, and D-penicillamine.

VII. **Central pontine myelinolysis (CPM)**
1. Neurologic disorder first described in alcoholics but subsequently found to occur also in patients with rapid correction of chronic hyponatremia.
2. Patients with CPM may remain in a coma for long periods and yet have excellent recovery.
3. Magnetic resonance imaging (MRI) is the single best diagnostic test, although it may be normal if obtained < 3 weeks after onset of findings.

Key References: Solenski NJ, Bleck TP: Managing secondary neurologic dysfunction in the ICU. J Crit Illness 9:843–853, 1994; Solenski NJ, Bleck TP: Neurologic disorders in the ICU: Common metabolic encephalopathies. J Crit Illness 9:770–782, 1994.

Coma

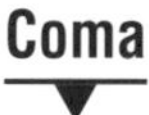

I. **Definitions**
   1. **Delirium:** acute confusional state characterized by disorientation, fear, and irritability.
   2. **Stupor:** unresponsiveness from which the patient can be aroused.
   3. **Coma:** unarousable unresponsiveness.

II. **Emergent management**
   1. Airways, breathing, circulation (**ABCs**): Ensure airway protection; intubate if necessary. Support circulation, address trauma issues, especially head and cervical spine.
   2. Draw blood for glucose, electrolytes, calcium, blood urea nitrogen, creatinine, and toxicology screen. Check arterial blood gas to assess SaO_2, $PaCO_2$.
   3. Infuse thiamine (100 mg IV), glucose (25 gm), and naloxone (0.4 mg). If indicated, start O_2, IV fluids or blood products, and pressors.

III. **Initial diagnostic assessment**
   1. **Level of consciousness**
   2. **Brainstem function**
      a. **Respirations:** the anatomic level that correlates with each type of breathing pattern is the highest level of function.
         - **Cheyne-Stokes respirations:** cortical/metabolic
         - **Central neurogenic hyperventilation:** lower midbrain–upper pons
         - **Apneustic breathing:** lower pons
         - **Biot's or ataxic breathing:** medulla

      b. **Pupils**
         - **Midposition and fixed:** midbrain lesions or glutethimide
         - **Pinpoint and slightly reactive:** pontine lesion (e.g., pontine hemorrhage) or opiates
         - **Dilated:** medullary lesion or anticholinergic overdose

      c. **Ocular movements**
         - **Oculocephalic reflex (doll's eyes) lost** with midbrain/pontine tegmental lesions.
         - **Oculovestibular (caloric) response lost** with various brainstem lesions. Normal caloric response is nystagmus with rapid phase away from cold stimulation or toward warm stimulation (**COWS** = **c**old–**o**pposite, **w**arm—**s**ame). **Warning:** Barbiturates and phenytoin may abolish ocular movements.
   3. **Motor tone**
      a. **Variable resistance** seen in metabolic encephalopathy.
      b. **Chorea, athetosis, and ballismus** are seen in basal ganglia lesions.
      c. **Decerebrate rigidity** (arms and legs extended, internally rotated) occurs with herniation, midbrain compression, and hypoglycemia/hypoxia; rare with hepatic coma.
      d. **Decorticate rigidity** (arms flexed) occurs with higher lesions in white matter, internal capsules, and thalamus.
   4. **Laboratory tests:** liver, renal, endocrine (thyroid/adrenal), and respiratory (arterial blood gas) function tests. Urine toxicology screen is mandatory; blood, urine, and sputum cultures should be obtained, because infections can be primary or secondary. Lumbar puncture if CNS infection or subarachnoid hemorrhage is suspected.
   5. **Imaging:** CT is useful if focal or lateralizing signs are present and if bleeding is suspected. In this setting, contrast should be given only after non-contrast

studies have been performed. MRI is preferable when a lesion of the brain parenchyma is suspected.

IV. **Differential diagnosis**

1. **Coma with focal or lateralizing signs**
   a. Intracerebral hemorrhage: sudden onset, headache, history of hypertension.
   b. Stroke (thrombotic or embolic): associated edema may increase intracranial pressure.
   c. Hypertensive encephalopathy: headache, other signs of malignant hypertension.
   d. Subdural hematoma: may have history of trauma and headache.
   e. Brain abscess: headache, fever; cerebrospinal fluid (CSF) with increased protein and cells, normal glucose.
   f. Fracture, concussion: trauma, bleeding from nose and ears.
2. **Coma without focal signs but with meningismus**
   a. Meningitis: fever; CSF is diagnostic.
   b. Subarachnoid hemorrhage: headache; bloody or xanthochromic CSF.
3. **Coma without focal signs or meningismus**
   a. Intoxication: syndrome varies with toxin. Carbon monoxide toxicity also causes coma.
   b. Endocrine: chemical and clinical evidence of hyper- or hypoglycemia, thyroid or adrenal disorders.
   c. Hepatic or renal failure: chemical and clinical evidence of either hepatic or renal dysfunction.
   d. Sepsis: fever or hypothermia, hypotension.
   e. Epilepsy: metabolic acidosis, characteristic EEG.

Key Reference: Adams RD, Victor M, Ropper A: Principles of Neurology, 6th ed. New York, McGraw-Hill, 1997.

Neuroprotective Measures Following Brain Injury

I. **Two basic types of central nervous system (CNS) injury**: focal injury or ischemia and global ischemia or anoxia.

II. **Ischemic stroke**

1. It is increasingly recognized that neurons are relatively tolerant to ischemia and that they can withstand hours of low or no flow and still survive. Thus, the approach now should be to restore circulation to ischemic areas before infarction is inevitable using thrombolytics after a CT scan rules out subarachnoid or intracerebral hemorrhage.
2. **Intravenous tissue plasminogen activator (TPA)** has been approved for use in ischemic strokes in selected patients. However, the risk of intracranial and extracranial bleeding is significantly more likely to occur. Contraindications to thrombolysis in ischemic stroke:
   a. Absolute contraindications: blood on CT scan, rapidly improving or only minor symptoms, suspicion of subarachnoid hemorrhage with normal CT scan, internal bleeding within 3 weeks, known bleeding disorder, cranial surgery stroke, or head injury within 3 months, and serious trauma or major surgery within 2 weeks.
   b. Relative contraindications: hypertension (systolic > 180, diastolic > 110), lumbar puncture within 7 days, arterial puncture, past history of head injury or intracranial bleed, past history of cerebral aneurysms, recent seizure, and recent acute myocardial infarction.

3. **Glucose-containing fluids should NOT be administered** in ischemic injury and hyperglycemia should be avoided.
4. General measures such as maintaining a patent and ensuring adequate oxygenation and prevention of aspiration are critical.
5. In general, **hyperventilation is NOT recommended** because it may reduce cerebral blood flow. Although hyperventilation may help in patients with acute elevations in intracranial pressure, routine use of sustained hyperventilation in ischemic stroke or other CNS injury should be avoided.
6. Prevention of any fever because elevated temperature may be deleterious to ischemic brain tissues.
7. **Blood pressure management** should be cautiously undertaken in ischemic strokes because of the loss of autoregulation in the cerebral blood vessels and the shift toward a higher cerebral perfusion pressure in chronic hypertensive patients. Thus, a common mistake is to reduce blood pressure to "normal" levels, which leads to further reduction in cerebral perfusion and worsening ischemia. There is suggestion that elevated blood pressure should not be treated in the acute ischemic stroke although the threshold level for treatment is not absolutely known. If it is decided upon that the elevated blood pressure requires treatment, then intravenous labetalol or enalapril, beginning at smallest doses, is recommended.
8. **Serial examinations is crucial** because remedial actions may be taken prior to any irreversibility.
   a. **Elevated ICP from edema**. CT findings: midline shift, small ventricles, gyral effacement. Possible treatment: osmotherapy to increase serum osmolality to 290-310 mOsm/L (or mmol/kg) (e.g., mannitol), steroids, infarctectomy, decompressive craniectomy).
   b. **Hydrocephalus**. CT findings: enlarged lateral ventricles, gyral effacement, transtentorial herniation. Possible treatment: ventriculostomy, high-volume spinal taps.
   c. **Intracranial hemorrhage**. CT findings: clotted blood, mass effect. Possible treatment: normalize coagulation factors, clot removal, decompressive craniectomy.
   d. **Extension of infarct**. CT findings: increase in hypodense areas, no change from previous scans. Possible treatment: anticoagulation, supportive care.

III. **Head and spinal cord injury**

1. A major change in treatment of severe CNS injury is to avoid hyperventilation, unless herniation is imminent because of elevated ICP.
2. Seizures should be aggressively treated to prevent further neurologic deterioration due to hypoxia and hyperthermia. The use of prophylactic phenytoin is common but unproven.
3. For head injury, identification and control of elevated ICP with sedation, osmotherapy, and decompressive craniectomy are the mainstays of treatment. Corticosteroids have not been shown to be helpful.
4. For spinal cord injury, methylprednisolone, 30 mg/kg within 8 hr of injury, followed by 5.4 mg/kg/hr for 23 hr, is associated with a better outcome.
5. **Fiberoptic bronchoscopy (FB) in patients with severe head injury:** a study of 15 patients with severe head injury revealed that FB "does not adversely affect neurologic status in patients with severe head injury." Both intracranial pressure and mean arterial pressure rose with FB, maintaining an adequate cerebral perfusion pressure.
6. **Epidural spinal cord compression due to cancer:** the most common causes are breast, lung, and prostate cancer. Back pain, weakness of lower extremities, sensory loss, and autonomic dysfunction (e.g., bladder) are clues to diagnosis.

Plain films and MRI are the preferred imaging studies. Treatment includes **dexamethasone** (50–100 mg bolus, then 4–24 mg every 6 hr), **radiation therapy** (30 Gy to region two vertebrae above and below lesion), and **surgery in selected patients**.

Key References: Byrne TN: Spinal cord compression from epiduralmetastases. N Engl J Med 327:614–619, 1992; Durbin CG: Neurological intensive care and cerebral protection. Crit Care Alert 6:28–32, 1998; Peerless JR, et al: The effect of fiberoptic bronchoscopy on cerebral hemodynamics in patients with severe head injury. Chest 108:962–965, 1995.

Nutrition

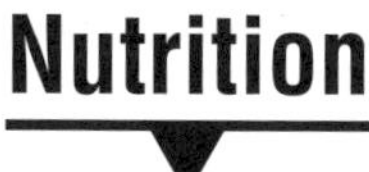

Marcie M. Chase, RD

Introduction

Malnutrition is a disease state induced by inadequate diet (oral, enteral, or parenteral) or altered nutrient utilization that results in organ dysfunction to the extent of increasing the risk of morbidity and that can be reversed only by aggressive nutritional support. Nutritional support was a "second thought" in the critical care setting until the era of cost containment. Malnutrition commonly occurs in the hospital setting and has been shown to add significantly to hospital costs. Surveys have found that 40–50% of hospital admissions are at risk for malnutrition and up to 12% are severely malnourished. The increased cost and poor outcomes associated with malnutrition have elevated nutritional support to a primary treatment modality.

Key Reference: Braunschweig C, Gomez S, Sheean P: Impact of declines in nutritional status on outcomes in adult patients hospitalized for more than 7 days. J Am Diet Assoc 100:1316–1322, 2000.

Nutritional Screening

I. **Nutritional screening** has become the primary tool to identify at-risk patients upon admission. Although a standard nutritional screening tool has not been established, several tools are available:
   1. **Nutritional Screening Initiative** (NSI): a bilevel tool that uses body mass index (BMI) and subjective data in the level I screen and BMI, anthropometrics data, laboratory data, clinical history, drug history, and eating habits in the level II screen to determine the risk for malnutrition.
   2. **Prognostic Nutritional Index** (PNI): this screening model calculates the risk of operative morbidity and mortality according to baseline nutritional status using the following parameters: PNI (percent) = 158 – 16.6 $\times$ albumin – 0.78 (triceps skin fold) – 0.20 (transferrin) – 5.8 (delayed hypersensitivity). PNI > 50% = high risk, PNI of 40–49% = intermediate risk, and PNI < 40% = low risk.
   3. **Nutrition Risk Index** (NRI): this screen calculates malnutrition using the following equation: 1.519 $\times$ albumin +1.417 $\times$ (current weight/usual weight) $\times$ 100.
   4. **Subjective Global Assessment** (SGA): nutritional screen and assessment based on an extensive history and physical examination.

II. **Nutritional screening within 24 hours of admission** is a standard of the Joint Commission on Accreditation of Healthcare Organizations (JCAHO). Patients considered to be at nutritional risk exhibit any one of the following:

1. **Actual malnutrition or potential for developing malnutrition**: (1) involuntary weight loss of 10% of usual body weight (UBW) within 6 months, 5% of UBW within 1 month, or < 20% of ideal body weight (IBW); (2) BMI < 18. BMI is calculated using the following equation: wt (kg)/ht (meter) $\times$ 2.
2. **Visceral protein depletion**: serum albumin <3 .5 g/dl, serum transferrin < 200 mg/dl, serum cholesterol < 160 mg/dl, serum prealbumin < 15 mg/ml, creatinine height index < 75%.
3. **Altered diet**: receiving total parenteral or enteral nutrition.

4. **Inadequate intake due to**: NPO status for 3 days, clear liquid diet for 5 days, malabsorptive disorder, impaired ability to ingest, increased metabolic requirements, gastrointestinal disturbances (nausea, vomiting, diarrhea, constipation).

Key References: Clinical Pathways and Algorithms for Delivery of Parenteral Nutrition Support in Adults. American Society of Enteral and Parenteral Nutrition, 1998. Malnutrition—A Hidden Cost in Healthcare. Ross Products, 1993.

Nutritional Assessment

I. **Nutritional assessment:** patients considered to be at nutritional risk are required to undergo a comprehensive nutritional assessment by a registered dietitian. Nutritional assessment includes evaluation of anthropometric and biochemical indices.

II. **Anthropometric evaluation**: height and weight are probably the most important vital statistics in nutritional assessment.

1. **Height**: height is the key component in determination of IBW, which can easily be determined using the Hamwi calculation: **Males**: 106 lb for the first 5 feet and 6 lb per inch thereafter (example: 5'10" = 166 lb); **Females**: 100 lb for the first 5 feet and 5 lb per inch thereafter (example: 5'10" = 150 lb).
2. **IBW** needs to be adjusted for frame size, spinal cord injury, and amputation.
   a. **Frame size**: small frame size: decrease IBW by 10%; medium frame size: no changes needed in IBW; large frame size: increase IBW by 10%
   b. **Spinal cord injury**: paraplegic: subtract 10–15 lb from IBW; quadriplegic: subtract 15–20 lb from IBW.
   c. **Amputation**: hand: – 0.7%, forearm and hand: –2.3%, total arm: –4.9%, foot: –1.5%, calf and foot: –5.8%, total leg: –16%.
3. **Weight**: admission body weight is probably the most reliable. Weights measured postoperatively or after admission to the intensive care unit tend may be unreliable because of the administration of fluids or edematous states.
   a. To determine weight to use for feeding calculations, first calculate %IBW:
      - %IBW = actual body weight/ideal body weight × 100
      - If actual body weight is < IBW, use actual body weight to determine nutritional needs.
      - If actual body weight is > IBW but < 120%, use IBW to determine nutritional needs.
      - If actual body weight is > 120% IBW, use adjusted (ABW) or relative body weight to calculate needs: IBW + (ABW – IBW × 0.25).
   b. Actual weight as a percentage of IBW can be used to categorize the nutritional status of patients as follows:

% of IBW	Classification	% of IBW	Classification
> 200	Morbidly obese	80–90	Mild malnutrition
> 150	Obese	70–80	Moderate malnutrition
> 120	Overweight	< 70	Severe malnutrition
100 ± 10	Normal		

III. **Evaluation of biochemical indices of nutritional status**.

1. **Serum albumin** is not a definitive measure of visceral protein status but reflects the complex relationship between synthesis, degradation, and distribution. Nonnutritional factors that may reduce albumin levels include (1) inadequate synthesis, as seen in cirrhosis, cancer, acute stress, congestive heart failure, and hypoxia; (2) impaired digestion, as seen in pancreatic insufficiency and malabsorption; (3) altered fluid status, such as edematous conditions and overhydration; and (4) chronic protein loss, as seen with nephrotic syndrome and burns.

a. **Key albumin levels: normal = 3.5-5.0 gm/dl.** Levels of 3.0–3.5 gm/dl (35–50 gm/L) are considered a medical decision point. Levels < 3.5 gm/dl correlate with poor surgical outcome, poor prognosis, increased cost of hospitalization, and prolonged intensive care unit stay. Levels <3.0 gm/dl often are associated with severe malnutrition. Levels < 2.5 gm/dl (< 25 gm/L) are associated with increased rates of morbidity and mortality.
b. **Limitations of albumin as a nutritional marker** are due to its long half-life of 21 days and the numerous factors that decrease albumin levels independently of nutritional status.

2. **Transferrin** resides almost completely in the intravascular compartment, where it serves as the transport protein for iron.
   a. Serum transferrin levels are determined primarily by synthesis. Its half-life of 8–9 days makes transferrin a better nutritional marker of visceral protein status. **Normal levels range between 200 and 400 mg/dl (2–4 gm/L)**; a level of 150 mg/dl (1.5 gm/L) is considered a nutritional decision point.
   b. Transferrin levels are **decreased** in situations of (1) impaired synthesis, such as acute fasting, chronic infection, and pernicious anemia; (2) increased excretion, as seen with nephrotic syndrome, inflammation, burns, liver damage, and overhydration; (4) increased iron stores, as seen with hemosiderosis, and hemochromatosis. Transferrin levels are **increased** in situations of (1) decreased iron stores, as seen with iron deficiency anemia and chronic blood loss; (2) increased protein synthesis, as seen in estrogen therapy and oral contraception; (3) dehydration; and (4) pregnancy (second and third trimesters). The serum concentration of transferrin is about 0.8 times the total iron-binding capacity (TIBC). Thus, transferrin level may be calculated indirectly from TIBC: transferrin = (TIBC × 0.8) – 43.
3. **Prealbumin** is also known as thyroxine-binding prealbumin and functions as a transport protein for thyroxine, retinal-binding protein, and vitamin A.
   a. It has a half-life of ~ 2 days, making it an excellent nutritional marker.
   b. **Normal values: 16–35 mg/dl (0.16–0.35 gm/L).** A prealbumin level < 11 mg/dl (< 0.11 gm/L) signifies malnutrition. The failure to increase prealbumin above 11 mg/dl (0.11 gm/L) is an indication that nutritional needs are not being met. Concentrations should increase by ~ 1 mg/dl/day (0.01 gm/L/day) or double in 1 week when adequate nutritional therapy is provided. Nonnutritional factors that decrease prealbumin include stress, inflammation, surgery, cirrhosis, hepatitis, and renal failure.
4. **Visceral proteins** in relation to the degree of malnutrition:
   a. **Albumin** (gm/dl): half-life = 21 days; normal level = 3.5–5 (35–50 gm/L); mild malnutrition = 2.8–3.5 (28–35 gm/L), moderate malnutrition = 2.1–2.7 (21–27 gm/L); severe malnutrition = < 2.1 (< 21 gm/L).
   b. **Transferrin** (mg/dl): half-life = 8–9 days; normal level = 200–400 (2–4 gm/L); mild malnutrition = 150–200 (1.5–2 gm/L); moderate malnutrition = 100–150 (1–1.5 gm/L); severe malnutrition = < 100 (< 1 gm/L).
   c. **Prealbumin** (mg/dl): half-life = 2 days; normal level = 16–30 (0.16–0.30 gm/L); mild malnutrition = 10–15 (0.1–0.15 gm/L); moderate malnutrition = 5–10 (0.05–0.1 gm/L); severe malnutrition = < 5 (< 0.05 gm/L).
5. **Retinol-binding protein (RBP)** is a small protein with a half-life of 12 hours, leading to a more rapid response to changes in protein and calorie intake.
   a. **Normal levels: 2.6–7.6 mg/dl (0.026–0.076 gm/L).** Levels < 1.6 mg/dl (< 0.016 gm/L) indicate malnutrition.
   b. Nonnutritional conditions leading to an **increase** in RBP are drug-induced hepatitis and renal disease. Conditions causing a **decrease** in RBP include stress, injury, hyperthyroidism, and vitamin A or zinc deficiency.

6. **C-reactive protein (CRP).** In contrast to albumin, transferrin and prealbumin, which are negative acute-phase reactants, CRP is considered a positive acute-phase reactant because levels rise hundreds or thousands of times above normal during inflammation. CRP is not considered an indicator of nutritional status, but its increase precedes change in nutritional status due to hypermetabolism. Levels > 0.5 are considered clinically significant.
7. **Creatinine height index (CHI)** relates the 24-hour urinary creatinine to an ideal value based on ideal weight for height as follows: CHI = (actual urinary creatinine/ideal urinary creatinine) × 100. CHI indicates the percentage of muscle deficit (or excess). CHI of 90–100% is considered normal. CHI of 60–80% indicates moderate muscle wasting. CHI < 60% indicates severe lean tissue loss. Standards for CHI may overestimate the severity of depletion in the elderly population due to their decreased lean body.
8. **Nitrogen balance studies.**
   a. Nitrogen balance studies measure the net change in the body's total protein. An estimate of nitrogen balance can be obtained by measuring urinary nitrogen (UUN) and comparing it with nitrogen intake during that same time.
   b. **Nitrogen balance = N_2 intake – N_2 excretion**
      - Grams of protein = 6.25 (gm N_2) because average protein is 16% nitrogen
      - **N_2 balance = (total protein intake [gm]/6.25) – (UUN + 4)**, where UUN = urinary urea nitrogen in gm/24 hr collection (keep cold); 4 = factor for skin and gastrointestinal protein losses.
   c. Normal adults are usually in nitrogen balance, i.e., nitrogen balance = 0. A **positive nitrogen balance** (nitrogen balance > 0) signifies that protein anabolism exceeds protein catabolism. It usually is seen with pregnancy, growth, and recovery from illness and/or nutritional repletion. The goal in nutritional repletion is a positive nitrogen balance of 4–6 gm/day. A **negative nitrogen balance** (nitrogen balance < 0) signifies that protein catabolism exceeds protein anabolism. It is seen in situations of starvation, increased catabolism due to trauma or surgery, and inadequate nutrition support.

Key References: Charney P: Nutritional assessment in the 1990's: Where are we now?. Nutr Clin Pract 10:131–139, 1995; National Academy of Clinical Biochemistry Laboratory Support in Assessing and Monitoring Nutritional Status, 1994.

Determination of Type and Degree of Malnutrition

I. **Marasmus** describes a typical starved patient. Malnutrition is characterized by deficiency in total caloric intake and depletion of somatic protein, skeletal muscle, and adipose stores, resulting in impaired muscle function. Cell-mediated immunity also is impaired. Visceral protein production is preserved.

II. **Kwashiorkor** describes a typical hypermetabolic or catabolic patient. Malnutrition is characterized by adequate calorie intake with protein deficiency, depletion of visceral protein pools, some depletion of somatic protein with relative preservation of adipose tissue, and immunodeficiency.

III. **Protein/calorie malnutrition** describes a marasmic patient who becomes hypermetabolic or catabolic. It is characterized by depletion of visceral protein pools, depletion of somatic protein and adipose tissue, and immunodeficiency.

Key Reference: A dietians guide to Diagnostic-Related Groups. Ross Laboratories, 1993.

Calculation of Nutritional Needs

I. **Energy needs:** energy requirements are assessed in a variety of ways.

1. **Harris-Benedict formula.** This formula has been considered the gold standard for predicting calorie requirements in hospitalized patients for many years. However, in the critical care setting it is somewhat time-consuming and has been said to overestimate energy needs. The basal energy expenditure (BEE) in kcal/day at rest is estimated by gender using the following formulas:
   a. **Male BEE** = 66.5 + 13.8(wt) + 5.0(ht) – 6.8(age)
   b. **Female BEE** = 655.1 +9.6(wt) + 1.8(ht) – 4.7(age)
   c. **The calculated caloric requirement (CCR)** = BEE × activity factor × injury factor

   Activity factor: Bed rest = 1.2
   Ambulatory = 1.3
   Injury factor: Anabolism = 1.5
   Cancer = 1.6
   Major surgery = 1.6
   Mild infection = 1.2
   Moderate infection = 1.4
   Starvation = 0.7
   Stress: low = 1.3, medium = 1.5, high = 2.0

2. **Body weight**. This approach uses body weight alone, omiting the variables of age, sex, and height. This type of estimate has been proved to be accurate and is time-efficient in the critical care setting.
   a. **Kcal/kg according to Jeejeboy**:

Status	kcal/kg
Basal energy needs	25–30
Ambulatory with weight maintenance	30
Malnutrition w/ mild stress	40
Severe injuries and sepsis	50–60
Extensive burns	80

   b. **Kcal/kg according to Cerra**

Status	kcal/kg
Simple starvation	28
Elective surgery	32
Polytrauma	40
Sepsis	50

3. **Indirect calorimetry**. Using a metabolic cart, this method allows measurement of oxygen consumption (VO_2) in relation to calculated 24-hour BEE. O_2 utilization is directly proportional to energy utilization in aerobic environments. Indirect calorimetry is useful in burn and septic patients because it enables the clinician to order specialized macronutrients based on utilization.
4. **Estimated caloric requirement based on hemodynamics**

$$\text{BEE (kcal/day)} = (\text{CO})(\text{Hb})(\text{SaO}_2 - \text{S}\bar{\text{v}}\text{O}_2)(95.18)$$

Reference: Liggett SB, St. John RE, Lefrak SS: Determination of resting energy expenditure utilizing the thermodilution pulmonary artery catheter. Chest 91:562, 1987.

5. **Obese patients**. Because of increased fat mass, formulas that have been developed specifically for this population.
   a. **Ireton-Jones**

   $$\text{Caloric needs} = 606(S) + 9(ABW) - 12(A) + 400(V) + 1444$$

   where S is sex (male = 1, female = 0), ABW is actual body weight (kg), A is age (years), and V is ventilatory status (ventilator dependent = 1, spontaneous breathing = 0).

   Reference: Ireton-Jones CS, Turner WW: Actual or ideal body weight: Which should be used to predict anergy expenditure? J Am Diet Assoc 91:193–195, 1991.

   b. **Ireton-Jones for ventilator-dependent patients**

   $$\text{Caloric needs} = 1925 - 10(A) + 5(ABW) + 281(S) + 292(T) + 851(B)$$

   where A is age (years), ABW is actual body weight (kg), S is sex (male = 1, female = 0), T is trauma (present = 1, absent =0), and B is burn (present = 1, absent = 0).

   Reference: Ireton-Jones CS, Borman KR, Turner WW: Nutrition considerations in the management of ventilator dependent patients. Nutr Clin Prac 8:60–64, 1993.

   c. **Owen et al.**

   $$\text{Men: RMR} = 879 + (10.2 \times ABW);\ \text{Women: RMR} = 795 + (7.2 \times ABW)$$

   where RMR is resting metabolic rate (kcal/kg) and ABW is actual body weight (kg).

   Reference: Owen OE, Kavil E, Owen RS: A repraisal of caloric needs in healthy women. Am J Clin Nutr 44:1-19, 1986.

II. **Protein needs:** many factors need to be considered when estimating protein needs including metabolic rate, body protein reserves, calorie intake, nutritional status, disease state, stress associated with critical illness, and age.

1. **Blackburn guideline** for protein needs based on stress level

Status	Estimated Requirements
Normal (RDA)	0.8–1.0 gm/kg/day
Moderately stress	1.0–2.0 gm/kg/day
Severely stressed	2.0–3.0 gm/kg/day

2. **Cerra guideline** for protein needs based on stress level.

Stress level	Setting	Protein/kg/day
0	Simple starvation	1.0
1	Elective surgery	1.5
2	Polytrauma	2.0
3	Sepsis	2.5

3. **Protein requirements per disease state.**

Disease state	Protein/kg/day
Catabolic	1.2–2.0
Hepatic encephalopathy	0.6, increase as tolerated to 1.0–1.2
Renal failure (not on dialysis)	0.6
Renal failure (on dialysis)	1.0–1.4
Chronic liver disease	1.0–1.5
Nephrotic syndrome	1.0–1.4
Ulcerative colitis	1.0–1.4
Acute burn/injury/trauma	2.0–4.0

Key Reference: Lang C: Nutritional Support in Critical Care. The Adult Patient. Aspen Publishers, 1987, pp 61–91.

Enteral Nutrition Support

I. Patients are candidates for enteral support when they will not, should not, or cannot take nutrition orally yet have a functional gastrointestinal tract. The benefits of enteral support include maintenance of GI structure/integrity, improved utilization of nutrients, cost-effectiveness, ease of administration, and lower hypermetabolic response.

II. **Feeding route**. The appropriate feeding route is the first consideration in enteral support. This decision is based on the duration of feeding, the patient's medical status, and the risk of aspiration. **Short term** (< 6 weeks): nasoenteric tubes are recommended. **Long term** (> 6 weeks): feeding gastrostomy tubes are recommended.

1. **Nasogastric route. Indication:** intact gag reflex, normal gastric motility, and gastric outlet. **Advantages:** low cost, easy placement and removal. **Disadvantages:** increased risk of aspiration, tube dislodgement, and sinusitis.
2. **Nasoduodenal/nasojejunal route. Indication:** high aspiration risk, delayed gastric emptying, gastroparesis, gastric dysfunction due to trauma or surgery. **Advantages:** lower incidence of nosocomial pneumonia. **Disadvantages:** requires endoscopy or fluoroscopy for placement, increased risk of tube migration and dislodgement.
3. **Gastrostomy. Indication:** normal gastric functions and no esophageal reflux or unavailability of nasal route. **Advantages:** optimal patient comfort, can be placed by endoscopy, laparascopy, or fluoroscopy. **Disadvantages:** increased risk of aspiration, fistula formation after tube removal, potential for tube dislodgement, and need for stoma care.
4. **Jejunostomy. Indication:** impaired gastric motility, gastroesophageal reflux disease, aspiration potential, and gastric dysfunction due to surgery or trauma. **Advantages**: decreased aspiration risk, can be placed via endoscopy, fluoroscopy, or laparoscopy. **Disadvantages**: potential for vovulus and intraperitoneal leakage.

III. **Method of administration**

1. **Continuous feedings.** Feedings are given over 16–24 hous. This method has been associated with lower residual volumes, decreased incidence of diarrhea, and decreased risk of aspiration; therefore, it is recommended for critically ill patients. Because the small bowel tends to be sensitive to large volumes, the continuous feeding method is recommended for postpyloric feeding.
2. **Bolus infusions.** Feeding via gravity or syringe is generally used in the non-critically ill patient. Feedings are given quickly, ~ 2 cans over 30 minutes 4–6 times/day, mimicking a regular meal. The maximal recommended amount is 400–500 ml per feeding. The most common infusion amounts are 250–400 ml.

IV. **Initiation and advancement schedule**

1. Administration of a promotility agent (unless contraindicated) 30 min before insertion increases the chances of transpyloric placement: metoclopromide, 20 mg IV, or erythromycin, 200–400 mg IV.
2. Before initiation of feeding via a nasoenteric tube, placement must be verified. Radiographic confirmation is the most reliable method.
3. **Initiation/advancement schedules** can be based on the type of feeding formula, location of the feeding, type of patient, and the patient's condition:
   a. **Feeding formula/location of feeding**
      - **Isotonic formulas or gastric feedings** can be initiated at full strength at a rate of 20–25 cc/hr and advanced every 8 hours in increments of 20–25 cc until the desired rate is achieved.

- **Hypertonic formula or small bowel feedings** should be initiated at full strength at 10–15 cc/hr and increased every 12 hours in 10–15 cc increments until the desired rate is achieved.

b. **Patient type**
- **Hypometabolic**. Patients are clinically unstressed and starved. Nutrition support should be cautious with the goal of rebuilding. Initiate tube feeding at a low rate, and advance conservatively because of the risk of refeeding syndrome.
- **Hypermetabolic**. Patients are clinically stressed from injury or trauma and considered catabolic. Nutrition support should be aggressive but not excessive.

c. **Patient condition**.
- **Altered mental status:** initiate and advance slowly because of increased risk of aspiration.
- **Recent use of gastrointestinal tract:** prolonged nonuse of gastrointestinal tract requires cautious initiation and advancement schedules.
- **Nutritional status:** can be more aggressive with patients of normal nutrition status.
- **Functional status of gastrointestinal tract:** partial vs. full function; if the gut works a little, use it a little.

V. **Formula selection**. The following formula catagories should be considered in selecting a product for enteral support:

1. **Polymeric** formulas require normal digestive and absorptive capacities. Most are lactose-free, gluten-free, low osmolality, and isotonic. They average 1–2 kcal/ml. Protein content is highly variable.
2. **Elemental/defined** formulas are generally indicated for patients with compromised digestive and/or absorptive capacities. Most are lactose-free, have low residue and low viscocity, and are hypertonic.
3. **Disease-specific** formulas have been modified in nutrient composition to meet the special needs brought on by injury or disease. They are expensive and controversial.
4. **Modular** products consist of a single nutrient that can be used to modify a standard formula. The advantage of a modular product is the ability to meet a specific substrate need. The disadvantage is the increased risk of bacterial contamination associated with mixing.
5. **Other considerations**

   a. **Water content**. Most enteral formulas contain a fair amount of free water. Free water needs can be calculated using the following formulas: 30–35 ml/kg or 1 ml/calorie (0.5 ml/calorie in patients with fluid overload). The amount of free water depends on the caloric density:
   - 1 calorie/ml: 85% free water
   - 1.2–1.5 calorie/ml: 70–82% free water
   - 1.5–2.0 calorie/ml: 69–72% free water

   b. **Osmolality**. Tube feeding formulas range from 300 to 700 mOsm/kg H_2O (or mmol/kg). An isotonic formula has an osmolality of ~ 300 mOsm/kg (or mmol/kg) water. Formulas with a higher osmolality were thought to induce diarrhea by causing a shift of free water into the intestinal space. This theory has not been proved. The greater influence is medications, because their osmolalities range from 450 to 10.950 mOsm/kg body weight (or mmol/kg).

VI. **Enteral formulations: Values for 1000 ml of Each Brand**

	Jevity	Deliver 2.0	Introlan	Immun-Aid	Vivonex TEN
Category	1 cal/cc, high fiber	2 cal/cc	½ cal/cc	1 cal/cc, immuno-modulating	1 cal/cc, elemental
Calories	1060	2000	530	1000	1000
Protein (gm)	44	75	22.5	37	38
Fat (gm)	37	102	18	22	2.8
Carbohydrate (gm)	152	200	70	120	210
Osmolality (mOsm or mmol/kg)	310	640	150	460	630
Volume to meet USRDA (ml)	1321	1000	2000	2000	2000
Sodium (mg)	930	800	345	1060	630
Potassium (mg)	1560	1700	585	580	780
Comments	Standard formula	May be used for dialysis, liver disease, cancer congestive heart failure, pulmonary disease	Half-strength product	Contains glutamine,* arginine, nucleic acids	100% free amino acids with glutamine; may be flavored for oral use

* Glutamine is the principal amino acid nitrogen carrier from the periphery to visceral organs. Gut consumption of glutamine increases in stress states, and with inadequate intake villous atrophy and bacterial translocation may occur.

Reference: Dove DE, Sahn SA: The technique of administering enteral nutrition. J Crit Illness 10:881–888, 1995.

VII. **Complications** associated with enteral support are largely preventable through formula selection, proper administration, and careful monitoring. Complications fall into three categories:

1. **Gastrointestinal**
   a. **Diarrhea** is the most common complication of enteral feeding. It is defined as 4 bowel movements/day or a large liquid stool (> 250 gm). The most common causes of diarrhea are medications (antibiotics, antacids, potassium supplementations, cimetidine, sorbiol-containing medications, or medications in the form of an elixer), hypoalbuminemia, malabsorption, bacterial contamination, lactose intolerance, lack of fiber, altered bacterial flora, and rapid enteral feed administration.
   b. **Constipation** is defined as no stools for 3 or more days. Possible causes include dehydration, lack of fiber, dysmotility, and gastrointestinal obstruction.
   c. **Vomiting**. Discontinue tube feeding if vomiting occurs to prevent possible aspiration. Aspiration is the most serious complication of enteral support. Potential causes include delayed gastric emptying, neurologic impairment, decreased intestinal motility, presence of a nasoenteric tube and tube migration. Preventive measures include use of a small-bore feeding tube (< 10 French), elevation of the head of the bed by 30° during feeding, ambulation whenever possible, monitoring for tube migration, postpyloric positioning of the tube, continuous vs. bolus administration schedule, positioning of the patient on the right side to facilitate passage of gastric contents through the pylorus, and use of promotility agents 30 minutes before feeding (metoclopramide, 10 mg 4 times/day PO, IM, or IV, or erythromycin, 250 mg PO 3 times/day or 200–250 mg IV).

- To determine aspiration of enteral feeding, the best test is to apply tracheal aspirate on a **glucose test strip**.
- Methylene blue is commonly used, but it is less specific because all body fluids may have a bluish tinge with absorption of the dye.

d. **Increased residual volumes**. There is no consensus about acceptable gastric residuals; however, if a residual volume is > 200 ml with a nasogastric tube or > 100 ml with a gastrostomy tube, it is prudent to hold the feeding.

2. **Complications of nasoenteric tubes.** Because of various forms of misplacement and unreliability of bedside technique to detect misplacements, it is recommended that a portable chest radiograph with upper abdominal views be obtained immediately after insertion and before use of feeding tubes. Potential complications include:
   a. **Bronchial insertion** with penetration of the parenchyma, pleural space, or mediastinum
   b. **Cephalad insertion** into the sinuses and cranial cavity
   c. **Esophageal perforation**
   d. **Massive aspiration** of enteral feed if the tube has reversed direction in the esophagus
3. **Metabolic complications**
   a. **Glucose intolerance. Causes:** diabetes mellitus, sepsis, trauma, metabolic stress, and refeeding syndrome. **Prevention or therapy**: control with oral hypoglycemics, insulin, or a change in tube feeding formula.
   b. **Dehydration. Causes:** inadequate fluid intake, excessive fluid losses, or use of hypertonic or high protein formula. **Prevention or therapy:** calculate free water needs and provide adequate free water based on tube feeding formula.
   c. **Overhydration. Causes:** excessive fluid and salt intake, cardiac-hepatic-or-renal failure, and refeeding syndrome. **Prevention or therapy:** calculate free water needs and use a more concentrated formula if necessary.
   d. **Hypokalemia. Causes:** refeeding syndrome, diuretic therapy, excessive losses from diarrhea, and insulin therapy. **Prevention or therapy:** supplemental potassium prior to advancement of tube feedings.
   e. **Hypophosphatemia. Causes:** refeeding syndrome, insulin therapy, phosphate-binding antacids. **Prevention or therapy:** supplemental phosphate prior to advancement of tube feedings.
   f. **Hyponatremia. Causes:** dilutional states, hyperglycemia, cardiac-hepatic-or renal insufficiency. **Prevention or therapy:** use more concentrated formula if necessary.
   g. **Hyperkalemia. Causes:** renal failure, excessive potassium in tube feeds. **Prevention or therapy:** adjust tube feeding formula.
   h. **Hypernatremia. Causes:** inadequate water. **Prevention or therapy:** calculate free water needs, use standard formula or less concentrated formula.

Key Reference: Skipper A: Monitoring and complications of enteral feeding. In Dietians Handbook of Enteral and Parenteral Nutrition, 1989, pp 293–310.

Parenteral Nutrition Support

I. **Parenteral nutrition support** is indicated for patients with a nonfunctioning gastrointestinal tract and inability to tolerate adequate oral or enteral nutrition. The two available routes are **peripheral parenteral nutrition** (PPN) and central or **total parenteral nutrition** (TPN). PPN is considered to be a short-term and adjunctive intervention. A time frame < 14 days is recommended. TPN is intended for full nutritional support and recommended for a minimum of 7 days for improvement in patient outcome.

II. **Parenteral access** depends on the duration of therapy as discussed above, the patient's medical condition, energy requirements, and fluid tolerance.
   1. **Peripheral access:** a standard venipuncture is used to access the peripheral circulation. The patient must have adequate peripheral veins and be able to tolerate hypertonic solutions. PPN solutions are generally 600–900 mOsm/L or mmol/kg. Peripheral access is difficult to maintain; hence the 2-week limit.
   2. **Central access**: is determined by the expected duration of nutritional support.
      a. **Short-term access**. Subclavian or internal jugular venipuncture is the most direct route to access the central venous circulation. Single-, double-, or triple-lumen catheters are available. The tip of the central catheter is positioned in the superior vena cava. Peripherally inserted central catheters (PICC) are also an alternative that can be placed by a trained nurse because they do not require a surgical procedure. The line is placed in the antecubital vein and threaded into the subclavian vein.
      b. **Long-term access**. Access is surgically placed and tunneled subcutaneously away from the insertion site. The exit site is the chest wall. Single-, double-, or triple-lumen catheters are available.

III. **Method of administration:** Parenteral nutrition is infused continuously over 12–24 hours. Cyclic infusion rates are reserved for more stable patients or patients who are likely to be discharged on TPN. Critically ill patients should receive a 24-hour infusion for optimal support and tolerance.

IV. **Initiation and advancement schedule:** Because PPN is restricted to a maximum of 10% dextrose (5% final concentration), patients can tolerate initiation at the target rate. TPN, with its higher concentrations of dextrose, requires an advancement schedule. The following are guidelines for the first 48 hours of TPN infusion:
   1. **First 24 hours: Volume** is based on patient tolerance. If fluid tolerance is unknown, begin with 1 liter or less. **Carbohydrate:** Dextrose can be maximally concentrated into 1 liter if glucose control is acceptable. With hyperglycemia, DB, or refeeding syndrome, begin with a 10–15% dextrose solution. **Protein:** maximal protein (60–70 gm) usually can be given. **Lipids:** administer lipids during this period if the baseline triglyceride level is < 400 mg/dl. **Electrolytes/minerals:** adjust as needed; replete deficiencies.
   2. **24-48 hours:** For most patients, the target rate can be achieved by the second day. **Volume**: increase to goal according to fluid tolerance. **Carbohydrate:** advance to goal if glucose level is < 200 mg/dl (< 11.1 mmol/L). **Protein:** if volume is not an issue, advance to goal. **Lipids:** maintain triglycerides < 400 mg/dl (4.51 mmol/L) during continuous feeds and < 250 mg/dl (< 2.82 mmol/L) 4 hours after infusion. **Electrolytes/minerals:** adjust as needed; replete deficiencies.

V. **Formula selection**
   1. **Nonprotein calorie (NPC) sources** are made up of two macronutrients: carbohydrates and lipids. The following is a summary of recommendations for infusion and general information:

	Carbohydrate	**Lipid**
Standard distriction	70–85% NPC	15–30% NPC
Maximal infusion	7 mg/kg/min	2.5 gm fat/kg/day (60% NPC)
Recommended infusion	< 5 mg/kg/min	<1.0 gm fat/kg/day
Calories/gram	3.4 kcals/gm	9.0 kcal/gm
Available concentrations	10–70%	10% and 20%
Optimal infusion schedule		Not less than 12 hours

2. **Dextrose is the carbohydrate (CHO) source as well as the major source of NPC in parenteral nutrition**. The CHO load should be adequate to spare protein for wound healing and metabolic demands without exceeding patient tolerance (hyperglycemia). The various dextrose concentrations, gm CHO, kcal/L, and indications are summarized below:
   a. **D10**, 50 gm CHO, 170 kcal/L, PPN
   b. **D20**, 100 gm CHO, 340 kcal/L, poor diabetes control
   c. **D30**, 150 gm CHO, 510 kcal/L, diabetes in fair control
   d. **D40**, 200 gm CHO, 680 kcal/L, considered a standard with no fluid issues
   e. **D50**, 250 gm CHO, 850 kcal/L, considered a standard with mild fluid restriction and possible lipid issues.
   f. **D60**, 300 gm CHO, 1020 kcal/L, increased needs with moderate fluid restriction.
   g. **D70**, 350 gm CHO, 1190 kcal/L, maximally concentrated for excessive nutritional demands.
3. **Lipids:** Intravenous lipid infusions are necessary as a source of essential fatty acids. The calories yielded depend on the concentration of lipid emulsion: 10% lipid = 1.1 kcal/cc, 20% lipid = 2.0 kcal/cc. Lipids are made up of egg phospholipid; therefore, patients with an egg allergy may not tolerate lipid emulsion.
   a. Common lipid schedules are as follows for 500 cc of lipid (*note:* when using 3-in-1 TPN, lipids are added to the TPN daily):

% Lipid	Schedule	Cal/wk	Weekly avg
10%	2×/week	1100	157
10%	3×/week	1650	235
10%	5×/week	2750	393
10%	Daily	3850	550
20%	2×/week	2000	286
20%	3×/week	3000	428
20%	5×/week	5000	714

4. **Amino acids**. Protein in TPN is in the form of crystalline amino acids that provide 4 kcal/gm. In a healthy population, protein should be provided as 11–20% of total kcal. In critically ill patients, 40% of the total kcal is recommended. An amount < 0.5 gm/kg protein does not promote positive nitorgen balance. All amino acid mixtures contain intrinsic electrolytes. Below is an example of the intrinsic electrolytes in some common amino acid formulation:

	10% Freamine	15% Aminosyn	6.9% HBC
Sodium (mEq/L)	5	31.4	7.5
Phosphate (mmol/L)		5	
Acetate (mEq/L)	45	53.8	43

5. **Electrolytes.** The available commercial electrolyte preparations are intended to meet normal-range requirements. The following chart summarizes requirements and standard amounts of electrolytes:

Electrolyte	24-hr requirement	Standard Liter TPN
Phosphorus (mMol)	20–45	15
Potassium (mEq)	60–100	30
Magnesium(mEq)	10–20	5
Sodium (mEq)	60–100	35
Calcium (mEq)	10–15	5
Chloride (mEq)	NA	NA
Acetate (mEq)	NA	NA

6. TPN can affect the metabolic acid–base balance; therefore, the chloride and acetate in the TPN can be adjusted. For metabolic acidosis, utilize maximal acetate, for metabolic alkalosis, utilize maximal chloride.
7. **Vitamins/minerals**: Parenteral supplementation of vitamins and minerals is recommended. The daily parental requirements are as follows:

Vitamin/mineral	Requirement for adults	Vitamin/mineral	Requirement for adults
Thiamine	3 mg	Ascorbic acid	100 mg
Riboflavin	3.6 mg	Vitamin A	3300 IU
Niacin	40 mg	Vitamin D	200 IU
Folic acid	400 μg	Vitamin E	10 IU
Pantothenic acid	15 mg	Chromium	10–15 μg
Pyridoxine	4 mg	Copper	0.3–0.5 mg
Cyanocobalamin	5 μg	Manganese	60–100 μg
Biotin	60 μg	Zinc	2.5–5 mg

8. **TPN calculation.** One of the most difficult tasks with TPN appears to be the calculation of the prescription. The following is a simplistic method that uses the information contained within this chapter:
   a. **Determine nonprotein calories (NPC)** required from dextrose per day = NPC/kg × kg body weight – weekly NPC estimate from lipids.
   For example: 25 NPC/kg × 70 kg = 1750 NPC/day – 500 NPC (from 20% lipids/day) = 1250 dextrose NPC needed/day.
   b. **Determine volume of dextrose** = dextrose NPC/(kcal/gm of CHO × % dextrose).
   For example: 1250 NPC/(3.4 kcal/gm × 70% dextrose) = 525 cc dextrose/ day.
   c. **Determine protein needs** = grams of protein/kg × kg body weight
   For example: 1.25 gm protein/kg × 70 kg = 88 gm protein
   d. **Determine volume of protein per day** = grams of protein/day divided by % amino acids = volume of amino acids per day.
   For example: 88 gm protein/day/15% amino acids = 586 cc protein/day.
   e. **Determine volume per day** = add together daily volume needs of dextrose and volume of amino acids needed.
   For example: 525 cc + 586 cc = 1111 cc/day.
   f. **Determine infusion rate** = divide volume needs by hours of infusion.
   For example: 111 cc/day divided by 24 hours = 46 cc/hr.
   g. **Determine grams of carbohydrate/liter** = dextrose NPC/day divided by NPC/gm CHO and divided by daily volume.
   For example: 1250 NPC/day/(3.4 NPC/gm CHO × 1.111 L) = 330 gm CHO/L.
   h. **Determine gram/liter of protein** = protein/day divided by daily volume.
   For example: 88 gm pro/day divided by 1.111 L = 79 gm pro/L.
   i. **Write TPN prescription as follows**:
      - 46 cc/hr
      - 330 gm CHO/L (70% dextrose)
      - 79 gm protein/L (15% amino acids)
      - 500 cc 20% lipid every other day
9. **Metabolic complications** associated with TPN
   a. **Hyperglycemia. Causes:** glucose load that exceeds endogenous insulin secretions, rapid infusion of dextrose, steroid treatment, underlying disease states such as pancreatitis, sepsis, diabetes, trauma, or surgery. **Treatment:** advance rate slowly; do not increase rate until hyperglycemia is controlled; add insulin to PN, provide fewer carbohydrate calories, and increase lipid calories.

b. **Hypoglycemia. Causes:** abrupt discontinuation of dextrose solution, amount of insulin in PN exceeds requirements. **Treatment:** treat hypoglycemia with IV bolus infusion of D50; avoid sudden cessation of PN. If PN is discontinued suddenly, give D10 infusion at the same rate, monitor glucose levels, and adjust insulin accordingly.
c. **Hyperkalemia. Causes:** decreased renal function, metabolic acidosis, excessive potassium in PN, low cardiac output, tissue necrosis and systemic sepsis, potassium-sparing medications. **Treatment:** discontinue PN and provide D10 replacement at the same rate; provide sodium bicarbonate, adjust electrolyte mixture to decrease potassium, adjust PN as needed, and assess for potassium-sparing medications.
d. **Hypokalemia. Causes:** potassium loss from diuresis, diarrhea, steroid treatment, potassium wasting medications. **Treatment:** increase amount of potassium in PN, and replete potassium peripherally.
e. **Hypernatremia. Causes:** dehydration from fever, inadequate free water, diuresis, ADH deficiency, and head trauma. **Treatment:** provide hydration with D5.
f. **Hyponatremia. Causes:** sodium losses from diuretics, diarrhea, and adrenal insufficiency; extracellular fluid overload as seen with CHF, renal failure, liver disease/cirrhosis. **Treatment:** for true sodium depletion, give normal saline or increase sodium concentration in PN by incresing dextrose concentrations.
g. **Hyperphosphatemia. Causes:** Excessive phosphorus in PN, renal insufficiency. **Treatment:** decrease amount of phosphorus in PN; consider the phosphate in lipid emulsions; give phosphate binders.
h. **Hypophosphatemia. Causes:** inadequate phosphorus in PN, increase in phosphorus needed during anabolism/protein synthesis, refeeding syndrome. **Treatment:** increase amount of phosphorus in PN, and replete phosphorus peripherally before advancing rate of infusion. Increase phosphorus in PN.
i. **Hypertriglyceridemia. Causes:** inability to clear lipids from bloodstream, sepsis, multisystem organ failure, idiopathic hyperlipidemia. **Treatment:** decrease lipid volume, and lengthen lipid infusion.
j. **Prerenal azotemia. Causes:** excessive protein provided, dehydration, inadequate NPC provided. **Treatment**: decrease protein load, increase fluids provided, and increase NPC.
k. **Abnormal liver function tests. Causes:** excessive glucose or lipid load. **Treatment**: ensure that the patient is not being overfed.
l. **Overfeeding: Causes:** excessive protein and NPC. **Treatment:** decrease protein and NPC.

Key References: American Dietetic Association Manual of Clinical Dietetics, 6th ed. Parent Nutr pp 619–636, 2000; Nutritional Advisory Group on Standards and Practice Guidelines for Parenteral Nutrition: Safe practices for parenteral nutrition formulations. J Parentl Ent Nutr 22:49–66, 1998.

Consequences of Overfeeding

I. **Carbohydrate > 5 mg CHO/kg/min**
  1. **Lungs:** increased CO_2 production, possible respiratory failure in patients with limited pulmonary reserve, prolonged mechanical ventiation.

2. **Hyperglyemia**
3. **Hyperinsulinemia**
4. **Impaired phagocytosis and neutrophil chemotaxis**
5. **Increaed intracellular transport of potassium and phosphorus**
6. **Liver:** fatty liver infitration; increased aspartate aminotransferase, alanine aminotransferase, and alkaline phosphatase; hepatomegaly; cholestasis.

II. **Fat > 2 gm fat/kg/day**
1. Increased serum triglycerides

III. **Protein > 2 gm protein/kg/day**
1. **Kidneys:** ureagenesis and decreased renal function.

Nutrition in Liver Disease

I. **Hepatic encephalopathy (HE)**
1. **Recommendations for protein load vary**
   a. Start from a baseline of 40 gm/day with gradual increase of protein in 10-gm increments every 3–5 days as tolerated. Protein intake should not exceed 70 gm/day in patients with a history of HE and should not be lower than 40 gm/day to avoid negative nitrogen balance.
   b. Initiate at 50 gm protein/day with a decrease to 10–20 gm/day with intolerance of baseline recommendation. Advancement schedule is 10-gm increments every 2 days, if possible, until target is reached.
   c. ASPEN recommendations are based on a per kg chart: 0.6 gm protein/kg initially; increase as tolerated to goal of 1.0–1.2 gm protein/kg.
2. **Overall recommendation.**
   a. Rule out other causes of encephalopathy (e.g., sepsis, thiamine deficiency, meningoencephalitis).
   b. Treat the underlying disorder that may precipitate HE (e.g., gastrointestinal bleed, peritonitis, electrolyte abnormalities).
   c. Initiate NPO status for grades III and IV HE.
   d. When diet resumes, provide adequate calories (30–35 kcal/kg) to allow hepatic regeneration and to prevent endogenous catabolism of lean body mass.

II. **Cirrhosis**
1. The Harris-Benedict formula for calorie estimates may overfeed. Caloric needs should be based on urinary creatinine estimates: 1180 ± 260 kcal/gm. Provide protein based on normal requirements; adjust only if the patient has been diagnosed with HE.
2. Other restrictions are based on additional factors associated with cirrhosis: (1) ascites (restrict sodium to 2 gm/day with concurrent diuretic treatment and 250–500 mg without diuretics at fluid restriction of 1.5 L/day) and (2) edema (sodium restriction of 2 gm/day and 1.5 L fluid restrictions if necessary).

III. **Tube feeding patients with liver failure.** When tube feeding becomes necessary in this population, specialized formulas are often indicated. Liver-specific formulas tend to be more calorically dense than a standard enteral product, providing 1.50–2.0 calories/cc and limiting sodium to 1 gm per 2000 calories. The use of the high-branched chain amino acid formulas should be considered only after the failed trial of a standard product. One theoretical disadvantage of enteral nutrition is that protein intolerance appears to be more common with cirrhotics.

IV. **Parenteral support in liver failure** is indicated in the setting of gastrointestinal hemorrhage and coma secondary to HE.

1. Calculation of the TPN prescription is not unlike that in other populations; concentrations in the dextrose, fat, and protein solutions are based on the patient's fluid requirements.
2. Electrolytes are prescribed according to the patient's needs at initiation and adjusted as needed thereafter. Lower sodium concentrations are recommended. Copper and manganese should be provided (based on blood levels) and monitored closely in patients with biliary obstruction or cholestasis.
3. The use of high-branch chain amino acids should be considered only after an unsuccessful trial of standard amino acids.

Key References: Plaauth M, Merli M,Kondrup J, et al: ASPEN guidelines for nutrition in liver disease and transplantation. Clin Nutr 16:43, 1997; Skipper A. Nutritional management of the adult with liver disease. In Handbook of Enteral and Parenteral Nutrition, 1989, pp 61–86.

Nutrition in Renal Disease

I. Overall nutritional requirements vary based on the stage of renal disease as well as concurrent treatment. In other words, nutritional management is based on acute vs. chronic renal disease and whether or not the patient is actively receiving hemodialysis (HD) or peritoneal dialysis (PD). Below is a quick comparison of the nutritional requirements in renal failure.

1. **Acute renal failure on hemodialysis**
   a. *Calories (kcal/kg): 35–50
   b. Protein (gm/kg): 1.5–2
   c. Sodium (gm): 1–2
   d. Potassium (mEq): < 50
2. **Acute renal failure not on hemodialysis**
   a. *Calories (kcal/kg): 35–50
   b. Protein (gm/kg): 0.6–1.5
   c. Sodium (gm): 0.5–1.0
   d. Potassium (mEq): 20–50
   e. Phosphorus (mg): ≤ 700
3. **Chronic renal failure on hemodialysis**
   a. *Calories (kcal/kg): 30–35
   b. Protein (gm/kg): 1.1–1.4
   c. Sodium (gm): 2–3
   d. Potassium (mEq): 38–75
   e. Phosphorus (mg): 800–1000
   f. Phosphorus (mg/kg): 12–17
   g. Calcium (mg): 1400–1600
4. **Chronic renal failure not on hemodialysis**
   a. *Calories (kcal/kg): > 35
   b. Protein (gm/kg): 0.6–0.8
   c. Sodium (gm): 1–3
   d. Potassium (mEq): < 70
   e. Phosphorus (mg/kg): 8–12
   f. Calcium (mg): 1200–1600
5. **Chronic renal failure on peritoneal dialysis**
   a. *Calories (kcal/kg): 25–35
   b. Protein (gm/kg): 1.2–1.3
   c. Sodium (gm): 3–4
   d. Potassium (mEq): 70–90
   e. Phosphorus (mg): 1000–1200
   f. Phosphorus (mg/gm protein): 15
   g. Calcium (mg): 1000–1500

* The above calorie/kg values are based on weight maintenance needs.

II. **Tube feeding in patients with renal failure**

1. Without HD, a more concentrated product is necessary because of fluid restriction. A protein restriction is indicated; therefore, a carbohydrate modular may be necessary to meet the patient's caloric needs.
2. With HD, the fluid restriction may still be indicated, calling for a more calorically dense product. Protein is not as great an issue; therefore, a carbohydrate modular is not necessary.

III. **Parenteral support in renal failure**

1. In both acute and chronic renal failure, patients not actively undergoing dialysis require a concentrated TPN formulation and restricted amounts of amino acids and electrolytes. Liberalization of these substances is possible once dialysis is initiated. NPC needs can be met easily in a fluid-restricted environment with 70% dextrose and 20% lipids.
2. The literature about using essential amino acids rather than a combination of essential and nonessential amino acids is not well supported. The use of a standard amino acid solution is highly recommended.

Key References: American Dietetic Asociation Nutrition Care in End-Stage Renal Disease, 2nd edition, 1994. Skipper A: Renal function. In Handbook of Enteral and Parenteral Nutrition,1989, pp 87–102.

Nutrition in Pulmonary Disease

I. The respiratory quotient (RQ) is a volume ratio between the O_2 consumed and CO_2 produced. The three macronutrients affect this ratio:

Substrate	RQ
Carbohydrate	1.0
Lipid	0.7
Protein	0.8
Overfeeding	> 1.0

II. **Overall energy** and protein needs are based on the patient's goal. For weight maintenance, energy needs are estimated at 25–35 kcal/kg and protein needs mated at 1.2–1.9 gm/kg. For repletion, energy needs are estimated at 35–45 kcal/kg and protein needs at 1.6–2.5 gm/kg.

III. **Tube feeding in pulmonary patients**

1. Various costly, specialized enteral products cater to the pulmonary patient. Most are excessively high in fat based on the lower RQ that fat produces. The high-fat content makes these products hard to tolerate, especially in critically ill patients. The theoretical benefits of these products does not outweigh their increased cost. The principal factor to remember is not to overfeed a pulmonary patient because overfeeding drives the RQ above 1.0.
2. Another common mistake in tube feeding pulmonary patients is the fear of exacerbating pulmonary function, or increasing the risk of pulmonary aspiration. Underfeeding or not feeding only contributes to increased complication rates and potentially increases the patient's time on the ventilator.

IV. **Parenteral support in pulmonary patients**

1. The push to provide a higher percent of NPC from lipid than carbohydrate is unwarranted. The NPC breakdown can lean slightly toward lipid infusion, but not excessively. The standard not to exceed 1 gm fat/kg/day still applies. Parenteral support should be prescribed based on the patient's metabolic needs and adjusted on the basis of tolerance. Underfeeding or not feeding potentiates complications and increases time on the ventilator.

Key Reference: Skipper A: Respiratory disease and mechanical ventilation. In Dietians Handbook of Enteral and Parenteral Nutrition, 1989, pp 137–150.

Endocrinology

Drugs That May Affect Thyroid Function or Test

I. **Drugs that affect thyroid function *testing* (euthyroid)**
   1. **TSH suppression:** phenytoin, high-dose salicylates, glucocorticoids, octreotide, dopamine.
   2. **Increased TSH**: theophylline, dopamine antagonists, amphetamines.
   3. **Euthyroid hypothyroxinemia**: phenytoin*, carbamazepine*, phenobarbitol*, rifampin*, high-dose salicylates, androgens, niacin (*can cause hypothyroidism in patients with borderline basal function).
   4. **Euthyroid hyperthyroxinemia**: iodine-containing agents, amiodarone, beta blockers (propranolol), estrogen, heroin, methadone, clofibrate, amphetamines, furosemide (> 80 mg IV), 5-FU, heparin (transient).

II. **Drugs that affect thyroid *function***
   1. **Hypothyroidism:** amiodarone, iodine-containing agents, lithium, interferon, aminoglutethamide, vitamin A, retinoids.
   2. **Hyperthyroidism:** amiodarone, iodine-containing agents, cytokines.

Thyrotoxicosis and Treatment of Thyroid Storm

I. **Thyrotoxicosis** is a hypermetabolic state due to an excess of thyroid hormones. A patient may be thyrotoxic without being hyperthyroid (e.g., subacute thyroiditis or excessive intake of exogenous thyroid hormone).

II. **Thyroid storm** is a severe manifestation of thyrotoxicosis characterized by altered mental status and decompensation in one or more organ systems. Clues include disproportionately high fever or tachycardia and unexplained restlessness and tremor. If untreated, it may lead to pulmonary edema, hepatic failure, dehydration, and shock. It is often precipitated by trauma, surgery, or infection.

III. **Causes:** In general, it is essential to categorize a patient as hyperthyroid (increased radioactive iodine uptake [RAIU]) or nonhyperthyroid (decreased RAIU) once the diagnosis of thyrotoxicosis is made because patients who are not hyperthyroid (despite being thyrotoxic) should not be treated with antithyroid drugs, radioablation, or thyroidectomy.

Increased RAIU	Decreased RAIU
Graves' disease	Subacute thyroiditis
Toxic multinodular goiter	Silent thyroiditis
Toxic adenoma	Exogenous thyroid hormone intake
Hashimoto's thyroiditis	Hashimoto's thyroiditis
TSH-secreting pituitary tumor	Ectopic thyroid tissue
Choriocarcinoma	Iodine excess (Jodbasedow)
Hydatidiform mole (HCG)	
Follicular thyroid carcinoma	

TSH = thyroid-stimulating hormone, HCG = human chorionic gonadotropin.

IV. **Clinical manifestations:** nervousness, sweating, heat intolerance, palpitations, weakness, weight loss, diarrhea, tachycardia, atrial tachyarrhythmias, congestive heart failure, systolic hypertension, moist skin, fine tremor, upper eyelid retraction, and lid lag. Altered mental status varies from confusion to coma. Infiltrative ophthalmology or proptosis is specific for Graves' disease.

V. **Diagnosis**
   1. Suppressed or undetectable levels of TSH
   2. Increased free thyroxine (T_4) index and increased triiodothyronine (T_3) or normal free T_4 index and increased T_3 (T_3 thyrotoxicosis)
   3. Measure RAIU once a diagnosis of thyrotoxicosis is made to determine whether hyperthyroidism is present.

VI. **Treatment**
   1. **Thyrotoxicosis without hyperthyroidism:** close observation, antiinflammatory agents, beta blockers.
   2. **Hyperthyroidism**
      a. **Antithyroid drugs:** time required to achieve euthyroid state with propylthiouracil (PTU), 100 mg every 8 hr, or methimazole, 10 mg every 8 hr or every 12 hr, is about 2–4 months. Discontinue antithyroid drug about 3–4 days before radioiodine.
      b. **Radioiodine:** treatment of choice for most adults with Graves' disease.
   3. **Thyroid storm**
      a. **PTU**, 600–1000 mg oral load, then 200–250 mg orally every 4 hr. PTU is a good antithyroid drug because it not only blocks thyroid hormone synthesis but also inhibits conversion of T_4 to T_3.
      b. **Lugol's solution**, 10 drops every 8 hr *or* standard solution of potassium iodide (SSKI), 5 drops/6 hr with the first dose given at least 1 hr after PTU. Iodine, although a precursor for new hormone synthesis, blocks release of T_3 and T_4. **Lithium carbonate** (target level of 0.5–1 mmol/L) may be substituted for iodide in iodine-allergic patients. **Dose:** load, 1.8 gm in 2–3 divided doses or 30 ml of lithium citrate solution (~ 48 mmol/L); maintenance, 900–1200 mg/day in 2–4 divided doses.
      c. **Propranolol**, 40 mg orally every 6 hr *or* 1–2 mg IV every 15 min as needed, followed by 5–10 mg/hr IV infusion in the absence of contraindications; not only controls symptoms of hyperadrenergic state but also inhibits T_4 to T_3 conversion. Alternatively, esmolol IV may be given.
      d. **Aggressive replacement of volume deficits** (which may be quite high).
      e. **Glucocorticoids** are usually given until adrenal insufficiency is ruled out. Corticosteroids also may decrease the peripheral conversion of T_4 to T_3. Dose of hydrocortisone: 100 mg IV every 8 hr.
      f. **Treatment of infection**, if suspected.
      g. In refractory cases, thyroxine may be removed by plasmapheresis, peritoneal dialysis, or **charcoal hemoperfusion**.

Key Reference: Tietgens ST, Leinung MC: Thyroid storm. Med Clin North Am 79:169–184, 1995.

Myxedema Coma

I. Myxedema coma is due to severe thyroid hormone deficiency and is often precipitated in patients with moderate or unrecognized hypothyroidism by infection, sedatives, narcotics, or surgery. **It should be considered in all stuporous or comatose patients.** The usual signs of infection are often absent.

II. **Therapy for myxedema coma should be instituted when the diagnosis is seriously suspected** because (1) euthyroid persons tolerate the short-term administration of a large dose of levothyroxine (LT_4) well and (2) mortality may be as high as 30–50% without treatment.

III. **Manifestations**
 1. **Unresponsiveness, hypothermia, bradycardia, myxedema, hyponatremia, hypoglycemia**
 2. **Respiratory failure:** major cause of death in myxedema coma; due to decreased sensitivity of the brainstem respiratory centers to hypoxia and hypercarbia. Decreased respiratory muscle strength due to hypothyroidism may contribute to hypercapnic respiratory failure. Other respiratory alterations include obesity-sleep apnea syndrome, macroglossia, and myxedematous swelling of the upper airway. Pneumonia and chronic obstructive pulmonary disease exacerbations also may be precipitating causes.
 3. **Hypotension:** ominous and often resistant to adrenergic agents.
 4. **Cardiovascular changes**: diminished β-receptor responsiveness results in decreased stroke volume, bradycardia, and decreased cardiac output. Increased α-adrenergic responsiveness results in diastolic hypertension. Pericardial effusion is common.
 5. Elevation of aspartate aminotransferase (AST), lactate dehydrogenase (LDH), and creatinine phosphokinase (CPK).

IV. **Diagnosis**: low T4 and high TSH makes a diagnosis of hypothyroidism. Other laboratory abnormalities may include elevated CPK, hyponatremia, hypoglycemia, and hypercholesterolemia.

V. **Treatment**
 1. **Treat on suspicion** because diagnostic tests may be delayed.
 2. **Maintain adequate ventilation and oxygenation**; a large tongue may be encountered in long-standing hypothyroidism.
 3. **Treat shock with plasma expanders or isotonic saline** rather than adrenergic agents.
 4. **LT_4, 200–500 μg IV, then 75–100 μg/day IV** (begin oral therapy after stabilization at 50 μg/day of LT_4. Alternatively, T_3 (liothyronine = triiodothyronine = Cytomel), 50–100 μg orally initially, then 12.5–25 μg orally 2 times/day.
 5. **Hydrocortisone**, 100 mg IV every 8 hr, to prevent precipitation of adrenal insufficiency.
 6. Treat hypothermia with **passive warming**. Do **not** treat by external heat, which may worsen circulatory failure by increasing O_2 requirements and decreasing peripheral vascular resistance.
 7. **Treat precipitating illness** (e.g., antibiotics for infection), or discontinue sedatives.

Key References: Jordan RM. Myxedema coma. Med Clin North Am 79:185–194, 1995; MacKarrow SD, Osborn LA, Levy H, et al: Myxedema-associated cardiogenic shock treated with intravenous triiodothyronine. Ann Intern Med 117:1014–1015, 1992.

Diabetic Ketoacidosis

I. **Manifestations** may include weight loss, polyuria, polydipsia, vomiting, vague and nonlocalizing abdominal pain, hyperventilation, shock, or coma. **Laboratory findings** include hyperglycemia, anion gap metabolic acidosis, serum ketones, pseudohyponatremia, hyperkalemia, elevated blood urea nitrogen and creatinine, and hyperamylasemia.

II. **Precipitating factors** include insufficient insulin therapy (for many reasons, including noncompliance, drug overdose, stroke), infection, and myocardial infarction. Patients should be carefully evaluated for evidence of these factors.

III. **Treatment**

1. **Normal saline (NS) or lactated Ringer's solution**
   a. Normal cardiac function: 1 liter over first hr; then adjust to correct heart rate, blood pressure, and urine output.
   b. Use hypotonic solutions (e.g., 0.45% saline) at 150–200 ml/hr when intravascular volume is restored or when sodium > 155 mmol/L.
   c. Infuse $D_5{}^1/_2$ NS when glucose < 300–400 mg/dl (< 16.65–22.2 mmol/L).
2. **Insulin** (use regular form)
   a. **Initial dose**, 10–20 units (U) IV as bolus
   b. **Infusion**, 100 U/500 ml 0.45% NaCl at 50–75 ml/hr (10–15 U/hr); adjust rate; taper to 1–2 U/hr when [HCO_3] > 15 mmol/L and anion gap resolves.
   c. **Alternative infusion method**, 0.1 U/kg/hr. Check blood sugar in 2 hr; if blood sugar has not fallen by 50 mg/dl, double infusion rate; if blood sugar has fallen by > 50 mg/dl in 2 hr, reduce infusion rate by one-half. After any change, recheck blood sugar in 2 hr, and repeat above steps. Begin subcutaneous insulin when patient is capable of oral intake and ketosis resolves.
3. Consider $NaHCO_3$ infusion for shock/coma, pH < 7.1, or severe hyperkalemia: 50–100 mEq/L (1–2 ampules) in 1 liter of 0.45% saline.
4. **Potassium chloride, 20–40 mmol/L.** Infusion rate up to 15 mEq/hr may be required with potassium concentration < 4 mmol/L. **Check urine output first.**

IV. **Monitoring**

1. Check glucose every 30–60 min, electrolytes every 1–2 hr, and arterial blood gases as needed.
2. The anion gap is a more reliable parameter of ketoacidosis than serum ketones unless lactic acidosis is also present.

V. **Complications**

1. **Lactic acidosis** may accompany ketoacidosis (due to sepsis or shock) and should be suspected when pH and anion gap do not respond to insulin.
2. **Cerebral edema** may occur with therapy.
3. **Arterial thrombosis** (strokes, myocardial infarction, organ dysfunction, or limb ischemia).

Key References: Eng S, Singer PA: Practical pointers for diabetic emergencies. Contemp Intern Med 8:51–66, 1996; Foster DW, McGarry JD: The metabolic derangement and treatment of diabetic ketoacidosis. N Engl J Med 309:159–169, 1983.

Diabetic Nonketotic Hyperosmolar Coma

I. Diabetic nonketotic hyperosmolar coma is **usually a complication of non–insulin-dependent diabetes mellitus**. It is characterized by severe hyperglycemia (glucose > 600 mg/dl [> 33.3 mmol/L]), hyperosmolarity (osmolality > 350 mOsm/kg or mmol/kg), dehydration (due to hyperglycemia-induced osmotic diuresis or inability to take oral hydration), and lack of significant ketoacidosis. Patients may have mild ketosuria and anion gap metabolic acidosis (due to volume depletion, lactate production, and prerenal azotemia).

II. **Pathogenesis** appears to be related to a relative or absolute insulin deficiency resulting in decreased glucose uptake and increased glucose output by the liver. A precipitating illness (e.g., stroke) also may result in the secretion of hormones that antagonize insulin's actions. Either intrinsic renal disease or prerenal azotemia is required for development of hyperglycemia. The reason for the lack of significant ketoacidosis is not exactly known, but free fatty acids levels are lower, thus limiting the substrate for ketone formation.

III. **Clinical presentation**

1. **The typical patient** is an elderly person who lives alone and, for one reason or another, is unable to take in sufficient fluids. Patients with neurologic diseases are susceptible.
2. **Precipitating factors** include strokes, drugs such as beta blockers and corticosteroids, infections (especially pneumonia and gram-negative sepsis), myocardial infarction, and pancreatitis.
3. **Central nervous signs** include confusion, focal neurologic deficits and seizures, and coma. In patients who do not improve neurologically with hydration and correction of hyperglycemia, a primary neurologic event, which may have triggered the hyperosmolar coma, should be sought.
4. **Patients with renal failure** may have dilutional hyponatremia (no osmotic diuresis) and be relatively asymptomatic.

IV. **Laboratory values**

1. Estimation of serum osmolality = 2 [Na] + [glucose/18] + [BUN/2.8], where Na = sodium (mmol/L), and BUN = blood urea nitrogen (mg/dl). Alternatively, serum osmolality = 2[Na] + glucose (mmol/L) + BUN (mmol/L).
2. Serum sodium is usually normal or elevated; given hyperglycemia, water deficit is present even with a normal serum sodium. However, total body sodium is also low, even with hypernatremia.
3. Serum potassium is usually normal or high, but again total body potassium is low.

V. **Treatment**

1. Fluid deficit may be ~ 10 liter. **Initially, treat with isotonic saline, 2–3 L over the first 1–2 hr until the patient is euvolemic; then one-half normal saline at 100–200 ml/hr.** As plasma glucose normalizes, change fluids to **D_5W at 100-200 ml/hr**. It is important to ensure that serum sodium does not become more hypernatremic while glucose is decreasing.
2. **Insulin:** initial dose of 10–20 U of regular insulin IV after fluid administration has begun, followed by an insulin drip to maintain glucose at ~ 200 mg/dl (~ 11.1 mmol/L). The dose of insulin needed is usually significantly less than with diabetic ketoacidosis because hydration causes glycosuresis.
3. Potassium replacement
4. **Caveat:** cerebral edema may occur with therapy.

Key References: Grace TW: Hyperosmolar nonketotic diabetic coma. Am Fam Physician 32: 119–125, 1985; Popli S, Leehey DJ, Dangridas JT, et al: Asymptomatic, nonketotic, severe hyperglycemia with hyponatremia. Arch Intern Med 150:1962–1964, 1990.

Adrenal Insufficiency

I. Adrenal insufficiency may be classified into primary and secondary causes, and each of these categories may be further divided into acute or slow in onset. Intercurrent illness or stressors may precipitate an adrenal crisis in patients with slow-onset adrenal insufficiency.

II. **Causes**

	Primary Adrenal Insufficiency	Secondary Adrenal Insufficiency
Acute	Adrenal hemorrhage, necrosis, thrombosis due to sepsis, coagulation disorders, antiphospholipid syndrome	Postpartum pituitary necrosis (Sheehan's syndrome), necrosis or bleeding into pituitary macro-adenoma, head trauma
Chronic	Autoimmune adrenalitis, tuberculosis, systemic fungal infections (e.g., histo-plasmosis), AIDS (e.g., cytomegalovirus, Kaposi's sarcoma), metastatic cancer, ketoconazole therapy	Pituitary, hypothalamic, or meta-static tumors, sarcoidosis, cranio-pharyngioma, histiocytosis X, long-term corticosteroid therapy

III. **Clinical manifestations**

1. **General:** weakness, fatigue, depression, anorexia, weight loss, orthostatic hypotension, nausea, vomiting, diarrhea, hyponatremia, hypoglycemia, normocytic anemia, lymphocytosis, eosinophilia (mild).
2. One important pearl is that the hypotension of severe adrenal insufficiency may **mimic either hypovolemic or septic shock**; therefore, adrenal insufficiency is in the differential diagnosis of both.
3. **Primary adrenal insufficiency:** hyperpigmentation, hyperkalemia, vitiligo.
4. **Secondary adrenal insufficiency:** amenorrhea, decreased libido, scanty axillary and pubic hair, small testicles, secondary hypothyroidism, diabetes insipidus, headaches, and visual symptoms.

IV. **Diagnostic tests**

1. **Basal hormone measurements.** Measure cortisol level between 8 and 9 AM.
   a. ≤ 3 μg/dl (≤ ~100 nmol/L)indicates adrenal insufficiency.
   b. ≥ 19 μg/dl (≥ ~500 nmol/L) rules out adrenal insufficiency.
   c. All other patients need further testing.
2. **Corticotropin (ACTH) stimulation test** is abnormal not only in patients with primary adrenal insufficiency but also in patients with secondary adrenal insufficiency because of adrenocortical atrophy due to lack of ACTH. Cortrosyn, 250 μg, is given IV or IM before 10 AM. Measure plasma cortisol level before and 60 min after. Adrenal function is normal if either value is at least 20 μg/dl (552 nmol/L).
3. **Radiologic evaluation**
   a. In cases of secondary adrenal insufficiency, MRI is superior to CT in imaging the hypothalamic-pituitary region.
   b. The adrenal gland is enlarged in patients with tuberculosis, fungal infections, metastatic cancer, lymphoma, and AIDS.

V. **Treatment**

1. **Replacement therapy** (given in divided doses in early morning and afternoon)
   a. Hydrocortisone, 15 mg, 10 mg orally, *or* cortisone, 25 mg, 12.5 mg orally.
   b. Fludrocortisone, 0.05–0.2 mg/day orally, for primary insufficiency.
2. **Emergency therapy**
   a. Saline
   b. Hydrocortisone, 100–200 mg IV bolus every 4–6 hr, then 50–100 mg IV every 6–8 hr.
3. **If diagnosis is in doubt** but suspected and requires empiric treatment, give dexamethasone, 5–10 mg IV, in place of first hydrocortisone dose and perform ACTH stimulation test.
4. **"Relative" adrenal insufficiency** describes the paradox of responsiveness to corticosteroids, despite the absence of biochemical or histologic evidence of

adrenal insufficiency. This diagnosis should be entertained and a trial of hydrocortisone (200–300 mg/day) considered in patients who are pressor-dependent or require prolonged mechanical ventilation. The cause of this phenomenon is not known but may be related to desensitization of glucocorticoid responsiveness at the cellular level.

Key Reference: Oelkers W: Adrenal insufficiency. N Engl J Med 335:1206–1212, 1996 (source of table); Shenker Y, Skatrud JB: Adrenal insufficiency in critically ill patients. Am J Respir Crit Care Med 163:1520–1523, 2001.

Pheochromocytoma

I. Pheochromocytomas produce catecholamines. About 90% of cases are derived from the adrenal medulla. They are most common in young and middle-aged adults and may occur in the setting of multiple endocrine neoplasia type IIA (MEN IIA) with medullary thyroid carcinoma and hyperparathyroidism.

II. **Signs and symptoms**
   1. **Classic triad** of presentation is headache, diaphoresis, and palpitations in the setting of hypertension. Severe apprehension and either pallor or flushing may occur. The hypertension may be sustained, may occur only during a paroxysm, or may be highly labile. Unusual blood pressure elevations after trauma or during surgery are suggestive.
   2. **Other manifestations** include cardiogenic pulmonary edema (due to sudden rise in blood pressure, ischemic heart disease even in the absence of coronary artery disease, and/or catecholamine-induced cardiomyopathy), noncardiogenic pulmonary edema (due to altered pulmonary capillary permeability or increased pulmonary venous tone), and orthostatic hypotension (due to decreased plasma volume and blunted sympathetic reflexes). Glucose intolerance is due to catecholamines.

III. **Certain drugs may precipitate a paroxysmal attack** by releasing catecholamine from the tumor: opiates, histamine, adrenocorticotropic hormone, saralasin, glucagon. Tricyclic antidepressants enhance the effects of catecholamines by inhibiting their neuronal reuptake. Serotonin reuptake inhibitors (e.g., fluoxetine) also may precipitate a crisis.

IV. **Diagnostic tests** (urinary samples should be 24-hr collection)
   1. **Urinary free catecholamines.** Upper limit of normal: ~ 590–885 nmol (100–150 μg)/day.
   2. **Urinary metanephrines** are falsely elevated by radiocontrast material and **vanillylmandelic acid (VMA)** by various foods such as bananas. Upper limits of normal in 24 hr: metanephrines, 7 μmol or 1.3 mg, and VMA, 35 μmol or 7 mg.
   3. **Plasma catecholamines** are more difficult to assay but helpful in borderline cases. Levels > 2000 pg/ml strongly suggest pheochromocytoma. Levels of 500–2000 pg/ml are borderline and best interpreted with the clonidine suppression test.
   4. **CT or MRI** is useful in locating the adrenal lesion once the diagnosis is made. Abdominal aortography, venous sampling of catecholamines at different levels of the inferior and superior vena cava, and ^{131}I-metaiodobenzylguanidine (MIBG) scintigraphy are further tests to localize the tumor before surgery.

V. **Control of acute hypertension and paroxysms with α-adrenergic blockade**
   1. **Phentolamine,** 5 mg IV every 4–6 hr, given slowly.
   2. Although beta blockers are useful for cathecholamine-induced tachyarrhythmia, they should not be used until adequate alpha blockade is in place.

VI. **Preoperative management**
1. **Phenoxybenzamine**, 10 mg orally every 12 hr with increase of 10–20 mg every few days until blood pressure and paroxysms are controlled. Severe orthostatic hypotension accompanies treatment and may require increased sodium intake and infusion.
2. **Prazosin**, 1–2 mg orally every 6 hr.

Key Reference: Sheps SG, Jiang NS, Klee GG, van Heerden JA: Recent developments in the diagnosis and treatment of pheochromocytoma. Mayo Clin Proc 65:88–95, 1990.

Hypoglycemia

I. Hypoglycemia is **traditionally defined as** (1) central nervous system symptom of confusion or coma, (2) simultaneous blood glucose < 40–50 mg/dl (< 2.22–2.77 mmol/L), and (3) relief of symptoms after administration of glucose.

II. **Causes:** insulinoma, exogenous insulin, sulfonylurea, hepatic dysfunction (especially in the setting of alcoholism), autoimmune disorders (antibodies to insulin receptors), tumors (sarcomas, lymphomas, benign mesotheliomas), hormonal deficiency syndromes (adrenal insufficiency, severe hypothyroidism), nesidioblastosis (β-cell hyperplasia, mostly seen in children but may be seen in adults), Reye's syndrome, postprandial syndrome, pentamidine, quinidine, and beta blockers.

III. **In-hospital causes** of hypoglycemia are mostly iatrogenic, due to excessive administration of insulin to diabetics in the setting of decreased caloric intake, treatment of hyperkalemia, and renal insufficiency. Other conditions associated with in-hospital hypoglycemia are liver disease, infections, shock, pregnancy, neoplasia, and burns.

IV. **Clinical manifestations** may be divided into **adrenergic** signs and symptoms (tachycardia, palpitations, sweating, anxiety, tremor, pallor) and **neuroglycopenic** signs and symptoms (bizarre psychiatric symptoms, confusion, seizures, coma).

V. **Differentiating endogenous vs. exogenous insulin excesses**

Blood levels	Insulinoma	Insulin	Sulfonylurea
Insulin	+	+	+
Proinsulin	+	±	+
C-peptide	+	–	+
Sulfonylurea	–	–	+
Insulin antibody	–	+	–

VI. **Treatment.** The obvious treatment for hypoglycemia is glucose. In alcoholics or malnourished patients, thiamine, 100 mg IV, should be given just before administration of 50 gm of IV glucose. Depending on the cause of hypoglycemia, continuous administration of D_5W may be needed to prevent relapses in hypoglycemia. Further tests, such as determination of C-peptide and insulin level or a 72-hr fast, may be required unless the cause of the hypoglycemia is obvious initially.

Key References: Comi RJ: Approach to acute hypoglycemia. Endocrinol Metab Clin North Am 22:247–262, 1993; Fischer KF, Lees JA, Newman JH: Hypoglycemia in hospitalized patients. N Engl J Med 315:1245–1250, 1986; Service FJ: Hypoglycemia disorders. N Engl J Med 332:1144–1152, 1995.

Corticosteroid Therapy in Severe Illness

I. **Cortisol** has a vital role in maintaining vascular tone, endothelial integrity, vascular permeability, and distribution of total body water within the vascular compartment.

II. **Occult relative adrenal insufficiency**: In patients with critical illness or who have undergone surgery, the cortisol level may be quite high. The level of cortisol correlates with illness severity score. Although adrenal function is often tested by the corticotropin-stimulation test, the interpretation is more difficult in critically ill patients because the serum cortisol level may be inappropriately low, suggesting the presence of relative adrenal insufficiency. For patients with suboptimal responses to corticotropin (> 9 µg/dl *increase* in cortisol is considered an appropriate increase), the mortality rate may be higher.

III. **Factors contributing to the development of relative hypoadrenalism in crtically ill patients**
1. Preexisting or previously undiagnosed asymptomatic diseases of the adrenal glands: autoimmune adrenalitis, tuberculosis, metastases
2. Acute partial destruction of the adrenals: hemorrhage from massive retroperitoneal bleed, thrombocytopenia, or anticoagulant therapy; bacterial (meningococcal), viral, or fungal infections
3. Previously unknown hypothalamic-pituitary axis disease
4. Previously unknown corticosteroid therapy
5. Medroxyprogesterone
6. Increased metabolism of cortisol from phenytoin, phenobarbitol, rifampin
7. Alteration in cortisol synthesis by ketoconazole, etomidate, aminoglutethimide, metyrapone, mitotane, trilostane
8. Interference with corticotropin action with suramin
9. Peripheralglucocorticoid-receptor blockade: mifepristone

IV. **Signs and symptoms that raise the suspicion for hypoadrenalism in critically ill patients**
1. Unexplained circulatory instability
2. Discrepency between the anticipated severity of the disease and the present state of the patient, including nausea, vomiting, hypotension, dehydration, abdominal or flank pain, fatique, and weight loss.
3. Fever of unknown cause
4. Unexplained mental status changes (apathy or depression)
5. Vitiligo, altered pigmentation, loss of axillary or pubic hair, hypothyroisism, hypogonadism
6. Hypoglycemia, hyponatremia, neutropenia, eosinophilia.

V. **Conditions in which corticosteroids may be beneficial**
1. *Pneumocystis carinii* pneumonia
2. Acute spinal cord injury
3. Fibroproliferative phase of acute respiratory distress syndrome
4. Typhoid fever
5. Early treatment of patients suspected of having a gram-negative bacterial infection: some studies have shown that administration of corticosteroids in the first few hours after the onset of shock may be beneficial in this subset of patients. Unfortunately, the meta-analyses showing that corticosteroids are not helpful did not address the issue of early treatment because of the lack of information about timing of administration in most trials. Moreover, benefits in gram-negative infections were offset by increased mortality rates in patients with gram-positive infections.

VI. **Cortisol replacement for patients taking oral corticosteroids for inflammation**

1. The daily rate of cortisol production in normal people is ~ 5.7 mg (15.7 μmol) per square meter of body surface area. This corresponds to ~ 10–12 mg of oral hydrocortisone equivalent per square meter per day, taking into account the first-pass hepatic metabolism of hydrocortisone.
2. Elective surgery or noncritical acute illness: continuation of the current doses of corticosteroids is sufficient to maintain cardiovascular function. On the other hand, overtreatment for 1–2 days is unlikely to cause any harm.
3. Prolonged or complicated surgery or critical illness: double or triple the current oral corticosteroid dose or give hydrocortisone 100–150 mg daily.

VII. **Cortisol replacement for patients taking oral corticosteroids for previously diagnosed hypothalamic-pituitary-adrenal insufficiency**

1. Hydrocortisone, 100–150 mg/day by continuous intravenous infusion during any severe illness or surgery.

Key Reference: Lamberts SWJ, Bruining HA, de Jong FH: Corticosteroid therapy in severe illness. N Engl J Med 337:1285–1292, 1997.

Environmental Critical Care

Hyperthermia

I. **Four clinical syndromes**, which may overlap, are associated with high ambient temperatures: **heat cramps, heat exhaustion, exertional heat injury, and heat stroke**. They occur with increased frequency in elderly people, alcoholics, and patients taking diuretics and drugs with anticholinergic effects.

II. **Heat stroke is generally the most severe form** of heat-related injuries. Classic heat stroke, which typically occurs in the elderly, is characterized by absence of sweating, paradoxical vasoconstriction, headache, vertigo, loss of consciousness, abdominal distress, confusion, hyperpnea, and severe pyrexia (rectal temperature > 41.4° C [106° F] is common), hot and dry skin, flaccid muscles, rhabdomyolysis, decreased deep tendon reflexes, shock, disseminated intravascular coagulation, seizures, and coma.

III. **Differential diagnosis**

1. **Central nervous system disorders:** acute hydrocephalus, hypothalamic hemorrhage or tumor, status epilepticus
2. **Endocrinopathy:** pheochromocytoma, thyroid storm
3. **Hyperthermic syndromes:** heat stroke (exertional, nonexertional), neuroleptic malignant syndrome, malignant hyperthermia, drug-induced hyperthermia, infection

IV. **Blood gases** drawn from hyperthermic patients falsely elevate the pH and falsely lower the $PaCO_2$ and PaO_2. For correction of each 1° C rise above 37° C, increase PaO_2 by 7.2% and $PaCO_2$ by 4.4%, and decrease pH by 0.02 units.

V. **Avoid** using dopaminergics and alpha agonists because they may cause vasoconstriction.

VI. **Cooling** should be done on an emergent basis in patients with heat stroke.

1. Place in a cool environment.
2. Remove patient's clothing.
3. Cool to 102.2° F (39° C) using evaporative fans, wetting the skin with water, cold water immersion, or shower (71.6° F, 22° C), gastric/colonic lavage, peritoneal lavage, axillary or perineal ice packs. Massaging the patient with heat stroke (particularly the torso and neck) decreases vasoconstriction.
4. In refractory cases, hemodialysis or cardiopulmonary bypass may be tried.

Key Reference: Aiyer MK, Crnkovich DJ, Carlson RW: Techniques for managing severe hyperthermia. J Crit Illness 10:643–646, 1995.

Hypothermia

I. **Definition:** core body temperature < 95° F (35° C).

II. **At risk** are people who are elderly, very young, immobilized, comatose, or poisoned (ethanol, phenothiazines, tricyclic antidepressants, benzodiazepines, morphine, heroin, organophosphates, carbon monoxide, barbiturates, vasodilators), people who exercise to exhaustion in the cold, and people with underlying illness, such as hypothyroidism, diabetic ketoacidosis, hypoadrenalism, hypopituitarism, hepatic encephalopathy, or CNS diseases (strokes, tumors, Wernicke's syndrome, sarcoidosis, subdural hematoma).

III. **Moderate (slowing) hypothermia:** temperature < 90° F (32° C) but > 86° F (30° C)

1. **Vital signs.** Initially heart rate, blood pressure, and cardiac output increase because of increased catecholamines. With progressive hypothermia, heart rate, blood pressure, and cardiac output decrease.
2. **Electrocardiogram:** prolonged PR, prolonged QT, inverted T waves, ST elevation, and **Osborn (J) waves**; bradycardia, atrial fibrillation, and ventricular tachycardia or fibrillation are seen with increased frequency with temperature < 30° C.

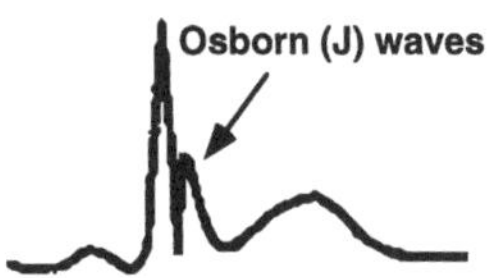

3. Hypothermia causes **shift of O_2 dissociation curve** to the left and tissue hypoxia, which causes metabolic acidosis and shift of O_2 dissociation curve to the right. Thus, aggressive resuscitation with hyperventilation and/or HCO_3 causes further shift to the left and increased tissue hypoxia.
4. As temperature decreases, solubility of O_2 and CO_2 decreases and pH rises; though in vitro measurement of $PaCO_2$ and pH at 37°C best reflects in vivo acid–base status regardless of body temperature.
5. **Central nervous system effects:** confusion, loss of voluntary motion, stiff muscles, dilated and fixed pupils, decreased reflexes, cranial nerve deficits, cerebellar signs, lack of shivering, and coma due to enzyme slowing, increased blood viscosity, decreased O_2 availability, and microcirculatory dysfunction induced by edema and vasoconstriction.
6. **Respiratory effects:** initially increased respiratory rate, then decreased respiratory rate and tidal volume.
7. **Renal effects:** initial peripheral vasoconstriction leading to increased central volume and diuresis. Decrease in tubular enzymatic activity leads to more diuresis and severe dehydration. In severe hypothermia, renal blood flow decreases.
8. **Hematologic effects:** impaired coagulation; however, prothrombin time and partial thromboplastin time may be falsely normal because the tests are performed on blood warmed to 37° C.

IV. **Severe (poikilothermic) hypothermia:** temperature < 86° F (30° C). The differential diagnosis is death.

V. **Treatment.** Because blood volume is reduced, cardiac arrest may occur with rewarming (due to increased metabolism coupled with inadequate supply). The brain is often protected from ischemia; therefore, total circulatory arrest may be tolerated for > 1 hr with no neurologic sequelae after rewarming. Defibrillation may be difficult to achieve until the core temperature > 30° C.

1. **D_5NS (5% dextrose in normal saline) at 100–200 ml/hr.**
2. **Passive external rewarming:** warm room, intravascular fluid at 98° F.
3. **Active external rewarming:** immersion in hot water bath or electric blankets at 40–45° C (risky, especially in the elderly, because of resultant decrease in peripheral vascular resistance (PVR) and hypotension, leading to paradoxically decreased core temperature, precipitating shock and ventricular fibrillation).
4. **Active core rewarming:** inhalation of warm (40–45° C) O_2, warm IV fluids (40–42° C), peritoneal dialysis, colonic irrigation, or extracorporeal blood rewarming.
5. Vagotonic maneuvers (e.g., during intubation) may precipitate asystole.

Key Reference: Bartley B, Crnkovich DJ, Usman AR, Carlson RW: How to recognize hypothermia in critically ill patients. J Crit Illness 11:118–127, 1996.

Bites and Envenomation

Animal	Venom	Manifestations	Treatment	Comments
Snake (pit vipers and coral snakes in U.S.)	**Pit viper:** tissue necrosis **Coral:** neuro-toxicity **Both:** coagu-lopathy, shock	**Pit viper:** edema, necrosis, bullae, gangrene and fever, nausea, vomiting, shock, coagulopathy, cramping, miosis, disorientation, de-lirium, convulsions **Coral:** numbness, ataxia, ptosis, pharyngeal or res-piratory paralysis, seizures	Wide constriction band to slow lymphatic flow **Pit viper antivenin:** Progressive swelling without systemic symptoms: 5 vials IV Mild systemic symptoms or heme/coagulation abnormalities: 5–15 vials Severe envenomation: 15–20 vials Increase dose by up to 50% for children and small adults Reconstitute each vial in 10 ml water; place reconstituted antivenin in 500 ml IVF over 1–2 hr; then 5–10 vials in IVF every 2hr as needed **Eastern coral antivenin:** 3–5 vials in 250–1000 ml NS over 1 hr	Call Regional Poison Control Center for addi-tional as-sistance by the National Antivenin Index
Black widow spider (red hourglass on females)		Local cramps with spread; boardlike and painful (but non-tender) abdomen, nausea, vomiting, headache, sweating, tremor, increased deep tendon reflexes, paresthesias	**10% calcium gluconate,** 10 ml IV over 10–20 min for cramps **Antivenin:** 1 vial (2.5 ml) in 50 ml normal saline IV over 15 min; repeat × 1 as needed	Bites: April through October
Recluse spider (violin marking)		Pain, bullae, and necrosis at site; fever, myalgias, morbilliform rash; intravascular hemolysis may cause acute renal failure	No signs or symptoms within first 6–8 hr: no treatment **Antivenin:** not available Consider corticosteroids early in severe cases	Bites: fall to early winter

I. Local wound care in all cases with cool (not ice) compress, with or without surgical debridement and fasciotomy.
II. Tetanus toxoid or immune globulin.
III. Antibiotics for gram-negative organisms in snake bites.
IV. **Must test for horse sensitivity before antivenin administration.**
V. **Identification of the black widow spider** (3/8 inch in length): the female's abdomen is almost spherical, with a red hourglass mark (or two transverse red marks separated by black) on the ventral surface. Habitat includes fallen branches and under objects of any kind, including toilet seats. (See figure, next page.)

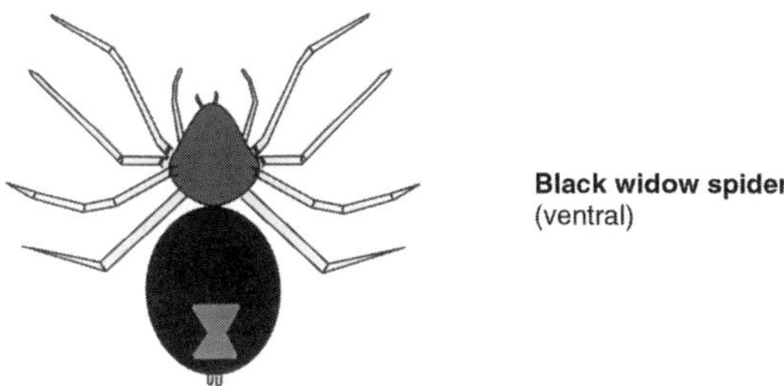

Black widow spider
(ventral)

VI. **Identification of the brown recluse spider:** also known as the violin spider, it is about ¼ inch (males) to ⅜ inch (females) in length. The thorax is orange-yellow with a dark violin pattern on the dorsal thorax. Habitat includes outdoor shelters and behind furniture or in clothing.

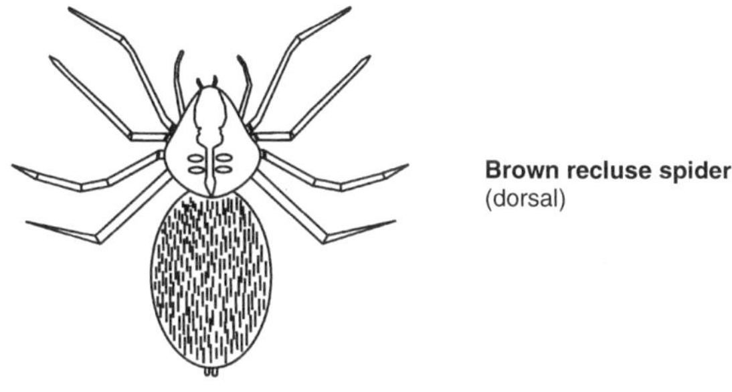

Brown recluse spider
(dorsal)

Scuba Diving-related Illnesses

I. **Mechanisms.** Besides trauma, hypothermia, and drowning, diving illnesses occur during ascent and arise from two basic mechanisms: (1) expansion of air in the respiratory system with resultant barotrauma or (2) formation of nitrogen bubbles in tissue or fluids as gas partial pressures decrease suddenly.

II. **Barotrauma**

1. **Pulmonary barotrauma.** Mediastinal and subcutaneous emphysema and pneumothorax may occur. Pneumothorax can be life-threatening.
2. **Air embolism.** Air may enter torn pulmonary vessels and the systemic arterial system with embolization of various organs. Most serious are brain emboli, which may lead to stroke symptoms immediately or within a few hours.
3. **Inner ear barotrauma** occurs with forceful efforts to equalize middle ear pressure that are unsuccessful because of blocked auditory canals. Vertigo, tinnitus, and sensorineural hearing loss are symptoms.
4. **Middle ear barotrauma.** Middle ear "squeeze" is common and results from edematous auditory tubes that prevent depressurization of the middle ear.
5. **Other.** Barotrauma may occur with other air-filled structures, including sinuses and GI tract.

III. **Decompression sickness ("bends").** When tissue nitrogen tension exceeds local tissue pressure, gas bubbles form and may cause symptoms by vascular or lymphatic compression or by activating inflammatory or clotting cascades. Symptoms start shortly after the dive but may be delayed for several days. Decompression sickness usually follows dives that require decompression and is accentuated by dehydration, alcohol, and obesity (nitrogen is more soluble in fat).

1. **Joint pain** is the most common symptom but usually resolves spontaneously.
2. **CNS involvement** is serious and may lead to spinal cord infarcts or neuronal injury, causing motor and sensory deficits. Cerebral involvement causes headache, visual and mental status abnormalities, and seizures. This is to be distinguished from CNS air embolism, which usually occurs more rapidly and with an uncontrolled ascent on dives that may not require decompression.
3. **Respiratory distress** may occur when gas formed in the systemic venous circuit is trapped in lungs ("the chokes"). The most severe manifestation resembles acute respiratory distress syndrome (ARDS).
4. **Inner ear decompression sickness** results from nitrogen bubbles forming in the perilymph or endolymph and may cause vertigo, tinnitus, and hearing loss. It should be distinguished from inner ear barotrauma, as noted above.
5. **Cutaneous manifestations** include pruritus, marbling (cutis marmorata), and rash. Marbling is associated with systemic involvement and warrants thorough evaluation.

IV. **Nitrogen narcosis.** Unrelated to decompression, the CNS malfunctions at high partial pressures of nitrogen, with consequent narcosis. This condition resolves as divers ascend above 100 ft (30 m) and is dangerous only insofar as impaired judgment at extreme depths precipitates accidents.

V. **Treatment**

1. **Administration of 100% oxygen** facilitates clearing of nitrogen from the body. IV rehydration improves tissue perfusion. Corticosteroids and mannitol are used to treat cerebral edema, although their use is unproven. Pneumothorax is treated with evacuation.
2. **Transportation by air should be at low altitudes** (1000 ft). The Trendelenburg position may decrease chances of cerebral embolism, although cerebral edema may be worsened.
3. **Repressurization** in a hyperbaric chamber is indicated for air embolism or serious decompression symptoms, especially symptoms referable to the CNS.
4. 24-hr consultative service is available through **Divers Alert Network** (DAN) at **919-684-8111**.

VI. **Near-drowning.** Because most victims aspirate < 10 ml/kg of water, treatment should be directed at restoring ventilation and circulation rather than attempting to empty fluid from the lungs. A particularly unique risk factor (termed shallow-water blackout) is caused by hyperventilation before submersion to such a degree that hypoxemia-induced unconsciousness occurs before the $PaCO_2$ reaches a break point.

1. **Aspiration**
   a. Salt water—hypertonicity causes irritation and exudation of fluid into the alveoli, resulting in ARDS.
   b. Fresh water—removes surfactant, which results in alveolar collapse and ARDS.
2. **Laryngospasm.** Although it prevents further aspiration, it causes hypoxia by asphyxiation.
3. **Metabolic acidosis** is a common finding.

Key References: Clenney TL, Lassen LF: Recreational scuba diving injuries. Am Fam Physician 53:1761–1766, 1996; Melamed Y, Shupak A, Bitterman H: Medical problems associated with underwater diving. N Engl J Med 326:30–35, 1992

High-altitude Pulmonary and Cerebral Edema

I. **High-altitude pulmonary edema (HAPE)**

1. Illnesses due to altitude include a spectrum of disorders from the minor (acute mountain sickness manifested by malaise, headache) to the more serious disorders such as HAPE and high-altitude cerebral edema (HACE). The cause of HAPE is not clear, but it appears that both an accentuated vascular response to hypoxia and increased permeability of the pulmonary endothelium to hypoxia and subsequent inflammation are required.
2. **Risk factors:** rapid ascent, strenuous activity on arrival, obesity, male gender, or history of HAPE. HAPE rarely occurs below 8,000 ft; it typically occurs 1–4 days after arrival at altitude.
3. **Clinical manifestations:** decreased exercise tolerance, fever, cough, tachypnea followed by frothy pink sputum production, dyspnea, and cyanosis. Later, obtundation and coma may develop. Chest radiographs typically show patchy peripheral infiltrates.
4. **Treatment**
   a. **Oxygen and descent** to lower altitude are the best forms of treatment.
   b. **Nifedipine** has been shown to be useful in both treatment and prophylaxis of HAPE. Begin with 10–20 mg sublingual nifedipine; acetazolamide and dexamethasone may be useful in the prophylaxis of acute mountain sickness but have not been shown to be effective in established cases of HAPE.

II. **High-altitude cerebral edema (HACE)**

1. HACE is the least common of high-altitude illnesses. It almost always occurs above 12,000 feet and within 2–3 days of arrival at altitude. If descent is not made quickly, permanent neurologic sequelae or death may ensue.
2. **Clinical manifestations:** severe headache, ataxia, loss of coordination, confusion, hallucination, and diplopia, progressing to lethargy and coma. Papilledema may be seen.
3. **Treatment:** descent and supportive therapy with oxygen. If descent is not possible, use portable hyperbaric chamber at 2 psi (13.8 kPa). At 2 psi, the equivalent altitude is ~ 2000 meters lower than the ambient altitude. If descent, oxygen, and hyperbaric chamber are not feasible or available, then give dexamethasone 8 mg po, IM, or IV initially, then 4 mg every 6 hrs. If dexamethasone is unavailable, give acetazolamide 250 mg twice daily. If all treatment options are unavailable, descent of only 500–1000 meters may be helpful.

III. **High-altitude flatus expulsion (HAFE):** due to increase in volume of gas in intestinal lumen, due in part to lower ambient pressure at high altitude, as described by Boyle's Law ($V \alpha \frac{1}{P}$). An annoyance, it is not known to be life threatening.

Key Reference: Hackett PH, Roach RC: High-altitude illness. N Engl J Med 345:107–114, 2001.

Procedures

General Note

This section is not intended to be an encompassing guide for learning how to do the procedures. Rather it is intended to be a reminder for operators who already have experience. As always, the best method of learning is to read about the procedure, to observe, and then to be taught by a skilled operator. Informed consent should be obtained except in emergency situations. The following are general reminders for a successful outcome:

I. **Aseptic technique and universal precautions**
II. **Adequate sedation and local anesthesia** (for the patient)
III. **Preprocedure preparation of all necessary equipment**
IV. **Rehearsing in one's mind the sequence of the procedure** before the actual performance
V. **Anticipation and treatment of complications**
VI. **An occlusive dressing should be applied over the insertion site after an intravenous catheter is removed** because air embolism may occur through the fistulous tract that forms. Insert **and** remove central venous catheters in a Trendelenburg position to prevent air embolism to the central nervous system.

Central Venous Catheters

I. **External jugular (EJ) vein insertion.** Patient is placed in Trendelenburg position, and the head is turned away. A dilator is not needed for EJ insertion. After cannulation with the needle, having the patient return his or her head slowly back to midline may facilitate guidewire placement if it does not advance easily.
II. **Internal jugular vein insertion.** Patient is placed in the Trendelenburg position with the head turned away. For the **middle approach**, the site of insertion is the apex of the triangle formed by the sternal and clavicular heads of the sternocleidomastoid muscle. Alternatively, the insertion site is approximately three fingerbreadths from the head of the clavicle while the operator "grabs" the sternal head with three fingers (see figure below). This method is useful for locating the site of insertion when landmarks are ill defined. Aim the needle (you may use a small finder needle first) for the ipsilateral nipple at 45° from the skin surface. The internal jugular vein is generally lateral and slightly posterior to the carotid artery. For the **posterior approach**, the insertion site is the junction where the EJ vein

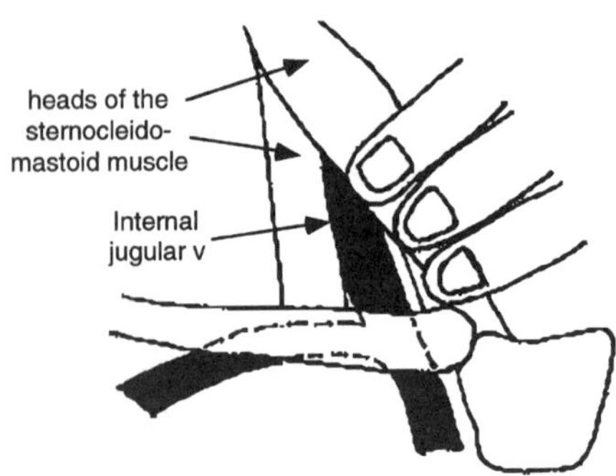

crosses the posterior edge of the sternocleidomastoid muscle. The needle is aimed for the suprasternal notch

III. **Subclavian vein catheter insertion.** Patient is placed in Trendelenburg position with the head turned away. Two simple but effective maneuvers may facilitate placement: (1) a rolled-up towel may be placed longitudinally between the scapulae, and (2) an assistant may pull gently the ipsilateral arm and shoulder down toward the floor. The insertion site is the inferior margin of the clavicle between the middle and distant thirds (or two-thirds the clavicle distance from the clavicle head). Aim needle for the suprasternal notch, and insert it beneath the clavicle, keeping it parallel to the posterior surface of the clavicle. It is important to keep the needle parallel to the chest surface (not angled downward) to lessen the risk of pneumothorax. Insert needle with the bevel up, but once it is in the subclavian vein, rotate needle 180° before guidewire insertion to facilitate thoracic (rather than cervical) insertion.

IV. **Femoral vein catheter insertion.** Patient's knee is extended with the foot rotated 15–30° outward. The site of insertion is approximately 2–3 cm inferior to the inguinal ligament and 1–2 cm medial to the femoral pulse (artery). A mnemonic for order of structure is **NAVY** for **n**erves, **a**rtery, **v**ein.

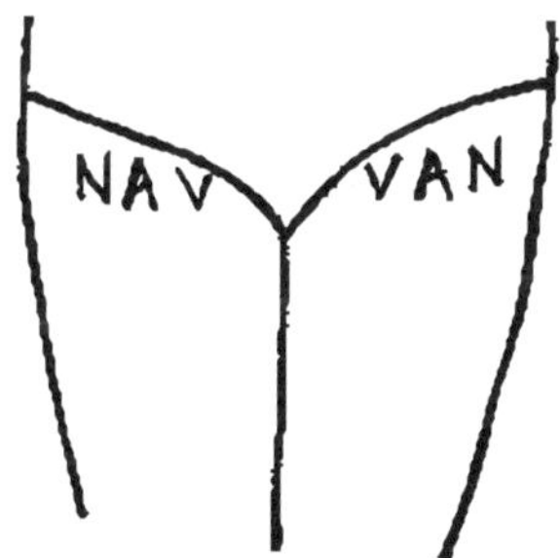

Key Reference: Agee KR, Balk RA: Central venous catheterization in the critically ill patient. Crit Care Clin 8:677–686, 1992.

Arterial Catheterization

I. The preferred sites for arterial cannulation are the radial, femoral, and dorsalis pedis arteries.

II. Before **radial artery cannulation**, the Allen test should be performed to confirm adequate blood supply to the hand by the corresponding ulnar artery. To facilitate radial artery cannulation, place a folded towel beneath the supine wrist to keep it at maximal extension. Taping the hand and forearm to the bed surface may help to stabilize the wrist. Radial and dorsalis pedis artery cannulations may be performed by either a catheter-over-needle or Seldinger technique with a needle and guidewire.

III. For **femoral artery cannulation**, confirm good distal pulses and perfusion. Femoral artery cannulation is best achieved by the needle-and-guidewire method.

IV. **It is of paramount importance to monitor the patient for the following complications and to document the results in the chart** (at least on a daily basis). If any are present, the arterial catheter should be removed.

1. Inadequate pulses and circulation distal to the site of insertion
2. Signs of infection
3. Lack of a medical need for the arterial catheter

V. It is also important to ensure **adequate hemostasis** after catheter removal (especially femoral catheters) because serious hematomas and life-threatening bleeding may result.

Key Reference: Clark VL, Kruse JA: Arterial catheterization. Crit Care Clin 8:687–697, 1992.

Pericardiocentesis

I. **Indications.** Pericardiocentesis may be required emergently in patients with clinical evidence of a life-threatening cardiac tamponade in whom delay in drainage may be fatal. Otherwise, echocardiogram and CT scan are the most accurate methods not only of diagnosing the presence and significance of the pericardial fluid but also of guiding drainage.

II. **Contraindications.** In the nonemergent setting, uncorrected coagulopathy is the major contraindication. Small or loculated effusions need echocardiographic or CT guidance. In the emergent setting there is no absolute contraindication.

III. **Technique.** Before performing the procedure, the patient should have adequate volume resuscitation and, if required, respiratory support. The **subxiphoid approach** is the safest and most widely used method: the needle passes through the skin, subcutaneous tissue, diaphragm, and then the parietal pericardium.

1. The area just left of the xiphoid tip is sterilized and locally anesthetized.
2. Attach an alligator clip (that leads to the V lead of the EKG monitor) to the needle hub of a 16–21 gauge cardiac or spinal needle (with a short bevel and attached to a syringe filled with a local anesthetic). Insert the needle perpendicular to the skin until it passes beneath the inner aspect of the rib cage. Then angle the needle toward the left shoulder, and advance with gentle suction.
3. Epicardial contact occurs when there is a palpable or audible "ticking" sensation from the syringe-needle and/or a current of injury on EKG tracing (ST or PR segment elevation). If this occurs, withdraw the needle a few mm, and reangle it more medially.
4. For relief of acute (life-threatening) tamponade, only about 50 ml of pericardial fluid needs to be removed. Once the needle is in the pericardial space, use the Seldinger technique to place a catheter over a guidewire into the space for additional drainage.

IV. If available in a timely fashion, **echocardiographic guidance** (with an experienced assistant) increases the rate of a successful pericardiocentesis.

Key Reference: Kirkland LL, Taylor RW: Pericardiocentesis. Crit Care Clin 8:699–712, 1992.

Identification of the Difficult Airway

I. **Factors associated with difficult mask ventilation:** full beards, facial dressing or scarring, edentulous patients, and repeated laryngoscopies.

II. **Factors associated with difficult direct laryngoscopy**

1. **Abnormal oropharyngeal anatomy** (small mouth, prominent maxillary incisors, large tongue, oropharyngeal closed space infections, inhalational injury)
2. **Temporomandibular disease** (arthritis of the TMJ joint: rheumatoid arthritis [RA], psoriatic, degenerative, or ankylosing spondylitis [AS])

3. **Abnormal laryngeal anatomy** (anterior larynx, RA, epiglottitis, trauma, tumors/cysts)
4. **Abnormal cervical anatomy** (arthritis, RA, AS, degenerative; fracture)

III. Visualization of the glottic opening requires alignment of the oral, pharyngeal, and laryngeal axis. **Put a towel under the occiput and extend the neck** ("sniffing position").

IV. **Mallampati classification** of tongue size in relation to the oral cavity. Have patient open the mouth as wide as possible and protrude the tongue. It is not a totally accurate method for assessing the degree of difficulty in intubation because of failure to consider neck mobility and size of the mandibular space. In general, difficulty with intubation is rare in class I and increases in frequency with the Mallampati class. The important point to remember is that difficulty may be encountered with any class; anticipatory measures must be thought out in advance.

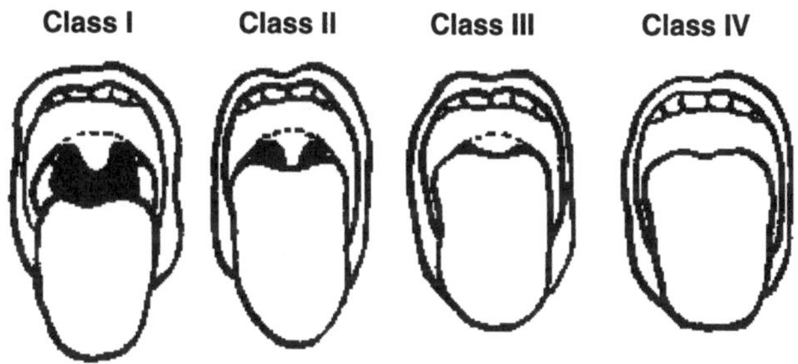

V. The space anterior to the larynx (**distance between the tip of the chin and thyroid notch with the neck extended**) correlates with ease of intubation (if < 6 cm, difficulty increases).

VI. In the patient with a difficult airway, a frequent mistake is repeated attempts at direct laryngoscopy, which create more trauma and edema, making intubation even more difficult. In such circumstances, consider the following options: (1) **early assistance**, (2) **intubation via fiberoptic laryngoscopic or bronchoscopic guidance**, or (3) **cricothyroidotomy**. **Transtracheal jet ventilation** allows one to oxygenate the patient temporarily while measures are taken for a definitive airway.

Key Reference: Marks JD, Bogetz MS: New concepts in the management of the difficult airway. Clin Anesth Updates 5:1–11, 1994.

Endotracheal Intubation

I. For the conscious or semiconscious patient, **adequate sedation** with a narcotic and amnestic is usually necessary before the procedure. A typical starting dose is **morphine sulfate, 1–3 mg IV, and midazolam, 2–3 mg IV**, titrating to sedation and monitoring blood pressure. An alternative regimen is **etomidate, 0.3 mg/kg (typical dose: 20 mg IV)**. Before intubation, a patent airway and adequate oxygenation must be ensured; most likely mask-bag ventilation with 100% oxygen and proper technique will be required. Patient's vital signs (including SpO_2) must be monitored at all times by an assistant.

II. **Technique**

1. Place the patient's head in a **sniffing position if there are no contraindications** (e.g., cervical spine injury). A reliable method for obtaining this position

is to **place about 2–3 inches of padding beneath the occiput and then extend the head back**. Do not place the padding beneath the neck because it will displace the tracheal axis away from the pharyngeal axis.

2. Using the scissor technique to open the mouth with the right hand, gently **insert the no. 4 or no. 3 curved laryngoscope blade** (McIntosh) with the left hand, and **sweep the tongue to the left**.
3. The tip of the blade is moved until it is front of the epiglottis. Then lift the blade up at about a 45° angle from the patient, aiming the end of the laryngoscope handle for the far end of the ceiling. **Do not cock the blade back**; this is not only ineffective but may injure the teeth.
4. **Visualize the cords**, and insert the endotracheal tube (ETT) between the cords into the trachea.
5. **Examine for clinical evidence that the ETT is in the trachea** and not in the right (or left) mainstem.
   a. Although not completely reliable, signs that the ETT is in proper position are condensation on the walls of the ETT with each expiration (may be misleading if there is a lot of gas within the stomach and the ETT is in the esophagus), breath sounds in the lungs, and absence of sounds over the stomach with each bag-delivered breath.
   b. A more reliable indicator is using an $ETCO_2$ monitor or a hand-held $ETCO_2$ detector (e.g., Capnocheck®) that changes color with the presence of CO_2.
   c. If unsure, one can reinsert the laryngoscope blade to confirm whether the ETT inserts between the vocal cords.
6. **Tape the ETT securely** (about 23 cm for women and 25 cm for men at the front teeth) when one is certain that it is in the airway.
7. Obtain a **chest radiograph** immediately to confirm position, and adjust accordingly.
8. The **straight laryngoscopic blade (Miller)** is more difficult to learn than the curved blade. It is good for the patient with a small mouth. The blade is placed in the middle of the mouth with the tongue draped over either side and is advanced to the tip of the larynx, thus touching and lifting the tracheal surface of the epiglottis.

III. **Helpful hints for successful visualization of the vocal cords and intubation**

1. Have all necessary equipment and personnel ready. If needed, suction out secretions, and mask-bag ventilate the patient to ensure adequate oxygenation before intubation. Have a **back-up plan** in mind (e.g., needle cricothyroidotomy or surgical cricothyroidotomy) in case the initial attempts at intubation fail. Remember that repeated attempts often make subsequent attempts more difficult because edema (and possibly bleeding) result from trauma due to the laryngoscope blade.
2. Do not put your head too close to the patient because this may decrease depth perception. In addition, insert the ETT at such an angle that it does not obstruct your view of the vocal cords.
3. Advancing the curved blade too far (a common mistake among aggressive intubators) may make visualization of the vocal cords more difficult.
4. Having an assistant **pull down the corner of the patient's mouth** may help to visualize the vocal cords.
5. If the epiglottis is visualized but the vocal cords are not, the **tip of the ETT may be used to lift up the epiglottis** to see the vocal cords that are "underneath."
6. **External laryngeal manipulation** (push the thyroid cartilage superiorly and dorsally) helps to visualize the vocal cords by displacing the larynx dorsally.

7. A **stylet in the ETT** often makes the insertion easier by angling the ETT favorably and produces a rigid tip for easier maneuverability.

IV. **Double-lumen endotracheal tubes** are endotracheal tubes with a distal bronchial port and a proximal tracheal port with a cuff above each opening. Left-sided tubes (in which the left lung is ventilated by the bronchial port and its corresponding cuff is in the left mainstem bronchus) is preferred over right-sided tubes because of a lower risk of right upper lobe obstruction. The intrinsically small caliber of the tube increases the risk of auto-PEEP. For independent lung ventilation, synchronization simplifies pulmonary artery catheter interpretation. The ideal setting for independent lung ventilation is unilateral lung disease in which application of PEEP results in worsening perfusion to the good lung and/or worsening barotrauma or chest tube leaks. The tube (about 39 French for women and 41 French for men) is advanced through the glottis with the curved tip positioned anteriorly. The tube is rotated 90° toward the bronchus to be intubated as the tip approaches the carina. Once mild resistance is met, the cuffs are inflated and position is checked by auscultation with or without bronchoscopy.

Key Reference: Hines D, Bone RC: The technique of endotracheal intubation. J Crit Illness 1:59–65, 1986.

Steps in Rapid-sequence Intubation

I. **Rapid-sequence intubation** requires technical skill and familiarity with the use of neuromuscular blocking agents. The main indication for this technique is a "full-stomach" situation or other propensity to aspiration (e.g., esophageal disease). It should not be performed by novices.

II. **Steps in rapid-sequence intubation**
1. Preoxygenate patient with 100% oxygen through a face mask or Ambu-Bag, but mask ventilation is *not* provided unless unsuccessful intubation necessitates it.
2. Make sure that working suction equipment is at hand.
3. Begin pulse oximetry monitoring and measure vital signs.
4. Perform the **Sellick maneuver** (cricoid pressure) to prevent gastric insufflation and regurgitation.
5. **Administer sedative of choice**:
   a. Midazolam, 1–3 mg IV or
   b. Etomidate, 0.3 mg/kg IV (~20 mg IV), is the sedative of choice for hemodynamically unstable patients or
   c. Fentanyl, 25–50 μg IV; repeat as necessary and as tolerated or
   d. Ketamine, 0.5–1 mg/kg IV.
6. **Administer succinylcholine**, 1 mg/kg, if there are no contraindications. Some physicians premedicate with a non-depolarizing agent such as curare, 3 mg IV, or rocuronium, 5 mg IV, to prevent facsciculations. If a nondepolarizing agent is used,the dose of succinylcholine is generally increased to 1.5 mg/kg. If muscle relaxant is required and succinylcholine is contraindicated, give rocuronium 0.6–1.2 mg/kg (onset is ~ 2 min and duration is 30 min).
7. If the patient has trauma, perform in-line cervical spine immobilization. In patients with suspected head injury, premedication with **lidocaine, 1.5–2 mg/kg IV,** can prevent the increase in intracranial pressure during endotracheal intubation.
8. Perform **orotracheal intubation**.

Transtracheal Ventilation

I. Percutaneous catheter placement through the cricothyroid membrane and surgical cricothyrotomy are options in cardiac arrest patients in whom endotracheal intubation is unsuccessful.

II. **Percutaneous catheter placement (needle cricothyroidotomy)**
1. Use a 14-gauge angiocatheter attached to a saline-filled syringe.
2. Insert the needle through the cricothyroid membrane directed caudally.
3. Confirm placement in the trachea by aspirating air into the syringe.
4. Advance the catheter over the needle. An assistant should hold the catheter in place because of difficulty in securing the catheter.
5. The oxygen tubing should be noncompressible, and all connections must be secured because of the very high pressures.
6. Allow 1 second of inflation and 4 seconds of exhalation. Typically a 14-gauge catheter and a 50-psi driving pressure deliver 500 ml of O_2 per second.

III. **Surgical cricothyrotomy**
1. Make an initial vertical or horizontal incision through the skin over the cricothyroid membrane (see figure below).
2. Incise horizontally through the membrane.
3. Insert the scalpel handle into the incision, and rotate 90° to open the airway.
4. Insert an endotracheal tube, tracheostomy tube, or any rigid cannula of appropriate size. When a cannula is not available and the patient is spontaneously breathing, any rigid object can be used to stent the airway open. But if a patient is not spontaneously breathing, a cannula must be used for positive pressure ventilation.

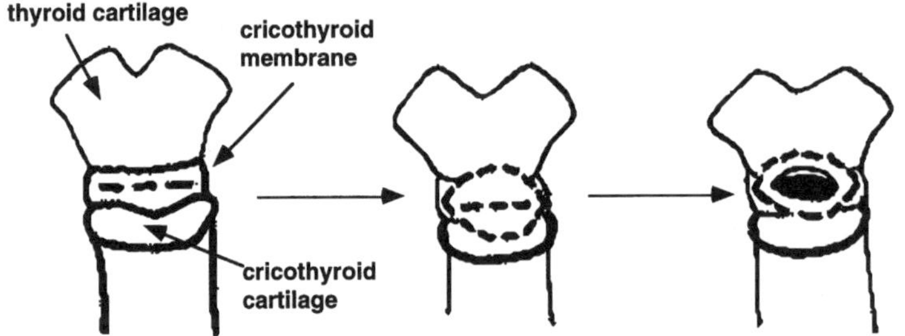

Key Reference: Reed AP: Current concepts in airway management for cardiopulmonary resuscitation. Mayo Clin Proc 70:1172–1184, 1995.

Closed Chest Tube Thoracostomy

I. **Indications**
1. **Pneumothorax.** Patients with minimal symptoms and a pneumothorax < 20–25% without evidence of an increase over several hours probably do not require a chest tube (CT). Patients on mechanical ventilation almost always require a CT for pneumothorax of any size.
2. **Complicated parapneumonic effusion** (see p. 19)
3. **Hemothorax** (see Thoracic Trauma)

II. **Technique.** Tube diameter varies from 16–40 French (5–11 mm internal diameter) for adults.

1. Most CTs, whether for pneumothorax or nonloculated (free-flowing) effusions, may be **inserted into the 5th or 6th intercostal space and then tunneled upward** to the next higher space along the anterior axillary line. Some recommend a small CT (16–20 Fr) through the second intercostal space at the midclavicular line for pneumothoraces, but this method is less efficient and more tissues may have to be penetrated.
2. Infiltrate the skin, subcutaneous tissue, and along the superior aspect of the rib (periosteum) over which the tube will pass with **1% lidocaine**; the needle also may be used as a finder needle to aspirate for fluid or air. Make an incision 2–3 mm larger than the index finger.
3. Using blunt dissection with a small and then medium (or large) Kelly clamp, **dissect through the subcutaneous tissues and intercostal muscle**. Additional local anesthetic may be required. Then use the tip of the clamp to enter the pleural space, using a spreading maneuver.
4. Grasp the CT with a medium clamp, and insert into the pleural space, angling it **toward the anterior apex for a pneumothorax** and **toward the posterior-basilar portion for fluid drainage**. Insert the CT with the last side hole 2–3 cm into the chest. Rotating the clamp 120° helps to direct the tube toward the anterior-apical part of the chest.
5. **Clinical evidence of correct placement:** expected drainage of fluid or air and condensation on the sides of the tube with each expiration.
6. Fasten the chest tube to the skin with **1-0 or 2-0 silk suture** and connect to suction bottle. Secure suction tubings well with adhesive tape.
7. Obtain **chest radiograph** for confirmation of placement.

III. **Recommendations for specific disorders**

1. **Empyema or complicated parapneumonic effusion.** Direct large tubes (28–36 Fr) posteroinferiorly or into the area of loculation. The CT may be removed once the patient is afebrile, pleural drainage is serous and < 50 cc/day, and minimal fluid is seen on chest radiograph.
2. **Malignant effusion.** Insert a moderate-sized tube (20–28 Fr). When drainage is minimal (< 50–100 cc/day) and chest radiograph shows complete reexpansion, inject sclerosing agent through CT; clamp CT for 1–2 hr, and reapply suction for 2–3 days. CT may be removed when drainage is minimal and chest radiograph shows complete reexpansion on water seal. Intrapleural sclerosing agents include:

Technique	Dose	Response Rate	Comment
Doxycycline	500 mg	88%	Add lidocaine (10 cc, 1%)
Bleomycin	60 IU	63–85%	Contraindicated in renal failure
Talc	5 gm	72–100%	Slurry or aerosol forms
Pleurectomy	—	88–100%	

3. **Hemothorax.** Bleeding > 100 ml/hr for 6–8 hr or > 200 ml/hr 2–4 hr is an indication for surgery.

IV. **CT removal.** Opinion is divided as to the necessity of clamping for 12–24 hr before CT removal. Clamping allows identification of persistent air leaks or reaccumulation of fluid. Remove suture in 3–5 days.

V. **Complications**

1. The diaphragm may rise as high as the 4th intercostal space on full expiration. **Insertion of the CT into the abdominal cavity** can be a catastrophic complication.

2. **Risk factors for reexpansion pulmonary edema:** chronic collapse, endobronchial obstruction, trapped lung, rapid removal of air or fluid, and increased intrapleural negative pressure due to suction.
3. **For transporting patients with CTs**, either continue the suction with a portable system or place the CT on water seal. The CT circuit should not be clamped because of the risk of tension pneumothorax.

Key References: Cohen R, Barbers RG: Thoracostomy: Our approach to tube placement and follow-up. J Respir Dis 15:1082–1092, 1994; Iberti TJ, Stern PM: Chest tube thoracostomy. Crit Care Clin 8:879–895, 1992.

Abdominal Paracentesis

I. Paracentesis may need to be performed **diagnostically** to help determine the cause of ascites or **therapeutically** to relieve symptoms caused by large amounts of ascitic fluid.

II. **Technique**
1. Paracentesis may be performed with the patient in the supine or upright sitting position, but generally success rates are higher in the more dependent areas. Localization of ascitic fluid by ultrasound may be required. A relatively avascular area is the linea alba.
2. Locally anesthetize the skin with 1–2% lidocaine by first causing a subcutaneous wheal; then stretch the skin about 1 cm before advancing the needle for further anesthesia (this technique provides a "Z track" to prevent leakage of ascitic fluid).
3. For therapeutic drainage, an 18–20-gauge angiocatheter may be used, followed by drainage by gravity or suction bottles.

III. **Diagnostic tests for ascitic fluid**
1. White cell count > 500/ml (> 0.5×10^9/L) or **neutrophil count > 250/ml (> 0.25×10^9/L)** is diagnostic of spontaneous bacterial peritonitis.
2. **Gram stain**
3. **Cultures:** inoculation into blood culture bottles increases the yield.
4. **Serum–ascites albumin gradient**
   a. A wide gradient (> 1.1 gm/dl or 11 gm/L) is consistent with cirrhosis, liver metastases, venoocclusive disease, and cardiac origin.
   b. A narrow gradient (< 1.2 gm/dl or < 12 gm/L) is consistent with peritoneal carcinomatosis, tuberculosis, fungal peritonitis, nephrotic syndrome.
5. **Amylase** (pancreatitis), **bilirubin** (pancreatitis or bile duct leak), **triglyceride** (chylous leak) may be elevated in various disorders.

Key Reference: Gerber DR, Bekes CE: Peritoneal catheterization. Crit Care Clin 8:727–742, 1992.

Lidocaine During Bronchoscopy

I. Much of the lidocaine administered in the upper airway is actually swallowed and undergoes first-pass metabolism in the liver. However, the potential toxicity of lidocaine given via the lower airways should be strongly considered because the lidocaine given by this route is directly absorbed into the systemic circulation without undergoing first-pass metabolism through the liver. More drugs are absorbed from the lower airways because of increased vascularity. The elimination half-life is about 100 min but may be 300 min in patients with chronic liver disease. The time to reach peak plasma concentration is 40–90 min after nasopharyngeal application and 5–20 min after oropharyngeal, laryngeal, or tracheal application.

II. **Toxicity of lidocaine** includes seizures, respiratory arrest, and methemoglobinemia.

III. Some recommend **maximal lidocaine dose** for local anesthesia of 200 mg or 6 mg/kg (~ **400 mg for a 70-kg patient**). Early signs of CNS toxicity include lightheadedness, tremors, or hallucinations. Use lower dose in patients with congestive heart failure or liver disease. **Lidocaine 1% = 10 mg/ml; lidocaine 4% = 40 mg/ml.**

Perioperative Assessment

Assessment of the Trauma Patient

I. **Approach to patients with major mechanism of injury**

1. **ABCDEs**
   a. Assess and secure **airway** while maintaining cervical spine and complete spine immobilization.
      - Apply oxygen
      - Bag mask ventilation and intubation for patients who meet the following criteria: (1) shock, (2) inability to maintain of control airway, and (3) Glasgow Coma Scale (GCS) score ≤ 8.

   b. Assess **breathing**. Use needle decompression for tension pneumothorax (tympanitic hemithorax, absent breath sounds, deviated trachea and evidence of shock). Apply 16-gauge needle in second intercostal above rib in the midclavicular line, and follow with chest tube insertion in the fourth to fifth intercostal space in the midaxillary line. Chest tube should be at least 28 French; a 30–32-French tube is preferred for adults. A useful landmark is to stay at or above the nipple in men and above the inframammary fold in women to avoid inadvertent abdominal placement.

   c. Assess **circulation**.
      - Early signs of shock are tachycardia, narrowed pulse pressure, and cool extremities with weak pulses. Hypotension is a late finding suggesting ≥ 30% blood loss.
      - Establish two IV lines, including 16-gauge antecubital line, and begin bolus with 2 liters of crystalloid.

   d. Assess and document neurologic **disability**, including pupil size and reactivity as well as best estimate of GCS score.

Score	**6**	**5**	**4**	**3**	**2**	**1**
Eyes			Spontaneous	Speech	Pain	None
Verbal		Oriented	Confused	Inappropriate	Incomprehensible	None
Motor	Obeys	Localizes	Withdrawal	Flexion	Extension	None

   e. Assess **extremities**.

2. Expose patient, and apply **direct pressure** to any areas of obvious bleeding.
3. Draw initial **arterial blood gases (ABG) and blood work**, including complete blood count (CBC), prothrombin time (PT), partial thromboplastin time (PTT), international normalized ratio (INR), blood-type crossmatch, electrolytes, creatinine, lipase, and glucose.
4. Order **initial x-rays**.
   a. First priority: chest x-ray
   b. Second priority: pelvic x-Ray)
   c. Third priority: lateral view of cervical spine
   d. Follow with complete spinal x-rays and extremity x-rays, as indicated.
5. Insert **Foley catheter** after ruling out urethral injury. In male patients with blood at the meatus, scrotal hematoma, or high-riding prostate, perform urethrogram first.

6. Insert **nasogastric (NG) tube**. In patients with evidence of basal skull fracture (raccoon eyes, otorhinorhea, Battle sign, facial smash), insert orogastric tube instead to avoid passing NG tube intracranially through cribriform plate.
7. **Reassess** airways, breathing, and circulation.
8. Complete and document **head-to-toe secondary survey**.
9. **Exclude** occult hemorrhage and major injury.
10. **Review chest x-ray**. (*Note:* A wide mediastinum is not an explanation for shock.)
11. **Review pelvic x-ray**. Tile class B and C fractures may be associated with massive blood loss.

Tile Classification of Pelvic Fractures

Tile class A	Stable
Tile class B	Rotationally unstable
Tile class C	Rotationally, vertically and posteriorly unstable

12. **Assess intra-abdominal compartment.** Computed tomography (CT) is used for hemodynamically stable patients. For hemodynamically unstable patients, use focused abdominal sonography in trauma (FAST) protocol or perform diagnostic peritoneal lavage (DPL).
13. **Asssess the patient for shock.**
    a. Head injury is not an explanation for shock.
    b. Use large-volume resuscitators for early blood transfusion and warmers for hypotensive hemorrhagic shock.
    c. Consider the possibility of other causes of shock: tamponade, tension pneumothorax, neurogenic shock.
14. Assess and evaluate for **blunt aortic injury** (loss of aortopulmonary window, depression of left mainstem bronchus, apical cap, deviation of NG to right). If the chest x-ray and mechanism of injury are suspicious for aortic injury, perform an aortic angiogram. If the chest x-ray is equivocal, perform contrast enhanced CT scan of the chest to evaluate for mediastinal hematoma. Transesophageal echocardioigraphy may be used to rule out damage to thoracic aorta instead of angiogram.
15. **Assess immobilized thoracic, lumbar, and cervical spines.** Patients who are alert and cooperative without a distracting injury (multiple rib fractures, long bone fracture) may be cleared clinically. In all other cases with significant mechanism of injury, a complete spinal series should be obtained: anteroposterior (AP) and lateral views of the thoracic and lumbar spines and AP lateral odontoid views of the cervical spine. The cervical spine must demonstrate full C7 and T1 vertebral bodies.
16. **Antibiotic prophylaxis** for compound fractures
17. **Tetanus prophylaxis** if immunizations are not up to date (initial series of 3 shots and booster within past 10 years): administer 0.5 cc of tetanus toxoid. If the wound is prone to tetanus and immunizations are unknown or the patient has had < 3 initial series, administer 250 units of tetanus immunoglobulin (separate site).
18. **CT head scan** for patients with GCS score <15 or significant loss of consciousness (> 5 minutes).
19. Document **neurologic exam**, including cranial nerves, sensory-motor exam of all four extremities, deep tendon reflexes, and Babinski sign.
20. Document **pulses in all four extremities**.
21. Examine **all major joints.**
22. Document **all penetrating wounds**. Do not list as entry/exit wounds; you may be wrong.
23. **Suture lacerations and splint fractures.** Major joint dislocations require immediate orthopedic consultation and reduction.

24. Initiate early consultation and communication with ICU, orthopedics, anesthesia, neurosurgery, plastic surgery, vascular surgery, and other disciplines as required. Emergency medicine and general/trauma surgery should be involved in initial assessment and resuscitation in trauma centers.
25. Perform **head-to-toe tertiary survey** within 24 hours. Injuries are missed on initial assessments in up to 15% of patients with major trauma.

II. **Pitfalls**
   1. Abdominal exam is frequently unreliable in patients with major trauma.
   2. The patient's condition often evolves and changes—you *must* reassess.
   3. Elevated hemidiaphragm = ruptured hemidiaphragm until proved otherwise. Direct visualization is often required.
   4. Alcohol intoxication and major head injury frequently coexist. In patients with a major mechanism of injury, perform a CT head scan.
   5. Patients with hemorrhagic shock require surgical control. Delaying surgery to perform multiple diagnostic maneuvers places patients at risk.

Key Reference: Trunkey D: Initial treatment of patients with extensive trauma. N Engl J Med 324:1259, 1991.

Preoperative Assessment of the Pulmonary Patient

I. **Postoperative pulmonary complications** include pneumonia, bronchospasm, respiratory failure, atelectasis, exacerbation of underlying lung disease leading to lengthened hospital stay or worsening morbidity morbidity rates.

II. **Risk factors**
   1. **Surgical location**
      a. Upper abdominal surgery is associated with complication rates of 19–33%.
      b. Lower abdominal surgery is associated with complication rates of 5–16%.
      c. Thoracic (nonresective) surgery is associated with complication rates of 10–19%.
   2. **Chronic obstructive pulmonary disease (COPD)**
      a. Relative risk of complications based on COPD alone = 2.7–4.7%.
      b. Patients with symptoms of bronchospasm, physical findings consistent with undertreated bronchospasm, or complaints of impaired exercise tolerance compared with baseline are especially at high risk for bronchospasm. Spirometry values aid little in assessing risk for surgical complications.
   3. **Age** is weakly related to high complication rates in poorly designed studies. When adjusted for overall health, mortality is consistent across all ranges of age.
   4. **Smoking**
      a. Relative risk of complications for smokers compared with nonsmokers is between 1.4 and 4.3.
      b. Smoking cessation 8 weeks before coronary aretery bypass grafting reduced pulmonary complications from 33–14.5%. Patients that stopped smoking less than 8 weeks before CABG were at higher risk for pulmonary complications.
   5. **General health status.** The Goldman criteria and the American Society of Anesthesiologists classification predict increasing incidence of pulmonary complications. The ability to exercise even minimally (heart rate of 99 beats/minute after 2 minutes) reduces the risk for pulmonary complications.
   6. **Anesthesia**
      a. Pancuronium should be avoided because of its association with prolonged neuromuscular blockade and concomitant hypoventilation.

b. Epidural/spinal anesthesia is likely to be beneficial. Retrospective studies demonstrated higher mortality rates secondary to respiratory failure in patients undergoing general anesthesia compared with patients undergoing epidural anesthesia.
c. Regional anesthesia reduces the risk even more than epidural anesthesia.
d. Surgery longer than 3 hours is associated with a complication rate of 15–33%.

III. **Preoperative evaluations**
1. **History and physical examination**
   a. Search for evidence of bronchospasm.
   b. Complete work-up of unexplained cough, dyspnea, or poor exercise tolerance.
   c. Include chest x ray if not done recently.
2. **Spirometry** is *not* indicated in all patients. It may be helpful in the following cases:
   a. Symptomatic patients with no previous history of bronchospasm
   b. Symptomatic patients with previous history of bronchospasm (to assess if patient is near baseline status)
   c. Spirometry measurements alone should not be used to exclude a patient from a procedure.
3. **Arterial blood gas analysis**
   a. Hypercapnea was identified as a risk factor for complications in earlier studies, but newer prospective studies have failed to find a relationship.
   b. May be helpful in defining hypercapnea if clinically indicated.
4. **Pulmonary risk indexes**
   a. Epstein Cardiopulmonary Index assesses risk based on clinical evaluation, spirometry and blood gas analysis.
   b. Recent analysis evaluating risk in abdominal surgery noted four independent risk factors: abnormal chest exam, abnormal chest x-ray, high score on the Goldman criteria, and high score on the Charlson Comorbidity Index.

IV. **Reducing complications**
1. **Goals:** reduce bronchospasm and air flow limitation, avoid atelectasis, stop smoking, maximize exercise tolerance, and maximize pain control.

The Diagram

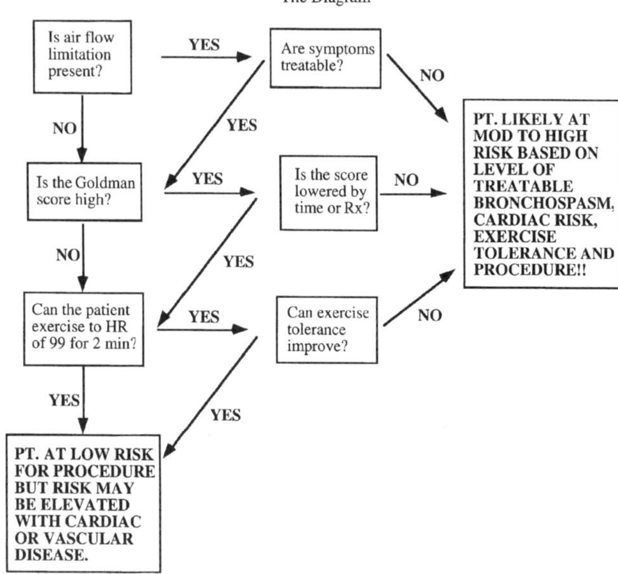

2. **Preoperative strategies**
   a. Use bronchodilators, gluccocorticoids, antibiotics, and theophyline to maximize pulmonary function in patients with air flow limitation.
   b. Complete treatment of pulmonary infections.
   c. Quit smoking more than 8 weeks before surgery (if possible)
   d. Maximize exercise tolerance.
3. **Operative strategies**
   a. Discuss use of epidural anesthesia.
   b. Use laproscopic procedures if possible.
   c. Use atracurium, not pancuronium.
   d. Minimize the time required for the procedure.
   e. Avoid upper abdominal or thoracic surgery if possible.
4. **Postoperative strategies**
   a. Lung expansion maneuvers with incentive spirometry (IS) or deep breathing. If unable to use IS, patients may benefit from continuous positive airway pressure (CPAP) or biphasic positive airway pressure (BIPAP).
   b. Effective pain control with epidural anesthesia, if needed.

Key References: Lawrence VA, et al: Risk of pulmonary complications after elective abdominal surgery. Chest 110:744–750, 1996; Smetana GW: Preoperative pulmonary evaluation. N Engl J Med 340:937–944, 1999; Zibrak JD, et al: Indications for preoperative pulmonary function testing. Clin Chest Med 14:227–236, 1993.

Preoperative Assessment of the Nonpulmonary Patient

I. **Identify risk factors.**
   1. In an attempt to identify the patient at risk for adverse perioperative cardiovascular complications, Goldman et al. performed a multivariate analysis and identified **nine variables** that were independent predictors for the development of perioperative cardiac events:

Variable	Points
Age > 70 years	5
Recent myocardial infarction (< 6 months)	10
Aortic stenosis	3
S3 gallop or elevated jugular venous pressure	11
Arrythmia	
Rhythm other than sinus or premature atrial contractions on last EKG	7
> 5 premature ventricular contractions/minute at any time	7
Poor medical condition	3
PaO_2 < 60 mmHg; potassium < 3.0 mEq/L; bicarbonate < 20 mEq/L; blood urea nitrogen > 50 mg/dl (18 mmol/L); creatinine > 3 mg/dl (260 mmol/L); abnormal aspartate aminotransferase; signs of chronic liver disease; bedridden from noncardiac causes	
Type of surgery	
Emergency	4
Intraperitoneal, intrathoracic, or aortic surgery	3
Total points possible	53

2. Goldman et al. defined **four classes of risk** based on point score:

	Life-threatening complications*	Cardiac death
Class I (0–5 points)	0.7%	0.2%
Class II (6–12 points)	5%	2%
Class III (13–25 points)	11%	2%
Class IV (> 26 points)	22%	5–6%

* These included intraoperative or postoperative myocardial infarction, pulmonary edema, or ventricular tachycardia without progression to cardiac death.

3. Because the risk for patients with peripheral vascular disease is underestimated using the Goldman criteria, Detsky et al. derived a **modified multifactorial risk index** to include the presence of angina to determine perioperative cardiac complications in noncardiac surgery. In the modified index, points assigned as follows:

Variable	Points
Coronary artery disease	
Myocardial infarction ≤ 6 months	10
Myocardial infarction > 6 months ago	5
Canadian Cardiovascular Society (CCS) Angina Classification	
Class III angina (angina on 1–2 flight exertion)	10
Class IV angina (angina at rest or with minimal exertion)	20
Unstable angina within 3 months	10
Pulmonary edema	
Within 1 week	10
Ever	5
Suspected critical aortic stenosis	20
Arrythmias	
Atrial premature beats or rhythm other than sinus on last EKG	5
Ventricular premature beats > 5/minute at any time	5
Poor health status	5
PaO_2 < 60 mmHg; potassium < 3.0 mEq/L; bicarbonate < 20 mEq/L; blood urea nitrogen > 50 mg/dl (18 mmol/L); creatinine > 3 mg/dl (260 mmol/L); abnormal aspartate aminotransferase; signs of chronic liver disease; bedridden from noncardiac causes	
Age > 70 years	5
Emergency operation (prior to optimization)	10
Total points possible	105

Using a nomogram with plotted odds ratios, a post-test probability or % risk for cardiac complications is then derived. The risk of cardiac death is 0.3 times the % risk of cardiac complications.

4. Detsky et al. derived **three risk classes** for adverse cardiovascular events based on likelihood ratios:

Risk Class	Likelihood Ratios		
(Points)	Major Surgery	Minor Surgery	All Surgery
Class I (0–15)	0.42	0.39	0.43
Class II (15–30)	3.58	2.75	3.38
Class III (> 30)	14.93	12.20	10.60

5. Although preoperative risk stratifications are useful to approximate the degree of risk, **low scores do not guarantee an event-free postoperative course.**

Expertise of the anesthesiologist and surgeon and type of procedure also influence outcome.

II. **Consent.** Discussion of usual risks, benefits, and alternatives should be documented. If the patient is incapable of informed consent, refer to institutional consent protocols.

III. **Nutrition.** Hold feedings or diet preoperatively (NPO status), usually for at least 6 hours.

IV. **Risk factors for deep venous thrombosis (DVT)**

1. Age > 40 years
2. History of prior thromboembolic disease
3. Immobility
4. Obesity
5. Congestive heart failure or myocardial infarction
6. Varicosities
7. Major surgery, particularly hip and knee surgery and surgery for major trauma

Risk of Proximal DVT	
Elective general surgery (moderate risk)	7%
Elective hip surgery (high risk)	20%

Risk of Fatal Pulmonary Embolism	
Elective general surgery	0.1%
Elective hip surgery	2%

V. **DVT prophylaxis**

1. Low risk (e.g., appendectomy): early ambulation
2. Moderate risk (e.g., major abdominal surgery): heparin 5000 IU subcutaneously 2 hours preoperatively and every12 hours or low-molecular-weight (LMW) heparin (with or without stockings)
3. High risk (multiple trauma or spinal cord injury): LMW heparin (with or without stockings)
4. High risk (hip fractures): LMW heparin or warfarin preoperatively; then adjust to international normalized ratio (INR) 2–3 times control

VI. **Laboratory tests and investigations**

1. Reassess volume status, central venous pressure, urine output, and hemodynamics when appropriate.
2. Coagulation profile
   a. INR, partial thromboplastin time
   b. Platelets: for major surgery platelet count should be > 100,000/mm^3 (> 100 × 10^9/L) (*Note:* 1 unit of platelets raises the count by approximately 10,000/mm^3 or ~ 10 × 10^9/L).
3. Reassess complete blood count, electrolytes, and glucose; correct any abnormalities.
4. Blood type and screen
5. Crossmatch for surgeries with anticipated risk of transfusion > 10%
6. Documentation of comorbidities, preoperative EKG and chest x-ray

VII. **Steroid coverage**

Equivalent doses			
Cortisone acetate	38 mg	Prednisolone	5 mg
Hydrocortisone	30 mg	Methyprednisolone	4 mg
Prednisone	5 mg	Dexamethasone	1 mg

2. For patients with potential **chronic adrenal insufficiency**: hydrocortisone, 30 mg every 24 hr (20 mg AM and 10 mg PM)

3. For **major stresses** (major surgery, sepsis, trauma), use hydocortisone, 100 mg IV every 8 hr

VIII. **Antibiotic prophylaxis**

1. Recommended for contaminated or dirty procedures with high infection rates or for major prosthetic implants.
2. Final choice of agent is determined by institutional resistance patterns (e.g., methicillin-resistant *Staphylococcus aureus*).
3. **Suggestions for prophylaxis**
    a. Upper gastrointestinal surgery: cefazolin (G-bacilli, G+cocci)
    b. Colorectal surgery: cefazolin + metronidazole (G-bacilli, anaerobes, enterococci)
    c. Cardiac surgery: cefazolin, cefuroxime, or vancomycin (*Staphylococcus epidermidis, S. aureus, Corynebacterium* spp., G-bacilli)
    d. Oropharyngeal surgery: clindamycin + gentamicin (*S. aureus,* anaerobes, G-bacilli)
    e. Craniotomy, vascular prosthesis, thoracic surgery, total joint surgery: cefazolin or vancomycin (*S. aureus, S. epidermidis*)
    f. Ruptured viscus: cefoxitin + gentamicin or clindamycin + gentamicin (G-bacilli, anaerobes, enterococci)
4. **Endocarditis prophylaxis** for patients with valvular heart disease.
    a. Upper respiratory tract procedures: ampicillin, 2 gm IV preoperatively; in penicillin-allergic patients, clindamycin, 600 mg IV
    b. Gastrointesintal or genitourinary procedures: ampicillin, 2 gm IV, + gentamicin, 1.5 mg/kg; in penicillin-allergic patients, vancomycin, 1 gm, + gentamicin

IX. **Beta blocker prophylaxis**

1. Postoperative ischemic events appear to be related to the persistently exaggerated sympathetic response associated with increases in heart rate throughout hospitalization.
2. Mangano et al. reported a randomized, double-blind, placebo-controlled trial comparing the effects of atenolol and placebo on overall survival and cardiovascular morbidity in patients with or at risk for coronary artery disease (CAD) who were undergoing noncardiac surgery.
    a. In patients with a heart rate ≥ 55 beats/min, systolic BP ≥ 100 mmHg, and no evidence of congestive heart failure, third-degree heart block, or bronchospasm, atenolol (5 mg) was given intravenously immediately before and immediately after surgery (5 mg IV) and orally (50 or 100 mg) daily thereafter for the duration of hospitalization.
        - Overall mortality rate at 6 months: 0% (atenolol) vs. 8% (control); $p < 0,00$)
        - Mortality rate at first year: 3% (atenolol) vs. 14% (control); $p = 0.005$
        - Mortality rate after 2 years: 10% (atenolol) vs. 21% (control); $p = 0.019$
    b. Therefore, in patients at risk for CAD who must undergo noncardiac surgery, treatment with a beta blocker to control heart rate during hospitalization can reduce mortality and the incidence of cardiovascular complications for as long as 2 years postoperatively. Perioperative beta blocker use appears to be well tolerated and safe.

X. **Pitfalls**

1. Major changes in ventilation strategies for patients with acute lung injury and acute respiratory distress syndrome
2. Loss of lines during transfer
3. Interruption or change in infusion rates of inotropes and vasoactive drugs
4. Loss of information during transfer to operating room and anesthesia team

5. In assessing patients, remove prosthetics, caps, implants, and contact lenses (if at all possible).

Key References: Detsky A, et al: Predicting cardiac complications in patients undergoing non-cardiac surgery. J Gen Intern Med 1:211, 1986; Goldman L, et al: Multifactorial index of cardiac risk in non-cardiac surgical procedures. N Engl J Med 297:845, 1977; Jones H, de Cossart L: Risk scoring in surgical patients. Br J Surg 86:149, 1999; Mangano D, et al: Effect of atenolol on mortality and cardiovascular morbidity after noncardiac surgery. N Engl J Med 335:1713, 1996.

Assessment of the Postoperative Intensive Care Patient

I. **Review the following:**
   1. Intraoperative findings and procedures
   2. Intra- and perioperative anesthetic notes, including fluids, blood products, and drugs (e.g., type of anesthetic, paralytics)
   3. Physiologic variables, including urine output
   4. Preoperative notes or consultant notes

II. **Follow the DAVID protocol**
   1. **D = Diet** (place the patient on NPO status or appropriate oral, enteral. or parenteral nutrition)
   2. **A = Activity**
      a. Order appropriate activity level with restrictions as indicated.
      b. Include instructions for chest and other physiotherapy.
   3. **V = Vital signs**
      a. Order specific vital and neurovital sign monitoring.
      b. Frequency and parameters for central venous pressure, hemodynamics, and urine output should be established and monitored hourly for critically ill patients.
      c. In cases of severe ongoing instability, continuous bedside attendance and monitoring may be required (patients in the intensive care unit).
   4. **I = Investigations**
      a. Order serial hemoglobin assessments; coagulation profiles; platelet counts; evaluations of electrolytes, glucose, and creatinine; arterial blood gas analyses; chest x-rays; and EKGs, as indicated.
      b. Review immediately Gram stain results for any culture material submitted intraoperatively.
      c. For clinical coagulopathy in patients with major trauma and hemorrhagic shock, do not wait for return of coagulation profiles, but continue resuscitation with fresh frozen plasma and platelets. Consider cryoprecipitate and calcium if more than 6 units of blood have been transfused.
   5. **D = Drugs, dressings, and tubes**
      a. **Intravenous fluids**
         - In general, 2 cc/kg/hr of crystalloid for adults with normal renal function is appropriate.
         - Patients with ongoing blood loss, extensive peritonitis, retroperitoneal surgery (e.g., for abdominal aortic aneurysm) may require significantly more fluid.
         - Order IV fuid replacement of large-volume outputs. Replace nasogastric tube output with 0.45 normal saline with 10 mEq/L potassium chloride. High output from fistulas and stomas also should be replaced. If you are not certain what to replace it with, measure it!

b. **Fistula and drainage guidelines**

	Na (mmol/L)	K (mmol/L)	Cl (mmol/L)	HCO_3 (mmol/L)
Gastric	20–100	10–15	90–120	0–25 (usually 0)
Biliary	140–150	5	90–110	30–40
Small Bowel	100–130	5	100–110	30–35
Pancreas	140	5	70	90

c. **Transfusion guidelines**. In general, a restrictive transfusion threshhold (hemoglobin of 7.0 gm/dl or 70 gm/L) is as safe as a liberal transfusion threshold (hemoglobin of ≥ 9.0 gm/dl or ≥ 90 gm/L) in critically ill patients, with the exception of patients with unstable angina. In the presence of ongoing or anticipated bleeding, a more liberal threshold should apply.

d. Specify **oxygen requirements and ventilator settings**.

e. **Order the following drugs**, as appropriate:
   - Inotropes, vasoactive agents, and cardiac medications
   - Antibiotics (see sections on Preoperative Assessment)
   - Bronchodilators
   - Steroid replacement (see sections on Preoperative Assessment)
   - Analgesics (in the intensive care setting, usually morphine, 2–10 mg/hr IV). *Note:* Avoid nonsteroidal anti-inflammatory drugs in patients with or at risk for renal dysfunction.
   - Insulin, as needed (sliding scale is appropriate)

f. **Prophylaxis for deep venous thrombosis** (see sections on Preoperative Assessment)

g. **Gastritis prophylaxis.** Risk factors include shock, burns, sepsis, mechanical ventilation > 48 hours, and recent GI bleed. If you are unable to establish enteral nutrition, follow the guidelines below:
   - If you are also unable to use the GI tract or anticipate gastroscopy, order ranitidine, 50 mg every 8 hours.
   - If you are able to use the GI tract and do not anticipate gastroscopy, order sucralfate, 1 gm 4 times/day by nasogastric tube.

h. **Review all preoperative medications.** Adjust all dosages for renal or hepatic dysfunction as required. If you do not know the dose, look it up!
   - Normal creatinine = 0.6–1.5 mg/dl or 53–133 µmol/L
   - Normal creatinine clearance = 95 ± 20 ml/min (women) or 125 ± 25 ml/min (men). Creatinine clearance is calculated by the following formula: urine creatinine × urine volume (ml/min) / plasma creatinine. Creatinine clearance can be estimated by the following formula: (140 – age)(weight [kg]) / 72 × plasma creatinine (mg/dl).

i. **List all drains with appropriate suction** (e.g., Foley with straight drainage, nasogastric tube with low suction, chest tube with 20 cmH_2O underwater seal). Determine frequency of monitoring, including drains and stomas.

j. **Review surgical instructions** for dressings, packings, and wound irrigations. Special precautions include the following:
   - Avoid vasoactive agents and diuretics with free flaps.
   - Discuss enteric nutrition with surgeon after GI or abdominal surgery.
   - Discuss chest tube and airway management with surgeon after thoracic and upper airway (ear-nose-throat/plastics) procedures.
   - Monitor and replace glucose and phosphate after hepatic resection.

   Note: Good communication with the surgeon is essential.

k. **Reassess.** In patients with ongoing requirements for large-volume resuscitation, always recheck the hemoglobin to rule out bleeding.

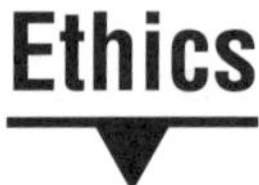

Ethics

Advance Directives

Several kinds of documents are called advance directives. The actual documents available and the laws for execution and direction of documents vary among the states. Each health care practitioner should be aware of the laws and standards of practice of his or her state. Types of advance directives include:

I. **Living will.** Living wills are documents that generally limit the use of artificial life support when the patient is terminally ill. In some instances the living will may also address whether the patient desires to receive nutrition (i.e., tube feedings or intravenous nutrition/hydration).

II. **Cardiopulmonary resuscitation (CPR) directive.** In many states, a CPR directive is available for patients. This document is signed by individuals who do not wish to have CPR performed if they sustain a cardiopulmonary arrest at any time.

III. **Medical durable power of attorney.** A medical durable power of attorney allows an individual to name the person empowered to make health care decisions if the individual is no longer capable of making the decisions. The patient does not have to have a terminal illness for the medical durable power of attorney to go into effect.

IV. **Substitute decision makers (medical proxies).** In many states the friends and family of a patient can designate a substitute decision maker, called a proxy, for the patient who cannot make decisions for him- or herself and who has no other advance directive document that addresses the relevant issues.

V. The following issues must be kept in mind in considering advance directives:
   1. The wishes of a competent patient are paramount and take precedent over any document or the wishes of any other person.
   2. People who complete advance directives such as living wills and CPR directives may change their mind when actually faced with a critical or terminal illness. Therefore, it is always a good idea to review the patient's wishes whenever possible.
   3. Often patients are competent and capable of making decisions on admission to the hospital, but as they become critically ill, they may no longer be able to participate in the decision-making process. Therefore, it is often helpful to encourage patients to elucidate how they want their advance directives followed and to name a proxy decision maker so that these issues do not need to be sorted out at a time of crisis.

Withdrawal of Treatment

Ethically there is no difference between the withholding of treatment and the withdrawal of treatment. In both instances the competent patient or appropriate decision maker for the patient as well as all members of the health care team should communicate about the decision. Although the most appropriate method for the withdrawal of treatment is debated, the following guidelines may be helpful:

I. Be certain that everyone involved in the decision communicates about the decision and the process.

II. Remember that the wishes of a competent patient take precedence.

III. Reassure the patient, family, and other health care providers that withdrawal of treatment does not mean withdrawal of care.
IV. Have a plan that addresses who will terminate treatment and how treatment will be terminated and identifies all likely scenarios, with plans for each.
V. It is wise not to say, "When treatment is withdrawn the patient will die." Although that may be the most likely scenario, we are sometimes surprised, and it is best to be honest ahead of time.

Futile Care

In general, it is believed that health care providers are not obligated to provide treatment that is not likely to benefit the patient (i.e., we do not offer open heart surgery if the patient has a cold). Currently, however, no definition of futile care is universally accepted, and no clear policy dictates how practitioners should deal with what they consider futile care.

Ethics Committees

A hospital ethics committee is usually a multidisciplinary committee (including not only health care providers such as doctors, nurses, respiratory therapists, and social workers but also members of the clergy, lay persons, and risk managers) that provides consultation for specific issues as well as serves as a forum for the discussion of ethical issues. The ethics committee may provide invaluable help when an ethical dilemma or concern arises.

Key Reference: Brody H, Campbell ML, Faber-Langendoen K, Ogle KS: Withdrawing intensive life-sustaining treatment—Recommendations for compassionate clinical management. N Engl J Med 336:652–657, 1997.

Appendix

Safety of Drugs for Pregnant Patients*

Categories A and B (no fetal risks demonstrated in first trimester; generally safe)	**Category C** (adverse effects in animals or inadequate data; use when benefits clearly outweigh risks)	**Categories D and X** (evidence for adverse effects to human fetus; use only in exceptional circumstances)
Amphotericin	Acyclovir	Acetylsalicylic acid
Cephalosporins	Albuterol	Angiotensin-converting enzyme inhibitors
Cimetidine	Aminoglycosides	Warfarin
Clindamycin	Atracurium	Tetracyclines
Erythromycin	Benzodiazepines	
Glycopyrrolate	Beta blockers	
Insulin	Bretylium	
Lidocaine	Bupivacaine	
Magnesium sulfate	Dantrolene	
Meperidine	Digoxin	
Methyldopa	Fluconazole	
Naloxone	Flumazenil	
Penicillins	Furosemide	
Propofol	Halperidol	
Ranitidine	Heparin	
Terbutaline	Hydralazine	
	Inotropes	
	Labetalol	
	Metronidazole	
	Midazolam	
	Nifedipine	
	Nitroglycerin	
	Nitroprusside	
	Pancuronium	
	Phenytoin	
	Prednisone	
	Procainamide	
	Suxamethonium	
	Thiopental	
	Vancomycin	
	Vecuronium	

* Food and Drug Administration classification.

Index